© Copyright 2015

The rights of Marc Draco, Kavin Senapathy, Mark Alsip, Kevin Folta, & Mike Petrik to be identified as authors of this work have been asserted by them in accordance with the Copyright Design and Patents Act, 1988.

No part of this publication may be reproduced, stored in a retrieval system or transmitted in any form or by any means, electronic, mechanical, photocopying, recording or otherwise, without prior permission of Senapath Press except as to the extent permitted by law.

Some text and images claim Fair Use for the specific purpose of comment, education or critique under United States Copyright act, 1976. 17 U.S.C.§107. For clarity and ease of digital search, some text has been reproduced from web sites/ books and may not reflect the exact formatting; however every possible care has been taken to ensure the correct context has been preserved.

Cover Photography and Ms. Senapathy's images by Patricia LaPointe. © 2015
Mr. Alsip's portrait by Sarah Bucknam, Pretty Pixels Photography. © 2014
Moulded bread images by Brian Jobson Photography. © 2015

Cover designed by John Girgus.

All rights reserved.

FOOD BABE is a registered trademark of Food Babe LLC

Citations from *The Food Babe Way: Break Free from the Hidden Toxins in Your Food and Lose Weight, Look Years Younger, and Get Healthy in Just 21 Days!* are abbreviated to The Food Babe Way and are taken from the First Edition (February 2015), Little, Brown and Company.

Published in the USA by Senapath Press (www.senapathpress.com)

ISBN: 978-0-692-50981-4

Late breaking errata will be published on the book's official Facebook page available at www.facebook.com/TheFearBabe. This is the reviewer's pre-release.

Epigraph

In the communication age, a lie could travel half-way around the world before the truth gets its pants on. Today, a lie can travel to all four corners[1] of the globe and get back in bed with a couple of smoking hot fallacies and a convenient obfuscation before the truth can fumble for the alarm clock.

[1] Wait—if it's a globe—how does it even have four corners?

To Carl Sagan, for making an infinite universe of possibilities accessible, Sir Terry Pratchett for making them funny; but most of all, for the dedicated scientists striving daily to make our world a better place against the tide of organized ignorance.—MD

To Jesse for holding down the fort, and to my beautiful children for tolerating mommy's writing time. And to my parents and sister, for fueling my love of science. My dear friend SA, thank you for always having my back. Finally, big love to the Senapath Crew for the inspiring conversations and laughter.—KS

To Melissa, mom and dad, Julie, Vicky, and Kelly. Your unconditional love and unwavering belief in me is a constant reminder that all things are possible.—MA

Contents

Preface

"Egotism is the anaesthetic that dulls the pain of stupidity."—Frank Leahy, American Footballer

To the Food Babe Army we say this: we understand much of this information is a direct contradiction to what you have been led to believe. This may cause feelings of anger or resentment. This is normal. We're not trying to get you to change your mind about what you consume, just trying to help you to question the information you've been presented and to understand why many people believe much of this information is wrong.

To *Vani Hari*: The evidence and the science is clear. If you were willing to accept your mistakes and move on, this book would not have been necessary. Our guess is you're in too deep to make those admissions now. If you choose to open up, the science community will probably welcome you. As crazy as it may seem, they are as interested in the truth as you claim to be. But some truths are harder to digest (no pun intended) and there's far less money in telling the truth.

There are invariably two sides to every story and often times the most convincing one, the one we like the sound of, is the wrong one. Even top academics–the smartest people in the world–are prone to this, so there's no shame in suffering from this most human of failures. To err is human, but to admit you've erred takes a special type of courage.

Some of history's greatest scientists have been wrong: Albert Einstein, for example, who detested the idea of the Quantum Entanglement and Lord Kelvin—most famed for his prediction of Absolute Zero—not only got the age of Earth horribly wrong (and tried to silence those who disagreed) but famously predicted man would never achieve powered flight. And just a few years later the Wright brothers did just that.

Science can be a challenging discipline. Although we have tried to keep the text in this book as simple as possible, we've occasionally had to resort to using some big words, simply because there aren't any small ones in common use. Many everyday chemicals have fancy names. Water, for instance, is the most abundant chemical (compound) on the Earth and many people are aware that it's also called H_2O.

However, were we to invite you to drink a beaker of fresh oxidane, you may think we'd gone mad. Oxidane is used to cool nuclear reactors and it's found everywhere as a simple, cheap solvent. The oceans are full of it; we are full of it and life cannot exist without it. It's just a fancy name for water and it's possible (if impractical) to make the stuff with no more than some hydrogen and a match!

Chemical compounds are everywhere and many of them have scary, long names which are hard to read, let alone pronounce. That last coffee you had probably had a dose of the heterocyclic aromatic organic compound and methylxanthine alkaloid 1,3,7-trimethylpurine-2,6-dione—which is an insecticide, herbicide, and psychoactive drug. It's better known as caffeine and it's harmless in the standard doses we consume in beverages such as coffee and tea.

Notice how easy it is to instill fear? That's how charlatans work. We're going to take you on a journey to show how you might have been fooled into believing that the people you thought had your back were really only there to rifle through your wallet while you were stunned, like a deer caught in the headlights.

We don't want you to take our word for it though. This book aims to teach critical thinking, and to demonstrate how vested interests may pretend to be your friend, only because they have something to sell. Is Monsanto evil? Of course not. It's a business and businesses exist to provide products and services, while making profits for the shareholders. Every organic manufacturer, every food supplier, everyone in the food chain is in business to make money. Even Food Babe LLC is a business and Food Babe is not about to let a few facts spoil a good scare story. After all, how is she going to make a living if you're not scared into buying what she happens to be selling?

Uniquely in the West, companies and organizations have a constitutionally protected right to bend the truth under the 1st Amendement. This book attempts to get to the truth by reporting on the consensus held by the world's experts.

Kavin Senapathy, Mark Alsip & Marc Draco. September 2015

Priming the Rise of Al Quesadilla

If you want to horrify a new mother, show her the website that says that the cereal bits on her daughter's high-chair tray are going to condemn her to a life with autism, cancer, and chronic obesity. Tell an elite triathlete that they can't trust that morsel on the end of their fork, and that published data confirm that it will destroy their performance if they elect to eat it. Teach affluent consumers that the options lining store shelves in that regular store are going to silently cause Alzheimer's disease and diabetes. Do you think they'll take another bite? The fear of dietary danger is penetrating, and potently changes food choices. Al Quesadilla knows that.

Food has a sacred place in the human experience. It is the thread in our cultural fabric. It is a traditional component when celebrating life's milestones, and is a staple of social functions. The meal is the true centerpiece when we gather for holidays. It is the bounty on the table between two old friends, catching up on time across a table. It makes sense. For 99.999% of humans that have ever lived there was not enough food. When you had it you were grateful, you gave thanks. You shared. It was the nutritional medium that connected us. Even my great aunt told me about times during the depression (only two generations ago) when the family would sacrifice their only scraps of bread for "Baby Edziu," a baby that would grow to become my grandfather. Food was scarce throughout human history, most fruits and vegetables were a rare treat, and most people would live their entire lives without luxury confections and specialty foods that we encounter almost every day today.

In all of human history, the food supply has never been more abundant, diverse or safe. Think of your last meal. Many in the world today will live a full life without eating something that good. In today's markets we enjoy a spectrum of colors and flavors never before known to humans. The choices and quality come from direct human dabbling in plant genetics, in shaping products by breeding, selection, and genetic modifications. New varieties of plants derived from clever combinations nature could never produce, anoint our store shelves at an affordable price. Better transportation, logistics and post-harvest handling allow novel fruits, vegetables and processed products to our markets from all around the world. Safe and well-tested chemistries help preserve the quality of food, enhance its sensory qualities, and ensure that it is safe to eat and less likely to be wasted.

We live in a time of great food safety and abundance in the Western world, where mundane medical maladies are few, and food is taken for granted. It is a perfect opportunity for Al Quesadilla to strike.

One definition of terrorism is, "Acts intended to intimidate or coerce a population to influence the policy of a government, or corporate or individual action, through intimidation or coercion." The same tactics are the basis of food terrorism, the preferred weapon of Al Quesadilla.

Who is Al Quesadilla?

Al Quesadilla is a moniker ascribed to a modern day elite and well-financed terrorist faction, sworn to use fear to force political change around food. Al Quesadilla has a central mission—to impose their beliefs about food and food production on the broader society. Their beliefs are religious in nature. They are deeply heartfelt and internalized. Their beliefs are grounded in a misinterpretation of nature, a mistrust of corporate culture, and a skepticism of modern science. Al Quesadilla's central holy tenets were not forged from rigorous hypothesis testing by trained scientists. Instead, they are kooky hunches spawned from abject ignorance, an activist crusade, or a hint of reality wrapped in fearful impossibility. This is a religion that wants your money, wants your vote, and wants you to change the fundamental way you eat. It is a movement fighting to install change, even if it harms the environment, brings hardship to the needy, destroys farmers, or results in fewer choices for the average consumer.

Al Quesadilla's leadership is handed down from a group of charismatic, wealthy and sometimes educated civilians that claim to know more than the rest of us. They seek to re-engineer social values to conform to a standard they define as acceptable. Their dream is an antiquated and impractical bucolic existence that didn't work well then, can't work now, and has no place in the future. They shun modern breakthroughs in genetics or food chemistry, and long for the way humans did things traditionally, like thirty to forty years ago. Most have never set foot on a farm or in a laboratory. Of course, these collections of well-funded and intellectually bankrupt know-it-alls can farm much better than farmers, know the science better than scientists, and know diet better than dietitians.

Al Quesadilla is an agile and sneaky terrorist group. Like all terrorists, they achieve their objectives through the implementation of fear and coercion. They plan careful strikes on vulnerable targets– American consumers. These are people that have few worries, where true first-world problems pinch their utopia. Even the least privileged enjoy a quality of life that the vast majority of people alive today will never know. When all is comfortable, bellies are full and wallets padded, the consumer presents itself as an easy mark for Al Quesadilla to make a buck or achieve a political motivation. The method is simple–use the tools of fearful rhetoric to frighten the average consumer, the concerned citizen that only wants the best for their families, their country, and their planet. Their central conduit is the Internet, exploiting social media and linkages to throngs of loyal legions to amplify the crooked message, spreading fear and disinformation about perfectly good food.

A Whole-y War

Al Quesadilla exploits an appeal to our core values. They know that we all want safe food, abundant food, and food produced with environmental sensitivity. We all hope for healthy children, humane treatment of animals, and a standard for the needy that satisfies their nutritional needs. From that core of agreeable and common values, Al Quesadilla advances its agenda, claiming that its twisted goals are simply extensions of the concepts we all hold dear. That's what makes Al Quesadilla so dangerous. We agree on so much, so what's the big deal with a few more little changes?

Take this platform of common concerns, and infuse it with a pretty face, the credibility of a TV doctor, Hollyweird's well-healed, and new effective agents of food terrorism are born. Here the sewage of anti-science can flow through friendly, approachable, seemingly credible yet crooked conduits of misinformation. The Internet then provides a means to polish these remarkably empty vessels as experts, transforming the daft edge of scientific illiteracy into perceived fountains of validated science.

One of these agents is a college-educated computer consultant that took an interest in diet and food, and in a strange twist of coincidence was catapulted into stardom. She appears attractive yet approachable. She is a skilled speaker, and uses the platform of social media to evangelize in the Church of Chemophobia, convincing her willing congregation that their food is poison and modern food production is a corrupt collaboration between evil corporations, patsy government regulators, and paid off professors. She uses coercive tactics to mobilize her loyal throngs, creating changes in food formulations not driven by evidence, but because these troops demand change at the knife point of clueless public opinion. She is the subject of this text, and is a charismatic leader within the cult of Al Quesadilla.

She has infected public consciousness by appealing to causes we all care about. We are certainly in a public health challenge centered on poor food choices, a lack of knowledge about nutrition and science in general. It is a place where fear of food can gain powerful traction.

Her actions become objectionable when they deny what we know from science. A desire to do what is right morphs into an anchor on progress and commerce when science slips into pseudoscience. Sadly, when corrected by experts she does not humbly accept criticism, step back, ask questions and learn. She screams that the experts are frauds, paid dupes of corporate food, and liars that question her expertise. If you dare to correct or question her via social media, your comments are erased, and your account is blocked from further interaction. Al Quesadilla must control the information flow, as its grip on the unwitting cannot be sustained if science, truth, and consensus are communicated and understood.

Effects of Mind Poison

Perhaps her heart is right and beats in the chest of a gifted speaker and network builder. But a well-intentioned, ambitious and connected heart operating without the guidance of an equally adept brain can do a lot of damage. This is why Ms. Hari is a central figure in Al Quesadilla's cult leadership. She takes a concern we share, overlays an ignorance of science to manufacture non-existent risk, and then stokes fear through a social-media-driven network of sworn warriors to misinform the public, defame good products, and imply danger where none actually exists. This approach then motivates angry action, forcing companies to make changes, not because of actual risk–but because they are threatened with damage to their image and reputation, driven by her internet-savvy followers that put her demands ahead of potential impacts. Reformulations bring no improvement to food safety. Zero. But they can negatively change quality, price and availability.

History will revere this jihadist as another non-expert that gained celebrity status and rode it into personal prosperity at the expense of the truth. She has exploited the climate that Al Quesadilla has created, manipulating a well-fed and malleable public to satisfy a screwy science-free mission, tarnishing reputations of good companies, and vilifying perceptions of safe food. It is exciting to see the scientifically sane stand up, recognize, and counter her crusade. The future of food will survive this blip of quack attack, it just has casualties along the way, through cost to those that can least afford food, and harm to brand reputation.

Al Quesadilla exploits soft spots in the understanding of food. We currently rest in a climate where we have so much, yet know so little about what it is genetically, how it is grown, or how it is produced. The strategy to fight back against Al Quesadilla is sharing knowledge, facts and hard science. It is to stand on common values and teach, to win hearts and minds, and identify the charlatans that find personal profit from exploiting the credulous. *The Fear Babe* exposes the errors that cultured a misunderstanding of food under the guise of improving it. It provides scientific dissection of the topics and sets straight the facts behind the fallacies. It is exciting to see authors and scientists take a stand against Al Quesadilla and the terror it creates against our understanding of food.

Forward Together

The modern phenomenon of food terrorism exists on a planet where almost a billion people do not have access to clean water. It exists on a planet where most do not have a reliable source of calories, they face scourges of incomplete nutrition and acute deficits where micrograms of vitamins lead to preventable blindness, death, and unfathomable suffering. It exists where deserts devoid of quality food have emerged even in our most affluent urban centers.

Instead of promulgating false information about food science, vilifying safe chemistry, and creating a growing list of first-world problems, what if Al Quesadilla's food terrorists used their energies to share our unprecedented access to safe food to these populations? What if the Food Babe Army traded hash-tags for hash browns, and invested their endless energy serving the underfed here in our own country? What if Al Quesadilla's leadership could demand their troops cease fire on science and scientists, and start supporting solutions for the lives that never will enjoy the luxury of walking into a Whole Foods or Trader Joe's?

Don't hold your breath. There's no money to be made in serving the ravaged poor, they don't buy science-less books or fear mongering documentaries. They don't buy defective diet plans or homeopathic remedies from Al Quesadilla's many websites. You can't scare people that have no food, into buying boutique food.

Again, we live at a time of unprecedented food abundance and quality. Instead of provoking needless hysteria about perfectly safe sustenance, what if Al Quesadilla could be convinced to love the least advantaged that share our planet? *The Fear Babe* is a good start to expose the harm of focusing food-safety energies on non-issues. It reveals the tremendous cost of forced reformulations and capitulation to food terrorism. It provides a platform to re-evaluate whether we should be following self-appointed "babes," or instead start following science.

Fear starves the mind, body and spirit. Food and truth feed them.

Kevin M. Folta, March 2015

1

Spread Fear, Babe!

"You can have the best vaccines for a woman or her child, but if you can't get her to come and get them then they won't work. What are the dynamics that motivate her to do that?."—Melinda Gates

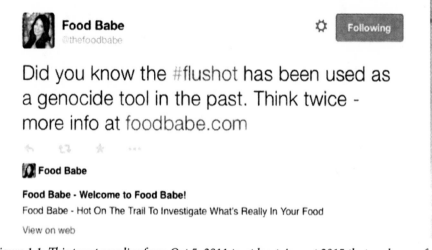

Food Babe
@thefoodbabe

Did you know the #flushot has been used as a genocide tool in the past. Think twice - more info at foodbabe.com

Food Babe

Food Babe - Welcome to Food Babe!
Food Babe - Hot On The Trail To Investigate What's Really In Your Food

View on web

Figure 1.1: This tweet was live from Oct 5, 2011 to at least August 2015 that we know of, creating a climate of fear around a safe and life-saving vaccination. (Twitter)

Vaccines were developed to help prevent death and serious illness. Many people alive today would not be here if it were not for the vaccines, including you. Even if you've never had a vaccination or a serious illness, your parents might have been protected by them or even by the herd immunity surrounding them and us. An example of just how lucky we are to be here appears on page 235.

The word vaccine derives from vacca, the Latin for cow—because the very first vaccine for smallpox was developed from cowpox. British doctor

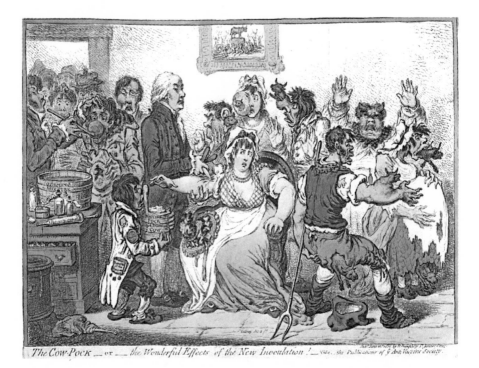

The Cow-Pock __ or __ the Wonderful Effects of the New Inoculation ! __ ...the Publications of ye Anti Vaccine Society.

Figure 1.2 In Jenner's day, vaccines were viewed with suspicion. People thought they would sprout cow's organs after treatment. Sadly, not much has changed. "The cow pock" by James Gillray—Library of Congress, Prints & Photographs Division, LC-USZC4-3147 (color film copy transparency)/Wikipedia

Edward Jenner (1749—1823) observed that milkmaids never contracted smallpox and hypothesized their protection derived from exposure to cowpox.

The girls caught cowpox, a much milder virus, from their charges and as a result didn't suffer from smallpox, the more virulent strain. Jenner took samples from an infected maid and tested them on patients to see if they developed disease. This sort of experimental medicine is outlawed today, yet ironically, is related to the techniques employed by vaccine fraud Dr. Andrew Wakefield. It's also one of the many reasons he was removed from the medical register in Great Britain.

When our bodies spot something that doesn't belong, they produce an army of specialist cells programmed to target it. A few of these cells hang around long afterwards just in case the invading organism comes back. Some viral strains are so powerful they overwhelm our defense mechanisms before our body can muster up an army. We get sick, and sometimes die.

Vaccines work by programming our body's defense mechanism by deliberately exposing them to a very weak form of the target pathogen. So rather than being overwhelmed, our natural defenses are able to identify and produce the antibodies we require. Once we're exposed to the real virus, our bodies are so well prepared we rarely even notice the invasion. Because viruses need living hosts to survive, if sufficient people are vaccinated the pathogens go extinct. This is one extinction that is actually a good thing.

Today's vaccines use what's known as an attenuated strain of the target pathogen. So a vaccine for H5N1 bird flu would contain a very weak form of that virus and one of the ways to weaken it is to add a minute amount of a natural chemical such as formaldehyde. Our bodies naturally produce formaldehyde and know how to deal with it. The small amount in the vaccine doesn't affect us but it cripples the virus sufficiently so our immune system can learn and build a defense.

The aluminum or other chemical adjuvants are there to irritate our tissue and trigger an immune response. They act like an emergency siren actively encouraging our immune cells to flock to the vaccination site—where they attack the weak virus and do their job. This is why we often see a small red swelling there. If the adjuvants were not present, we would have to give a much larger (more dangerous) dose of the virus and cause a much more uncomfortable response.

In mid April 2015, Australian Prime Minster Tony Abbott set out a plan to make vaccinations effectively compulsory by withdrawing financial support from anti-vaccination parents.

> *"The choice… is not supported by public policy or medical research nor should such action be supported by taxpayers in the form of child care payments," Mr Abbott told reporters in a statement.*

The Fear Babe

In a 2011 post, Food Babe takes aim at the flu shot—the influenza vaccination offered annually to people in the hope of stemming an epidemic of influenza among children, the elderly, and people with compromised immune systems.

> ***Disclaimer—This post is strictly based upon my opinion and consultation of my own health provider, I recommend you make the best choice for you and your family based upon your own due diligence and research on this topic. *** [1]

Disclaimers are all well and good, but that's a legal dodge to protect Food Babe LLC from potential legal action. We have to weigh that against the content that opens up almost immediately, with a terrifying list of claims.

> Before you consider jumping off the ledge with other lemmings and taking this years Flu Shot—Here are the questions I think you should ask yourself... What's exactly in the Flu Shot? To sum it up—A bunch of toxic chemicals and additives that lead to several types of Cancers and Alzheimer disease over time. [2]

Food Babe's vaccine additive list appears on page 2355.

She goes on to say:

> I won't eat any of these ingredients or even put them on my body[3]

But the first thing on that list is eggs. Scientists used eggs because they are a cheap, easy and reliable medium to grow the live virus. But Food Babe won't eat them… really? Strange to reflect that in 2013 she's creating a tasty recipe [4] using *eggs*. Her four serving Mini Fritatta looks delicious albeit eggy!

What's exactly in the Flu Shot?

Thimersol (Thimerosal) is a preservative. It is not mercury. Let's say that again. It is NOT mercury. It contains mercury in much the same way as

---

1   http://foodbabe.com/2011/10/04/should-i-get-the-flu-shot/

2   http://foodbabe.com/2011/10/04/should-i-get-the-flu-shot/

3   http://foodbabe.com/2011/10/04/should-i-get-the-flu-shot/

4   http://foodbabe.com/2013/11/22/are-eggs-yolks-good-or-bad/

- *Egg Products (including avian contaminant viruses)*
- *Aluminum*
- *Thimersol (Mercury)*
- *Monosodium Glutamate (MSG)*
- *Chick Embryo Cells*
- *Latex*
- *Formaldehyde*
- *Gelatin*
- *Polysorbate 80*
- *Triton X100 (strong detergent)*
- *Sucrose (table **sugar**)*
- *Resin*
- *Gentamycin*

Scientists have developed a seasonal flu vaccine. Jim Gathany Content Providers(s): CDC

Food Babe's "research" into the influenza vaccine trawled up this list of ingredients.

the food we eat contains, say, carbon. It also contains sulphur, oxygen and sodium.

The chemical formula, for those wondering, looks like this: C_9H_9Hg-NaO_2S, where:

C—Carbon	Na—Sodium
H—Hydrogen	O—Oxygen
Hg—Mercury	S—Sulfur

That's not to say that concerns haven't been raised about it because it does degrade into simpler mercury-containing compounds in the body. Perhaps you're thinking: "All the stories are right!"

A lot of research has gone into this field and the results are tricky to understand. In essence, Thimerosal breaks down into *ethylmercury* and *thiosalicylate* and it's the ethylmercury that was considered a problem based on some studies using the related compound, *methylmercury*. Both com-

Permitted Additives in the Influenza Anti-viral. (CDC)

Influenza (Afluria)	beta-propiolactone, thimerosol (multi-dose vials only), monobasic sodium phosphate, dibasic sodium phosphate, monobasic potassium phosphate, potassium chloride, calcium chloride, sodium taurodeoxycholate, neomycin sulfate, polymyxin B, egg protein, sucrose	April, 2013
Influenza (Agriflu)	egg proteins, formaldehyde, polysorbate 80, cetyltrimethylammonium bromide, neomycin sulfate, kanamycin	June, 2012
Influenza (Fluarix)	octoxynol-10 (Triton X-100), α-tocopheryl hydrogen succinate, polysorbate 80 (Tween 80), hydrocortisone, gentamicin sulfate, ovalbumin, formaldehyde, sodium deoxycholate, sucrose, phosphate buffer	May, 2013
Influenza (Flublok)	monobasic sodium phosphate, dibasic sodium phosphate, polysorbate 20, baculovirus and host cell proteins, baculovirus and cellular DNA, Triton X-100, lipids, vitamins, amino acids, mineral salts	December, 2012
Influenza (Flucelvax)	Madin Darby Canine Kidney (MDCK) cell protein, MDCK cell DNA, polysorbate 80, cetyl-trimethlyammonium bromide, β-propiolactone, phosphate buffer	October, 2012
Influenza (Fluvirin)	nonylphenol ethoxylate, thimerosal (multidose vial–trace only in prefilled syringe), polymyxin, neomycin, beta-propiolactone, egg proteins, phosphate buffer	January, 2012
Influenza (Flulaval)	thimerosal, formaldehyde, sodium deoxycholate, egg proteins	February, 2013
Influenza (Fluzone: Standard, High-Dose, & Intradermal)	formaldehyde, octylphenol ethoxylate (Triton X-100), gelatin (standard trivalent formulation only), thimerosal (multi-dose vial only) , egg protein, phosphate buffers, sucrose	April, 2013
Influenza (FluMist)	ethylene diamine tetraacetic acid (EDTA), monosodium glutamate, hydrolyzed porcine gelatin, arginine, sucrose, dibasic potassium phosphate, monobasic potassium phosphate, gentamicin sulfate, egg protein	July, 2013

pounds move fairly freely through our bodies and are eventually eliminated via our kidneys– more proof (if any more were needed) that our bodies are amazing at detoxing themselves entirely naturally—no "woo" required.

The precise contents of current flu shots are listed in table on page 6— sourced from the *Centers for Disease Control*.

MSG (see page 32) is harmless, despite an uninformed campaign based on a piece of non-science *ad hoc ergo propter hoc* self-diagnosis by a physician who should have known better… but wait a moment. Flu-mist isn't administered via injection– you put it up your nose (the clue is in the name).

Gentamicin/Gentamycin is an antibiotic in its own right and none of the vaccines the CDC list contained any MSG; nor latex (rubber) and not even aluminum. Gelatin is only used in Fluzone's trivalent formula and should be avoided by strict vegetarians/vegans.

Other ingredients are not there just for the sake of it. There's no commercial sense placing something in a vaccine for no reason. It costs the manufacturer money and does not benefit them. These additives are used as preservatives and adjuvants and make the vaccines safer and more effective.

A small percentage of people are allergic to eggs, and therefore, cannot use flu shots created from egg cultures in case they suffer from an allergic reaction.

> Long term effects of the combination of these toxic additives are very alarming—a very famous immunologist & geneticist has completed studies and research that shows in that every five flu shots a person receives over a ten year period they increase their risk of Alzheimer (sic) Disease by ten times! This is because of the ingredients above—Aluminum and Mercury—they slowly destroy your brain cells one by one. [5]

Aluminum isn't in any of these preparations and its effect on our brains is immeasurable at small doses. Mercury compound is removed from our bodies by a natural process; besides which it's not actually elemental mercury in the first place. Food Babe doesn't name this "very famous immunologist & geneticist" but even if she had, it's entirely possible the

---

[5]   http://foodbabe.com/2011/10/04/should-i-get-the-flu-shot/

research was biased, challenged, or just plain wrong. *Andrew Wakefield*, the infamous quack MD driven by greed, created another scare over the MMR vaccine that continues to rumble on even now. The claim:

> *"[people] increase their risk of Alzheimer's Disease by ten times!"*

Begs a closer look because even though we were unable to source the data, this is one of those weasel phrases that doesn't sound like one. When you see something like this, you need to ask yourself: 10x what? It sounds horrifying "TEN TIMES!"

Let's assume your lifetime chance of winning the lottery is about 1 in 13,983,816. If your chances increase 10 times, your odds of winning increase to 10 in 13,983,816, which are still stupefyingly long odds.

For anyone interested in reading more about this, *How to Lie With Statistics* (Huff, D. 1991) is probably the finest primer you could wish for, especially if mathematics is not your thing.

> Does the Flu Shot really protect me against the Flu? No, the CDC even admits it doesn't protect you because the virus mutates every year and they can't predict which strains will hit. Even when they do get the strain right, they can't prove it actually works. [...] In a couple of studies I read, The (sic) flu shot was compared to a placebo—The (sic) same number of people caught the flu regardless if they took the shot or not! [6]

Once again, this distorts the facts—perhaps from ignorance, perhaps to make a point. It's not clear. Like HIV, the virus that causes AIDS, influenza is a complex and evolving virus with strains coming and going each year. It's something of a crap shoot trying to figure out which one (two, or three) is going to hit. Rather like forecasting the weather, scientists have to take an educated guess. In another crushing display of her absolute ignorance, Food Babe continues:

> Why do I have to get a Flu Shot every year? Aren't vaccines supposed to immunize you for life? They have to continuously give you a flu shot, because it is not a real vaccine. Let's say for instance, you get a vaccine for another virus like Hepatitis A or B—you are immunized for life. Why isn't this the case with the flu

---

6   http://foodbabe.com/2011/10/04/should-i-get-the-flu-shot/

vaccine? Because the scientists have not developed a real vaccine for the flu and are continuously guessing on how to come up with a new chemical formula that could be effective. [7]

There are actually three types of flu virus—but classes might be a better word: A, B and C. (Scientists are not known for their snappy naming conventions).

- *Type A*: is spread by birds and animals and makes us fairly sick. It's spread by coughing and sneezing too. This variant, also known as bird flu, comes in Hn variants, where H9 is the least serious. It was one of the H5 class (H5N1) that caused the 2009 pandemic.
- *Type B*: is generally milder but can still be serious. It's only seen in humans.
- *Type C*: is the weakest form of the virus and causes mild symptoms in affected people. It's not part of the current vaccination program in the USA.

Within the sub-types, scientists separate out the virus using two proteins: *hemagglutinin* (the H part) and *neuraminidase* (the N part). As new versions of these proteins are discovered in the wild, the number is increased. So, for example: H5N1 was the fifth form of hemagglutinin and the first version of neuraminidase.

As of early 2015, H7N9 bird flu had already killed nearly 100 people in Asia.

So despite Food Babe's desperate and ignorant claims the flu vaccine is not "real" per:

> Because the scientists have not developed a real vaccine for the flu... [8]

It should be fairly clear that she has absolutely no clue just how complex this problem is. Indeed, it seems like she pulled her theory out of thin air. According to Food Babe, vaccines are there to make money for Big Pharma, not help us stay well. Not all viruses mutate like this. The very

---

7   http://foodbabe.com/2011/10/04/should-i-get-the-flu-shot/
8   http://foodbabe.com/2011/10/04/should-i-get-the-flu-shot/

fact that HIV mutates so often and at such high rates is what has made a simple and effective vaccine an almost impossible dream. Hepatitis A and B on the other hand, are relatively stable and the vaccines remain effective for life.

> Why is there so much pressure to get the Flu Shot year after year? Why does every drug store have a sign up promoting the shot? Why are shots available at work? And at school? Why is there so much propaganda each year around this time? There is only one answer—Money. The making, distributing, and administering of the flu shot is a 7 Billion Dollar Industry. Each year the pharmaceutical industry eyes glow with $ signs when it's time to make more as the American public become the guinea pigs again to try it out. [9]

Why is the Food Babe making such a fuss about this? Does she care about us protecting ourselves from highly infectious and potentially dangerous disease? Perhaps (as we'll see in a minute), but really she's doing this for the "holy sh*t" factor to drive more traffic to her web site and make more money.

> Why are Flu Shots recommended for children, women who are pregnant and the elderly? Because that group of individuals typically have weaker immune systems and if they catch the flu and don't treat it in time it can lead to other complications like pneumonia. However, why would you give a group with already weakened immune systems something that weakens their immune system systemically further? [10]

Once again, this demonstrates a total ignorance of basic immunology, and a dangerous one at that. Doctors don't go around injecting attenuated (effectively it's harmless but still "alive") viruses into immuno-compromized people to make more money from the drug companies; they do it because vaccination may be the only way such people are able to survive. Has Food Babe ever considered that there's more money for pharma in treating the already ill than in preventing disease?

> Can I immunize myself naturally from the Flu? Yes! You can build lifetime antibodies against the infection. Just Skip (sic) the

---

9   http://foodbabe.com/2011/10/04/should-i-get-the-flu-shot/
10 http://foodbabe.com/2011/10/04/should-i-get-the-flu-shot/

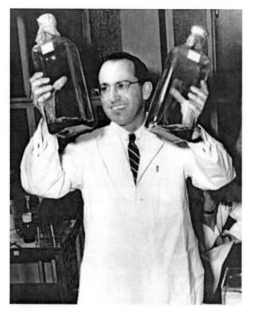

Figure 1.3: Jonas Salk created the first successful vaccine against poliomyelitis (polio). (Wikipedia/ University of Pittsburgh Digital Archives)

vaccine, boost your vitamin D intake, and encounter the flu naturally. If you encounter the flu—rest, take care of yourself, understand that your body needs a break and focus on getting better—This (sic) type of immunizing yourself works amazingly better than relying on an artificial injection that has been proven ineffective. You'll have these new antibodies for life that will ultimately protect you from similar strains of the virus better than any yearly shot could ever provide. [11]

There's so much wrong here it's difficult to contemplate. If Food Babe thought appendicitis was unpleasant, we suggest H5N1 might help her get some perspective. If you encounter a real A-class influenza, you're going to find yourself in a heap of trouble. Flu is not a cold nor is it a stomach virus. A cold is mild and rather unpleasant, but ultimately little more than a minor inconvenience. "Stomach flu" isn't an influenza virus at all, but the term has entered the vernacular and helps perpetuate the pesky misconception.

Flu kills thousands of people every single year. [12]

Those people who survive it are left in a weakened state for weeks or even months. Some are left with debilitating, sometime chronic post-viral syndromes. Just being a healthy, youthful person isn't enough to protect you. When Spanish flu (H1N1) hit in 1918 the highest mortality rates were among young, healthy adults. 500 million people are thought to have been infected with as many as 50 million ultimately succumbing and losing their lives.

---

11   http://foodbabe.com/2011/10/04/should-i-get-the-flu-shot/
12   http://www.who.int/mediacentre/factsheets/fs211/en/

The Fear Babe

Finally, Food Babe closes with this virtual "disclaimer," which is pretty pointless for people who take her at her word over the previous paragraphs.

> P.S. If you know someone who would like to hear about this perspective, please share this post with them.
>
> P.S.S. I am not "anti-vaccination", I choose not to take the flu shot for the ingredients they contain as stated above. [13]

Despite the disclaimer, this page contains a very powerful and disturbing message: the flu vaccine is bad for you. Followers of Food Babe, some of whom worship her almost as a deity, are potentially putting themselves *and others* at risk from a virus that can and does kill. And once you start questioning the flu vaccine, where do you stop? Melinda Gates' pointed question might well be answered right here. Fear is what motivates people more than anything else. It's a basic instinct that has kept our species alive for millennia; and this is why we call her *The Fear Babe*.

This entire affair is particularly disturbing because Food Babe's perspective is based on lazy research and a complete misunderstanding of how vaccines work. If she had to make a post about this at all, perhaps what she could have said was:

"I have decided, for personal reasons, not to partake in the flu vaccination program."

Period.

Instead she's created an entirely ludicrous post filled with baseless presumptions and stupid "advice" that people are bound to follow, potentially putting lives at stake.

Again. ∎

---

13   http://foodbabe.com/2011/10/04/should-i-get-the-flu-shot/

2

Shards

"In the land of the blind, the one-eyed man is king"—Desiderius Erasmus, 16th C., Dutch humanist and theologian

As of this writing there are probably few bloggers who can honestly claim to have the reach and power of Vani "Food Babe" Hari. In compiling this book—originally planned as a filmed documentary—we approached Ms. Hari for comment and spoke to a number of her most outspoken critics.

We have not received a response to requests for an interview and we're not the only ones. In the wake of the SciBabe/Gawker article [1] debunking many of her claims and launching the most widespread media backlash against her to date, multiple news sources have asked Ms. Hari for an interview. There was no response to these requests.

To some, this charismatic Indian-American daughter of a college professor is a self-styled food activist on a mission to get dangerous chemicals out of our food.

To others, Hari is a narcissistic, misinformed, fear-mongering bully who leads a zombie army of uncritical followers, refusing to engage with her critics and actively attacking anyone who doesn't agree—even to the extent of pre-banning some of her critics from her Facebook page and actively deleting comments from her blog.

Her story begins as a child of immigrant parents from India—who would consume the typical American diet.

> I grew up eating McDonald's and Burger King. My parents wanted us to be American. Indian food is so amazing and medicinal and organic... [2]

---

1   http://gawker.com/the-food-babe-blogger-is-full-of-shit-1694902226
2   Interview with Dr. Mercola

The Fear Babe

She was a spoiled child as she tacitly admits in her book, *The Food Babe Way: Break Free from the Hidden Toxins in Your Food and Lose Weight, Look Years Younger, and Get Healthy in Just 21 Days!* While her parents consumed a traditional fare, she and her older brother were allowed to indulge in whatever they fancied. She even admits, without any apparent remorse, to stealing the sweets her mother refused to buy her:

> I'd steal candy (because she [her mother] wouldn't buy it for me) and hide it my pockets until I got home. [3]

Describing her diet and spoiled upbringing:

> ...for me and my brother, anything we wanted. There were no rules. If we wanted McDonald's, we got it. If we wanted Wendy's, we got it. If we wanted mozzarella sticks from the FryDaddy, she made them. [4]

This self-described unhealthy child joined the high-school debate team and in the pre-Google days, recounts spending hours in the library learning how to debate while avoiding her homework. This is a person developing a competitive edge and isn't shy in coming forward or boasting about her achievements; a narcissistic trait that would serve her well in future.

Upon leaving college, Hari joined Accenture, which she describes as one of the top management-consulting firms in the country. But that came at a price.

> ...managing large–scale projects, mergers and acquisitions, integration work.... and they put me on a schedule where I was traveling Sunday through Thursday. 22–23 years old I became really sick. [5]

She goes on to relate how she was doing everything her co-workers were doing:

> ...not really paying attention to my health. Not working out because I was trying to work as many hours as possible. Show up

---

3   The Food Babe Way, p. 8
4   The Food Babe Way, p. 8
5   Interview with Dr. Mercola

before my boss, leave after my boss and tried to get promoted. [6]

After eating the free meals (steak, chicken parmesan) she ended up in the hospital with a severe stomach pain. Overdoing it with the hyperbole is something Hari does well—describing her fairly common ailments of asthma and eczema and alluding to an attack of appendicitis as:

> Then I got sick, really sick [7]

Appendicitis can be dangerous and even life-threatening. It's a common ailment with nearly 300,000 cases recorded in the United States during 2010, and remains the most common form of acute hospital admission requiring surgery. About 30% of those admissions are related to a perforated appendix, which is a more dangerous development as pus leaks into the abdominal cavity resulting in potentially life-threatening peritonitis. UK statistics suggest a lifetime risk of about 6% with a generally positive outcome.

She claims to have gained 25 to 30 lbs in just three months and the sickness provided "an awakening." Although doctors agree that appendicitis is an increasingly rare condition that can strike anyone, Hari made the connection that since the appendix is part of the digestive tract, toxins in her food must logically have caused hers to become inflamed.

Our lifetime risk of appendicitis is around 1 in 13 with a peak risk between 10 and 20 years of age. Although the exact cause is unknown, most infections are thought to originate when fecal matter [poop] becomes lodged in the organ or the entrance is blocked by a swollen lymph node following a respiratory tract infection.

So the evidence says that Vani Hari was struck by a common illness at a fairly typical age. Making the connection between diet and the illness is a case of *post hoc, ergo propter hoc* (from the Latin meaning "after this, therefore because of this") in essence making a connection without evidence to back it up.

Hari's claim that she was "really sick" is relative. But as anyone who has come through any one of a whole barrage of serious illnesses will tell you,

6   Interview with Dr. Mercola
7   The Food Babe Way, P. 6

appendicitis, while painful and disturbing, is rarely a death sentence. Full-blown influenza (not the common cold which is often errorneously called "flu") often kills elderly people and even healthy adults. Victims are left weakened for weeks and even months. Lifetime conditions such as Type I diabetes are serious, life-threatening illnesses. Many more are far more serious than an inflamed appendix and cannot be corrected by an everyday minor surgery.

By 2009 she had started researching food and two years later the blog was born—to a shaky start. Among early entries (long since deleted and even purged from the Google cache) two embarrassing moments really stand out: one on microwave ovens and another about air travel. Remember though, this is a person who claims to have been researching for two years. Admitting you're fallible is one of the first rules of science; correcting your errors and learning from them is a hallmark of maturity. Airbrushing them from history is deceitful.

Bending the facts is something Hari does with some panache. Here she is describing her fear of making the transition from a well-paid management consultant to a full-time blogger, quitting her full time job in December of 2012:

> I was terrified. I was worried about how I'd make my mortgage, have health insurance, and feed my family. [8]

Since she started blogging, Hari's professional profile lists her as "Program Manager—Global Information Security" for Bank of America from 2012-2013 and a Product Manager—Mobile Banking for Ally Financial from April 2009 to November 2011. [9] It does not, however, mention that she was also married to a successful and (presumably) very well-paid Finley Clarke– also known as Mr. Food Babe.

So unless Ms. Hari has dependants (i.e. children) she has never spoken about, the implication that she was risking everything for the sake of her blog is preposterous. But at face value, it's believable. As Hari tells it, she's prepared to risk everything for the greater good when the reality is she has a safety net the size of a small country.

---

8   The Food Babe Way, p. 27
9   Source: LinkedIn.com

The Food Babe Way or The Highway.

Perhaps the most accurate way to describe Food Babe's language is that of a cult leader. If that sounds a little overwrought, consider how charismatic cult leaders work. They sit at least one step removed from their followers who worship them like gods and do their every bidding without question. Food Babe even refers to her followers as the Food Babe Army, and while they are not an organized militia, they are hugely militant.

Food Babe uses a number of literary devices to distance claims from the science—most usually *weasel words*: ambiguous words or phrases meant to give the casual reader a sense of authority when no actual authority exists. She also employs liberal sprinklings of words and phrases (toxic, carcinogenic etc.) designed to instill fear (of death or serious illness) and these techniques are almost certainly products of her debating experience, where all that matters is winning the debate. Facts are a distant second.

She's not a toxicologist, oncologist nor even a food scientist (her degree is in computing) but as David Dunning and Justin Kruger demonstrated, the more ignorant a person is, the more confident they are of their facts, observing:

> "*The miscalibration of the incompetent stems from an error about the self, whereas the miscalibration of the highly competent stems from an error about others*"

Dunning and Kruger's work [10] can be briefly summarized with these traits:

- Fail to recognize their own lack of skill.
- Fail to recognize genuine skill in others.
- Fail to recognize the extremity of their inadequacy.

From reading the following pages you will soon begin to get a sense of how incompetence has lured Food Babe into the belief she actually knows a lot more than she does—leading to the level of frustration leveled at her by competent and trained people; particularly her outright and utter refusal to engage with people who actually know the subject or correct her own mistakes.

---

10   Kruger, J. and Dunning, D.."Unskilled and Unaware of It: How Difficulties in Recognizing One's Own Incompetence Lead to Inflated Self-Assessments," Journal of Personality and Social Psychology, 1999 (http://psych.colorado.edu/~vanboven/teaching/p7536_heurbias/p7536_readings/kruger_dunning.pdf)

Although a modern twist, this idea has been around for a very long time, as this saying from the 16th century shows:

> *"Young men think old men fools, old men know young men are."*—
> *William Camden, English Historian.*

With great power comes great responsibility. What started as an innocent blog is now shirking its responsibility by creating a fog of fear around harmless ingredients. In this chapter, we will examine some grouped quotations taken from Hari's work and see just what is going on behind the high-production value videos, professional photography, and terrifying and occasionally dangerous claims.

It's rather ironic that the woman who writes stuff like this:

> In Europe they use the precautionary principle—if there is significant evidence of harm, absolute proof is not required to act. Sadly in our country, the burden is on the public to prove safety instead of the food companies. [11]

Can be sufficiently or even willfully ignorant to espouse the consumption of raw milk, which is a very real risk to health:

> Raw dairy products are "alive" and have all of their probiotics, vitamins and enzymes intact, including phosphatase, which is necessary to properly absorb the calcium in milk. [12]

Oh, they're alive alright! This is what the experts at the CDC have to say about this sort of advice:

> *"Many people who chose raw milk thinking they would improve their health instead found themselves (or their loved ones) sick in a hospital for several weeks fighting for their lives from infections caused by germs in raw milk."* [13]

Pathogens potentially present in raw milk read like a nightmare. We present a short list adapted from information from the CDC and other sources, making it one of the world's most deadly pathogen lists.

---

11   http://foodbabe.com/an-open-letter-to-food-babe/
12   http://foodbabe.com/2014/10/29/organic-milk/
13   http://www.cdc.gov/foodsafety/rawmilk/raw-milk-questions-and-answers.html

Play The Raw Milk Lotto: It Could be You!

Brucella: the bacteria responsible for brucellosis and miscarriage in pregnant women.

Campylobacter jejuni: a common form of bacterial food poisoning, campylobacteriosis.

Coxiella burnetii: a fortunately rare, parasitic bacterium that causes Q-Fever in humans.

Escherichia coli: (a family of bacterium also known as e. coli with O157:H7 being the most likely to cause disease in humans) may produce the Shiga toxin leading to dysentery.

Giardia: a protozoan (larger than a bacteria) and the cause of Giardiasis (Beaver Fever.)

Listeria monocytogenes: the nasty blighter responsible for the rare, but extremely serious listeriosis. Primarily affecting people with a weakened immune system including children and expectant mothers and can cross the placental barrier resulting in fetal death. May cause death in up to one fifth of cases and can survive and reproduce even at the low temperatures found in a refrigerator.

Mycobacterium avium paratuberculosis: causes Johne's disease in cattle and may be responsible for Crohn's disease in humans.

Mycobacterium bovis: the pathogen behind bovine tuberculosis which can affect humans.

Salmonella: responsible for typhoid fever and serious food poisoning (salmonellosis) which may result in death and remains the most common cause of food-related deaths in the USA today. Salmonella can live in our guts and, therefore, is easily transmitted person-to-person through poor food handling.

Shigella: the bacteria responsible for Marlow Syndrome.

Yersinia enterocolitica: a bacteria thought to be associated with Crohn's disease. Causes diarrhea and can grow in refrigerated conditions.

Norovirus: commonly called the Winter Vomiting Bug in the UK, is the pathogen responsible for the highly contagious and unpleasant gastroenteritis that can sweep through a close community in a matter of hours as contaminated vomit and fecal matter spreads via air currents.

In the The Food Babe Way, Food Babe only sees the positives.

> Raw milk also contains several types of naturally occurring probiotics that help populate your digestive system with beneficial bacteria... Raw milk keeps seven to ten days in the fridge. [14]

What she doesn't seem to get—or conveniently ignores—is raw milk is not standardized. You could get it from the same farm, even the same cow, for years and then suddenly get a batch full of deadly bugs and you won't know until you find yourself running for the toilet or worse. A lot worse.

> It is unfortunate that the government can impose bans that override our rights as consumers to decide what we want to eat and drink, especially when they cut out something that is healthier than the alternative. [15]

There's a reason raw milk is restricted—if it wasn't our hospitals would be overrun by people suffering from preventable disease. Further, there is the potential to pass these microbes on to people who have not consumed the product. Raw milk consumption is playing Russian roulette with your health and it's simply not worth it.

> The heat also destroys enzymes your body needs for proper digestion. One of these is phosphatase. Without this enzyme the calcium lingers in your bloodstream and can accumulate in your arteries. As a result, your arteries get stiff and it's more difficult for them to pump blood. Stiff arteries give rise to hypertension (high blood pressure), chest pain, and heart failure. [16]

And there we were thinking it was our heart that pumps blood... This is the sort of thing the publishers—someone anyway—should have picked up on because it's so obviously stupid, no one would believe it ... would they?

Somewhat ironically, high blood pressure can also disturb the delicate lining of the arterial walls leading to a build-up of plaques and further stiffening of the walls; but phosphatase? Food Babe is referring to alkaline phosphatase, which is easily destroyed by heat and is something a lab can use to

---

14   The Food Babe Way, p. 112
15   The Food Babe Way, p. 113
16   The Food Babe Way, p. 111

ensure milk has been effectively and completely pasteurized. However, our bodies are already full of the stuff.

Enzymes are fascinating things—so much so that entire books have been written about them and we still don't know how many exist or what they all do. While enzymes themselves are not actually alive, they are essential to all life and perform functions completely automatically by binding to specific chemicals and doing their work (often breaking complex chemicals into simpler ones) without any effort on our part. All enzymes are proteins, but they are more complex than simple proteins. You might even think of them as tiny biological machines.

Broadly speaking, the names of enzymes end in -ase; with the first part of the name implying what the enzyme's target is like this: lipases target lipids (fats); proteases: proteins and so on. There are a lot of them with a wide range of functions.

There's an enzyme in your saliva called *amylase* that breaks down complex carbohydrates into simpler ones, and you can try this one for yourself and see how it works. Get a small piece of any bread and chew it; after a while you'll notice the "bread" taste starts to dissipate to be replaced by a pleasant, sweet flavor: glucose.

This is why, rather ironically, things like fries and chips (chips and crisps in the UK), can be bad for our teeth. Potatoes are primarily starch and when we eat those products, little bits get left behind. These tiny pieces are broken into glucose by the amylase in our saliva and metabolized by oral bacteria. The bacteria then poop out acids which attack the enamel on our teeth, resulting in dental cavities and even gum disease and bad breath.

Bon appétit!

Raw milk contains a bundle of "living" enzymes but for an enzyme to work, it has to be at least at the correct temperature and pH (acidity). Our saliva, for instance, is slightly alkaline but our stomachs contain strong acids and amylase is destroyed when it gets into our gut.

Biological molecules are fairly sensitive to temperature and many, such as lipoprotein lipase, are easily destroyed by heat. This is useful in milk production since if the lipase comes into contact with fats, it breaks them down resulting in unwanted side effects. *Plasmin*, another enzyme deactivated by pasteurization (and one of the few not ending in -ase) would otherwise break down proteins and cause milk to taste "off."

You might have heard there are anti-bacterial enzymes in natural milk and that's true up to a point; but the problem is twofold: Firstly, enzymes target very specific compounds and secondly one bacteria is very much like another. A bacteria that makes us seriously ill is no different than a harmless one so far as the enzymes are concerned.

Milk itself should be sterile when it leaves the cow—if not the calf would get sick. Despite the farmer's best efforts—viruses, bacteria and protozoans get in there; often from fecal matter that's gotten onto the cow's udders but it can come from anywhere; even the cleanest farm in the world is a pathogen's five star hotel.

Lactoferrin, probably the most potent anti-bacterial in milk is isolated using temperatures of up to 212°F/100°C meaning it's still present in normally pasteurized milk—which is known to spoil… so that pretty much writes that off. *Lactoperoxidase* has similar effects but is only operative in the presence of peroxide and thiocyanate (neither of which are present in milk) meaning that's essentially useless too.

> Calcium can also build up in plaque, the cholesterol–filled pouches lining the interior of the arteries. This process constricts the arteries and potentially chokes off the blood supply to the heart and other vital organs. Should a plaque rupture, you'd be at risk of a heart attack or stroke. [17]

The exact cause of atherosclerosis (hardening of our arteries) is still unknown although there are a number of risk factors including smoking, obesity, type I and II diabetes, raised blood pressure and high levels of LDL cholesterol.

LDL (bad) cholesterol is made in our livers and carried through our blood to the cells that need it. Although we call it "bad" cholesterol, we need a certain amount, just not too much. HDL (good) cholesterol is produced in our cells and either broken down in our liver or simply passed out as a waste product.

---

17   The Food Babe Way, p. 111

A chemical in cigarettes called *acrolein* (aka *propenal*) interferes with the transport of HDL cholesterol from our cells and leaves the LDL to run riot and cause our arteries to narrow. Smoking doesn't just cause cancer.

About 1 in 500 of us has an inherited condition called *familial hypercholesterolaemia* which causes our bodies to produce too much LDL cholesterol regardless of what we eat or how much we exercise. Even our ethnicity can affect us, with people from India, Pakistan, Bangladesh or Sri Lanka being at the greatest risk.

Other risk factors for elevated levels of LDL cholesterol (and triglycerides) are obesity, lack of exercise, poor diet (too much dietary fat and sugars) and drinking excess alcohol.

When our arteries narrow they cause effects such as shown in the panel "Narrowing Arteries... should I worry?" on page 24

The calcium connection is due to calcifications in the coronary arteries which can be spotted on a coronary calcium scan. We need calcium to build and maintain our bones. The idea that raw milk can somehow prevent atherosclerosis or maintain cardiovascular health is just very bad science and further promotes the potentially life-threatening consumption of raw milk.

Pretty Little Liars

One question continues to smolder: is Food Babe a liar?

The answer to this is more nuanced than might first appear because to tell a lie, one first has to know (or at least could reasonably deduce) the truth. Human memory is fragile—clinical neurologist and professor, *Dr. Steven Novella M.D.* refers to it as a construct. Every time we recall a memory we change it slightly.

"Did I remember to put the cat out? Where did I leave my keys? Do I need milk from the store?" You can be reasonably sure that you bought milk from the store (a belief: based on a memory) and you can go to the refrigerator and check (testing the evidence).

Narrowing Arteries... should I worry?

- A loss of effective blood supply to and from the bowels leading to progressive conditions like *ischemic colitis* and *mesenteric ischemia*.
- Slow but steady reduction of blood supply to the brain may also give rise to vascular dementia.
- Ruptured plaques cause clots which in turn cause the following conditions—aggravated by already narrowed arteries—which may be life-threatening.
- *Angina pectoris*: the four coronary arteries surrounding our hearts supply the heart muscle with blood and if the heart muscle cannot get enough blood during exertion, it causes severe chest pain which can be relieved with *glycerine trinitrate* (GTN). GTN causes the arteries to relax and resume normal blood flow but in severe cases, cardiac artery bypass surgery may be required.
- *Myocardial infarctions*: heart attacks—a major cause of death in the West and about a third of people don't even make it to hospital. A heart attack caused when a plaque ruptures and blocks the blood supply to our heart causing symptoms similar to angina but more severe as the heart muscle and nerves begin to die. Nerve damage can result in cardiac arrhythmia causing the heart to beat so fast it gives up. Cardiogenic shock where the muscle is so damaged the heart fails to pump blood and even heart rupture where the valves break down. These factors invariably result in a painful death.
- *TIAs* (transient ischemic attack sometimes, erroneously, called a mini-stroke) where a plaque breaks off and blocks blood flow to part of our brain resulting in a temporary loss of function.
- *Cerebrovascular insult*: the medical term for a full-blown stroke where sufficient brain tissue is damaged to cause paralysis, loss of speech and even death.

Every one of us forgets things from time to time. Even when we remember things we rarely remember them exactly and in some cases our memory can be primed. Imagine going into an office and asking everyone:

"Is the boss wearing a tie today?"

But prime that in some way, such as:

"What color tie is the boss wearing today?"

and people will assume the boss is wearing a tie even if he isn't.

This technique, called leading the witness, can be that subtle because it relies on the frailty of human memory. In the absence of strong, contrary evidence (for example, the boss stood right next to you wearing jeans and a tee-shirt) we tend to believe what we were first told and in rare cases, people dismiss even irrefutable evidence out of hand; something we'll look at later.

Scientists have designed a way around this by publishing their work and allowing other scientists to examine all their evidence even to the point of reproducing the same finding. Reproducibility is a central tenet of science, and this transparency allows scientists to declare things with very high degrees of certainty because they have tested them over and over again and always got the predicted results.

On the Internet many writers will pick up a story and run with it because it appeals to them (fits with their belief) and sounds plausible. Spreading half-truths and falsehoods like this isn't quite the same as instigating the lie but the effect is just as bad. It is, for example, widely believed Hollywood actress Hedy Lamarr invented a technique used in WiFi and Bluetooth and other radio-technologies. It's a lovely idea but the reality, as physics professor Dr. Tony Rothman discovered, is far more complex (not to mention dull and secretive) than people are willing to believe. Similarly, an anti-GMO site recently began re-spreading rumours that KFC was using GM chickens. It's not, of course, and like all good scares GM chickens actually exist (a little truth lends credence to a fantastical story) but they are not in the food chain. [18, 19]

---

18   http://www.hoax-slayer.com/kfc-fake-chickens-hoax.shtml
19   http://www.nytimes.com/2002/05/24/international/24CHIC.html

Food Babe isn't wrong about everything: a diet low in processed food, salt, red meat and alcohol, and high in fresh fruit, vegetables and fish is good for us.

We've known that for decades. It's not news.

The wheels come off when she parrots unreliable sources and people with agendas couched in language that is designed to curry fear and loathing—and, of course, sell product!

But how do you spot them? How does anyone spot them? It's actually pretty tricky as Food Babe notes herself in this late Jan 2015 tweet.

> A fake article titled "Cuckoo for Cocoa Puffs?" was accepted by 17 medical journals. [20]

Dr. Mark Shrime, the Harvard medic behind this obviously hoax article pointed out to author, *Dr. Liz Segran*, that very few people would know the difference between *International Journal of Pediatric Otorhinolaryngology* and *Global Journal of Pediatric Otorhinolaryngology*. One is a respected journal; the other is completely bogus—but which is which? We'll leave you to ponder that one.

Absolute truth can be very difficult to establish—not that this lets Food Babe off the hook. Journalists and bloggers alike are open to legal action for libeling or otherwise defaming other people, but is that OK because she's an investigator?

> I've never claimed to be a nutritionist," she says. "I'm an investigator. [21]

A claim that allows Food Babe to elevate herself to another generally accepted (but not protected) job title. Professional investigators invariably have many years of experience in their own field. For instance the National Transportation Safety Board (NTSB) or Air Accident Bureau (AAB) investigators who look into the causes of air accidents are frequently highly experienced pilots in their own right who have undertaken years of extra training in other aspects of aviation.

---

20 https://twitter.com/thefoodbabe/status/560458602126004224 (tweet removed)
21 http://www.charlotteobserver.com/news/local/article9140060.html

A proper investigator would, at the very least try to get to the source of a story and in the case of scientific evidence, you have to check that source to see if (a) it's in a respected journal and (b) if any other scientists agree. In common parlance, one should always "get your facts straight from the horse's mouth." A phrase that dates back to the 1920s and means you should always seek a reliable witness. Don't just believe the guy selling the horse that it's only two years old—look at its teeth and check!

Spotting a source with an agenda can be very tricky and requires an amount of background knowledge, not to mention a very open mind. Some websites promote intellectual flummery to lure you into a false sense of belief but others are just dishonest, couching their fictions in pseudoscience and diversion.

These techniques have been used by illusionists for centuries and they work, to some degree, because we want to believe them. Dr. Steven Novella produced a lecture course available as a video series and audiobook, to help break through this fog. Called "*Your Deceptive Mind: A Scientific Guide to Critical Thinking Skills*" [22] it's highly recommended for anyone who wants to pull back the curtains and see who is pulling the strings on the information war.

"If you can't convince them, confuse them."—Harry S. Truman

As an example the website: nongmoproject.org [23] offers a whole raft of facts on why GMOs are bad but can you trust it? Well, that depends—it's a nonprofit started by some concerned citizens in 2003 and has paid staff. Those staff are unlikely to be there because they're pro-GM.

Sites like nongmoproject.org will give you free fact sheets detailing the facts and fantasies of GMO but can you trust them? It's easy to distrust large corporations like Monsanto but we need to apply the same level of skepticism to all businesses, however innocent they may appear, that have sprung up on the other side of the fence.

They are still businesses and they still have agendas. The instant we assume either side is telling the truth, we lose any objectivity. Remember, even the mighty Monsanto was small once.

22 http://www.thegreatcourses.com/courses/your-deceptive-mind-a-scientific-guide-to-critical-thinking-skills.html
23 http://nongmoproject.org

The writing team behind this book grew out of a Facebook group of people banned by Food Babe and her moderators for daring to question the Food Babe version of things: this is an academic exercise and we're not asking you to take our claims at face value, after all we might be wrong.

Is Food Babe a liar or just a purveyor of lies? Our guess is she honestly believes what she says; but she's a very unreliable investigator because if she was any good, nothing in what you're about to read would make any sense. Science (and good investigation) is about following the rabbit hole wherever it goes.

For the rest of this chapter, we're going to look at the evidence for Food Babe's claims and, where possible, discuss the sources of the sometimes dangerous lies she so widely distributes.

On Yoga Mats

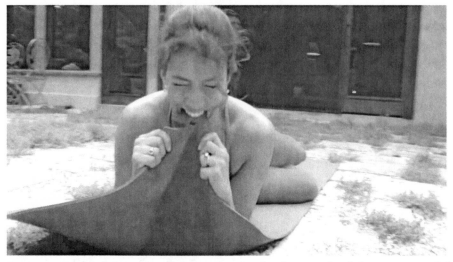

Figure 2.1: Food Babe's graphic demonstration involves biting a chunk from an expanded foam yoga mat. (Food Babe LLC/YouTube)

One of Food Babe's most visible campaigns and almost certainly one of those responsible for catapulting her to fame was her unbridled attack on Subway which went rather like this:

> Azodicarbonamide is the same chemical used to make yoga mats, shoe soles, and other rubbery objects. It's not supposed

to be food or even eaten for that matter. And it's definitely not "fresh." Subway is using this ingredient as a bleaching agent and dough conditioner which allows them to produce bread faster and cheaper without regard to the following health consequences and alarming facts: [24]

1. The World Health Organization [25] has linked it to respiratory issues, allergies and asthma.

2. When a truck carrying azodicarbonamide overturned on a Chicago highway in 2001, it prompted city officials to issue the highest hazardous materials alert and evacuate people within a half mile radius! Many of the people on the scene complained of burning eyes and skin irritation as a result. [26]

3. The U.K. Health And Safety Executive has recognized azodicarbonamide as a potential cause of asthma. [27]

4. When azodicarbonamide is heated, there are studies that show it is linked to tumor development and cancer. [28]

5. Not only is this ingredient banned in Europe and Australia, but you also get fined 450,000 dollars if you get caught using it in Singapore and can serve 15 years in prison. [29]

That looks like a laundry list of problems—and yet, expert chemists like *Dr. Joe Schwarcz* insist the chemical is safe—so who is right?

The first three claims here relate to pure azodicarbonamide (ADA) in its raw form and the effects on humans as an airborne dust. However, precisely the same allegation can be levelled at the other major ingredient in breads—flour.

Flour is a respiratory irritant that can cause the condition "Miller's Lung" [30, 31]

---

24 http://foodbabe.com/subway/
25 http://www.who.int/ipcs/publications/cicad/en/cicad16.pdf
26 Pandora's LunchBox by Melanie Warner (pgs. 103—104)
27 http://www.inchem.org/documents/cicads/cicads/cicad16.htm
28 http://www.ncbi.nlm.nih.gov/pubmed/21786817
29 http://www.kat-chem.hu/en/prod-bulletins/azodikarbonamid
30 http://www.sciencedirect.com/science/article/pii/S0422763813001994
31 http://www.merckmanuals.com/home/lung-and-airway-disorders/interstitial-lung-diseases/hypersensitivity-pneumonitis

An allegation to which one might reply, "ah, but we don't go around snorting it though!"

The only people exposed to flour dust like this are millers and factory workers where processed flour is produced and used: including bakeries. In much the same way, the only people at risk of asthma from the inhalation of ADA are workers in factories where it's employed. Looked at this way, ADA is no more dangerous than the flour that makes up the majority of the bread that we eat. This isn't a case of the dose making the toxin, rather the route of administration.

We don't inhale ADA any more than we inhale flour. The same could be said for water (another major component of breads)—water is deadly if we get lungs full of the stuff but we need to ingest large amounts every day just to survive.

When ADA is heated it decomposes primarily into common and broadly innocuous chemicals [32] (the dose is key here). Questions have been raised over one of the minor breakdown chemicals, semicarbazide or SEM and its carcinogenic effects in animal studies.

While this sounds scary, the reality is rather different than the simple claims made. SEM has been shown to cause tumors in female (not male) mice and had no effect in rats and in those studies, [33] SEM was fed to animals in far larger doses than we would normally be exposed to.

So why is it banned in Europe? Science is a slow process and the risk levels from SEM are thought to be extremely low [34] so it's expected these findings are a belt-and-braces approach on the assumption there may be some perceived danger, with the potential to damage consumer confidence. Naturally, bloggers like Food Babe aren't interested in this level of detail.

The reality is, ADA isn't banned in Europe as has been widely reported. During 2005 it was banned from use as a blowing agent in the production of plastic gaskets that come into contact with food; especially infant foods, as this quote from the EU press release demonstrates.

---

32 http://pubs.rsc.org/en/Content/ArticleLanding/1975/P2/P29750000046

33 http://www.fda.gov/Food/IngredientsPackagingLabeling/FoodAdditivesIngredients/ucm387497.htm

34 http://www.efsa.europa.eu/en/press/news/afc050701.htm

"The implementation of an EC Directive banning the use of azodicarbonamide in plastics used as food contact materials** which is due to enter into force on 2 August 2005 should eliminate this source of SEM in food. The Panel also concluded that other, lesser sources of SEM in food were not of concern." [35]

The claim that you're going to do 15 years in the pokey for using this stuff in Singapore is probably fallacious. We have written to Food Babe's source and the Singapore embassy in Washington, but at the time of going to press (more than six months after requesting clarification) we have not received a reply from either.

On The FDA

> The FDA is asleep at the wheel and the Food Industry is in charge. [36]

That's a pretty strong allegation. To really see just how the FDA is "snoozing" look at its enforcement letters. [37] Scan down the list to see that no one is free from its scrutiny—including organic manufacturers and overseas suppliers—even in the Far East!

The venom spitting doesn't stop at that though:

> The GAO [US. Government Accountability Office] concluded that there are GRAS [generally recognized as safe] ingredients currently on the market that may not be safe. [38]

May not be safe… you mean you don't know? Is the FDA the only food additive regulatory body in the entire world? Of course it isn't! Amazingly, food scientists do actually talk to each other. A better question might be to ask why do we (as the public at large) tend to believe the pen scratchings of self-styled "experts" like Food Babe and Jenny McCarthy while ignoring the evidence-based and duplicable findings of independent scientists?

---

35   http://www.efsa.europa.eu/en/press/news/afc050701.htm

36   http://foodbabe.com/2015/01/06/read-ingredient-lists/

37   http://www.fda.gov/ICECI/EnforcementActions/WarningLetters/

38   http://foodbabe.com/2015/01/06/read-ingredient-lists/

We've addressed this question throughout the book and the answers might surprise you. Food Babe gets up in arms about ingredients the FDA doesn't regulate even though they are not actually found in the final product.

> One of the main ingredients in fake beef and chicken is soy protein isolate. It's processed by soaking soybeans in a chemical called hexane, whose emissions are a main constituent of smog. Hexane is a known carcinogen and neurotoxin that has been linked to brain tumors. Despite this the FDA doesn't regulate it. [39]

Hexane (more correctly, n-Hexane) is a general name for the chemical with a formula of C_6H_{14} but that's not the whole story because hexane comes in five forms (called isomers). Each one is chemically different with boiling points ranging from about 122°F (50°C) to 156°F (69°C)

Removing hexane isomers from another product is simply a matter of boiling it off (the vapor can even be condensed back)—in much the same way as the original was "cracked" from crude oil. Hexane is also used in the production of cooking oils. This is similar to how we'd serve a meal cooked with sherry, or brats boiled in beer to a child. This doesn't mean we're serving them alcohol.

On MSG

> MSG is an ingredient that literally excites your brain cells to death.[40]

Monosodium glutamate has had a bad rap ever since someone got a headache after eating a Chinese meal. Despite being a naturally occurring compound (our bodies produce about 40 grams every day) it's one of Food Babe's favorite whipping boys along with gluten.

Food Babe derives her evidence directly from *Natural News,* a source known for its gratuitous fabrications. Natural News describes the product (with aspartame) as pernicious and Food Babe concludes that MSG must be evil and avoided at all costs.

> Kraft adds straight up Monosodium Glutamate, aka "MSG" to

---

39 The Food Babe Way, p. 173
40 http://foodbabe.com/tag/panera-bread/page/2/

create an addiction to processed food early in a child's life—they don't even try to hide it under the name "yeast extract" like some food companies do. [41]

MSG, the sodium salt of glutamic acid or glutamate, is a substance found widely in nature—it's present for example in potatoes, tomatoes, mushrooms, meats, and strong cheeses. There are two forms—bound, which we can't taste and free which we can.

> These ingredients also promote an addiction to pizza so that you keep coming back to order more. Repeat business keeps their pockets lined with lots of cash. Ever wonder why you can't stop at one slice? This is why. [42]

Free glutamate gives the familiar savory taste to traditional Chinese cuisine. It's so natural it's even found in human breast milk at 10x the concentration found in cow's milk—and this is where many of us get our first taste of the stuff.

> While it's true that tomatoes and cheese are naturally high in glutamates, they do not have the same effect on the brain as added manufactured free glutamic acid additives. When I talked to Papa John's, they admitted that these additives are used as a replacement for MSG by the food industry. [43]

As a distinct flavor, umami is one of the five basic tastes that humans are capable of detecting along with sweet, sour, salty and bitter. It's found culinary usage since ancient times but was first scientifically isolated by *Professor Kikunae Ikeda* of Tokyo Imperial University in 1908.

Food Babe claims that MSG is somehow addictive.

> MSG tricks your brain into believing that what you are eating tastes so great that you want more of it. Your taste buds sense that there is more protein in the food than there really is—which is great for food manufacturers that want to save money by using less or lower quality meat. [44]

41   http://foodbabe.com/2014/11/19/just-because-this-kraft-food-is-easy-doesnt-mean-you-should-eat-it/
42   http://foodbabe.com/2014/03/23/if-youve-ever-eaten-pizza-before-this-will-blow-your-mind/
43   http://foodbabe.com/2014/03/23/if-youve-ever-eaten-pizza-before-this-will-blow-your-mind/
44   http://foodbabe.com/2014/03/23/if-youve-ever-eaten-pizza-before-this-will-blow-your-mind/

The reality is MSG is no more addictive than salt. To turn this claim against salt: we add salt to our meals to trick our brains into thinking there are electrolytes present.

But is it bad? Put simply, it isn't—we've been eating it for thousands of years and it's never done us any harm at normal levels. The fear of MSG is an entirely Western phenomenon. It's an everyday ingredient in the Far East where it is to be found alongside other seasonings.

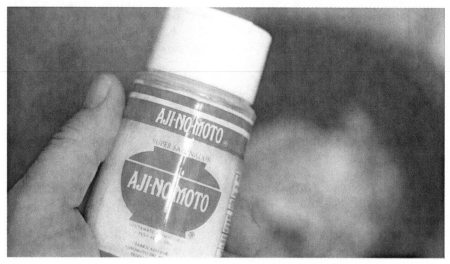

Figure 2.2: Ajinomoto—MSG produced by the Ajinomoto corporation of Japan. The name means "essence of taste." (Richard Masoner/flickr.com)

Food expert and critic *Jeffrey Steingarten* wryly observed in Vogue as far back as 1999:

"Why Doesn't Everybody in China Have a Headache?"

Physician *Dr. Michael Eades* lays the blame on a single article in a 1967 issue of the New England Journal of Medicine in which *Dr Ho Man Kwok* wrote a letter claiming that he suffered palpitations and numbness after eating a meal at a Chinese restaurant.

Since the only ingredient missing from the American diet at the time was MSG, Dr. Kwok assumed, ***entirely anecdotally***, that the MSG was to blame—and so Chinese Restaurant Syndrome was born—and that fear stays with us today.

> Utilizing filling ingredients such as lentils, that are packed with fiber and protein is a great way to lose excess pounds. Also, soups are super nourishing but easy on the waistline because they naturally help you eat less (if the soup doesn't have hidden MSG which can make you eat more!) [45]

MSG is a powerful flavor enhancer—English folks (including our editor, who uses it in soups) use dashes of it in a form of yeast extract called Marmite and their Australian friends have their own version, Vegemite, epitomized in the song "A Land Down Under" by Men at Work.

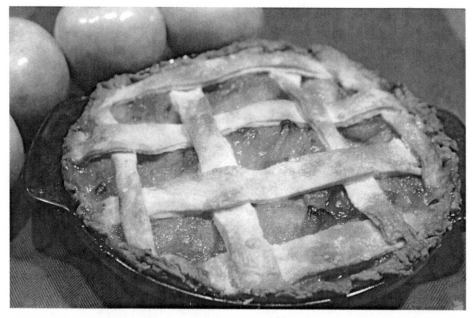

Figure 2.3: Some of this apple pie will naturally produce more methanol in your system than the aspartame in a can of soda—but it won't blind you. (Dan Parsons/flickr.com)

On Aspartame

> Aspartame is linked to diabetes, auto-immune disorders, depression (which can cause you to eat more—once again), birth defects, and several forms of cancer. [46]

---

45   http://foodbabe.com/2015/01/12/mexican-lentil-tortilla-soup/
46   http://foodbabe.com/2011/12/09/wanna-a-piece-of-gum/

Aspartame was created by accident in 1965 by chemist *James M. Schlatter* while attempting to synthesize a *tetrapeptide* (a combination of four amino acids) of the hormone gastrin. (Gastrin stimulates the natural production of gastric acid in our guts and the aim was to test the efficacy of a new anti-ulcer drug.) The story goes that Schlatter got some of the intermediate product (which we call aspartame) on a piece of paper and noticed the sweet taste when he licked his finger.

> *"Toxicology is based on the premise that all compounds are toxic at some dose." Dr. Lewis Stegink (reviewing aspartame)* [47]

Aspartame was originally declared safe by the US Food and Drug Administration in 1974. The FDA rescinded the approval the year later after doubts were expressed about Searle's testing program, and final approval wasn't granted until 1981. Further testing by the Centers for Disease Control concluded there was no risk from aspartame at the levels found in a typical diet.

The weight of hard scientific evidence continues to show aspartame safe, but thanks in part to the work of organizations like *Center for Science in the Public Interest* (CSPI) and *Mission Possible World Health International* (MPWHI) founded by "Dr." Betty Martini—a fear monger to rival Food Babe, the product is repeatedly rolled out as the singular toxin creating a shopping list of maladies, including death!

It might seem disrespectful to put "Dr." Martini's doctorate in quotes but we do so simply because the title is (a) purely honorific and (b) is in humanities. That has not stopped her from using her experience working with medical professionals to create the impression she has some medical expertise as this quote from her website shows:

> *"Dr. Martini has spent 22 years in the medical field. While working with a hematologist she supplied the CDC with reports on leukemia, which CDC said, were more than all the case histories submitted by the entire Emory University Hospital system combined, an indication of the low level of physician generated reports to the CDC. This*

---

47 http://www.ncbi.nlm.nih.gov/pubmed/3300262

reveals that only a small percentage of serious health threats are collected and statistically tabulated." [48]

This is an example of the *honor by association* fallacy—even a secretary or PA could reasonably claim to "work with a hematologist" but that no more makes them medically qualified than a cow can operate a telephone. Likewise, the claim about the CDC reports without documentation is a claim made without evidence and, using *Hitchen's Razor,* [49] it can be equally dismissed as such.

Don't do that—you'll go blind!

Breaking down the allegations against aspartame (and other artificial sweeteners) would take a book, but let's take a look at the main thrust of the arguments.

> Phenylalanine is added to the ingredient Aspartame and could seriously be dangerous if you have certain health conditions. Consuming this substance (if you have a condition that makes you sensitive to this additive) can cause mental retardation, brain seizures, sleep disorders and anxiety. [50]

When we ingest aspartame it's broken down into two amino acids, aspartic acid and phenylalanine (it's not "added" to it) plus a tiny amount of methanol. Amino acids are essential to our bodies because they are the building blocks of proteins. Methanol is a simple alcohol, similar to ethanol, the alcohol yeast excretes during the fermentation of sugars to make wines and beers. Methanol, however, is toxic in large quantities as it breaks down into formic acid.

Our bodies produce much larger amounts (relatively speaking) from consumption of everyday foods, fruit in particular, as the breakdown product of naturally occurring pectin. No one in their right mind would willingly drink methanol (it's been found as an adulterant in counterfeit vodka and gin and is often used in Asia).

> Another large study linked aspartame to an increased risk of lymphomas, leukemias, and transitional cell carcinomas of the

---

48   http://www.mpwhi.com/our_founder.htm

49   http://en.wikipedia.org/wiki/Hitchens's_razor

50   http://foodbabe.com/2011/12/09/wanna-a-piece-of-gum/

> pelvis, ureter, and bladder [51]

Death from accidental methanol intoxication, while still rare, is not un-heard of. Edinburgh resident Rebecca Dickson lost her life to it in 2003 and more recently, 21-year old beautician Cheznye Emmons died of methanol poisoning on vacation in Indonesia while consuming punch from a counterfeit branded gin. In smaller quantities, just a few shots of contaminated methanol may cause irreversible blindness as the formic acid attacks the nervous system where the optic nerves are particularly vulnerable. As little as six shots is thought to be sufficient to kill an adult.

Here lies aspartame's first bogeyman: formic acid—what the naysayers conveniently forget to mention is that the amount of formic acid produced by the levels of aspartame in food and drink is dwarfed by the amount produced when we digest ripe fruit such as apples. No one ever went blind eating too much of Mom's All-American Apple Pie.

PKU?—Bless you!

Aspartame's second bogeyman is, like the first, blown out of proportion by people out of pure ignorance or (dare we suggest) because they have a financial interest in selling some alternative like conventional sugar or even stevia (which has an interesting history of its own).

Phenylalanine is an essential amino acid—we must get it from a dietary source: babies get it from their mother's milk but a rare, inherited condition, phenylketonuria (PKU) exists where sufferers cannot correctly metabolise phenylalanine. This lifetime condition means that sufferers have to carefully monitor their diet, with children particularly vulnerable.

PKU is the condition from which the anti-aspartame lobby derive their other bogeyman. It causes disordered cerebral development, seizures and psychiatric disorders. Individuals with untreated PKU may also develop a musty aroma due to the levels of unprocessed phenylalanine, may have lighter skin and suffer from eczema (an auto-immune disorder).

Rates of PKU vary across populations with rates as low as 1 in 100,000 in Finland to 1 in 10,000 in the USA, and with screening at roughly two weeks (the heel prick test) sufferers are identified long before dietary prob-

---

51 http://foodbabe.com/2014/05/21/this-childhood-favorite-has-a-warning-label-in-europe-why-not-here/

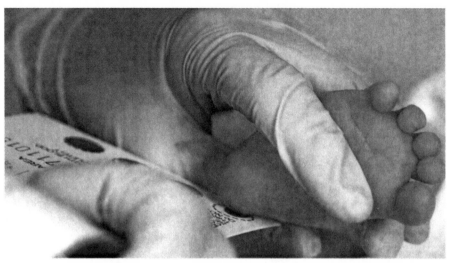

Figure 2.4: The heel prick blood test to screen for PKU on a two-week old child (U.S. Air Force photo/Staff Sgt Eric T. Sheler)

lems can become a factor. Since aspartame is considered to be a non-natural source of phenylalanine, some countries—quite reasonably—require foods containing aspartame to carry a warning on the label so PKU sufferers are not exposed by accident. Screening began in the 1960s so undiagnosed sufferers are now in their late forties and older.

While aspartame is singled out for containing phenylalanine, there are many other sources including milk, fish, eggs meat and cheese. [52]

Magnuson, Burdock et al. writing for a 2007 edition of *Critical Reviews in Toxicology* conclude:

> *"Critical review of all carcinogenicity studies conducted on aspartame found no credible evidence that aspartame is carcinogenic. The data from the extensive investigations into the possibility of neurotoxic effects of aspartame, in general, do not support the hypothesis that aspartame in the human diet will affect nervous system function, learning or behavior."* [53]

Food Babe's claims can be summarized into the following conditions—which we'll address using the assumption of normal intakes of aspartame:

---

52   http://www.nhs.uk/conditions/Phenylketonuria/Pages/Introduction.aspx
53   http://www.ncbi.nlm.nih.gov/pubmed/17828671

Auto-immune disorders
Eczema is a factor for PKU sufferers—but there is no compelling body of evidence that links this, SLE or asthma to aspartame consumption.

Birth defects (teratogenesis)
Undiagnosed maternal PKU is the most likely cause of this story. No evidence to support this in the greater population.

Cancer
5-benzyl-3,6-dioxo-2-piperazine acetic acid (DKP) produced when aspartame breaks down in storage. No evidence of carcinogenicity even at high-blood serum levels (Wistar rats) for 104 weeks.

Even natural food advocate *Dr. Joe Mercola* is unwilling to commit to this one preferring to avoid a hard conclusion—emphasis ours:

> *"DKP has been implicated in the occurrence of brain tumors. [Dr. John W] Olney noticed that DKP, when nitrosated in the gut, produced a compound that was similar to N-nitrosourea, a powerful brain tumor causing chemical. Some authors have said that DKP is produced after aspartame ingestion. **I am not sure if that is correct.**"* [54]

Diabetes
According to Sioned Quirke of the British Diabetic Association:

> *"There is no evidence to suggest that low calorie sweeteners, such as saccharin, aspartame and sucralose, are bad for you."* [55]

The Mayo Clinic says you can use most sugar substitutes [56] if you have diabetes, including:

Saccharin (Sweet'N Low)

Aspartame (NutraSweet, Equal)

Acesulfame potassium (Sunett)

Sucralose (Splenda)

Stevia (NuNaturals, Truvia)

---

54 http://articles.mercola.com/sites/articles/archive/2011/11/06/aspartame-most-dangerous-substance-added-to-food.aspx

55 http://www.bbc.co.uk/news/magazine-22758059

56 http://www.mayoclinic.org/healthy-lifestyle/nutrition-and-healthy-eating/in-depth/artificial-sweeteners/art-20046936

Depression
> *No known causative link found in reliable sources.*

Nothing. Nada. Nix. Zero. For now, aspartame can be considered safe.

On Sugar

This is from one of Food Babe's most invidious and successful campaigns in recent years—bashing the crap out of Starbucks for selling coffee with the stuff in it. This went viral so quickly, it even attracted the attention of urban legend specialists, Snopes. Not that that worried the Food Babe's dedicated followers. So what about the sugar?

> Order up a non-fat grande and you'll get served 50 grams of sugar. Is it a pick-me-up from the caffeine, or all that toxic sugar? [57]

It's toxic? Call the FDA, call the President, call your local moms' group—give the unqualified blogger a Nobel for discovering the toxic effects of sugar without ever performing a single experiment.

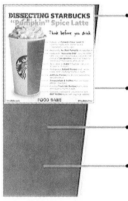

- Made with "**Monsanto Milk**" cows fed GMO corn, soy, and cottonseed or soy milk that contains **Carrageenan** stabilizer linked to intestinal inflammation and cancer
- Toxic dose of **Sugar** ("Grande" has over 50 grams of sugar)
- Ambiguous **Natural Flavors** that can be made from anything found on earth
- **Artificial Flavors** made from substances like petroleum

Figure 2.5: Close up this viral infographic proclaims a "toxic" dose of sugar. Inset: Orginal graphic. (Food Babe LLC)

In one breath Food Babe is implying the dose doesn't matter (toxicologically, it does) and in the next breath she's telling us that it does. Like much of Food Babe's later output, the visual quality goes up while the quality of

---

57 http://foodbabe.com/2014/08/25/starbucks-pumpkin-spice-latte/

the indignation stays about the same. The righteous outrage seems to stem from *Mark Bittman's* 2013 opinion [58] piece in the NYT which opens:

> *"Sugar is indeed toxic. It may not be the only problem with the Standard American Diet, but it's fast becoming clear that it's the major one."*

Problem is, Bittman had apparently misunderstood the study's finding:

> *"Mark Bittman's column on Thursday incorrectly described findings from a recent epidemiological study of the relationship of sugar consumption to diabetes... It did not find that "obesity doesn't cause diabetes: sugar does." Obesity is, in fact, a major risk factor for Type 2 diabetes, as the study noted." (Corrected: March 6, 2013)*

Sugar isn't toxic at this dosage—it's just not good for us—and 50g is around the maximum daily intake for a healthy adult (ouch!) A pure carbohydrate, it's a fantastic source of energy—which makes it a lousy food; but worse than that, sugar is a simple carb and 50% pure glucose, which is what our cells use for energy.

You can live on sugar and water for a short period but very soon you'll find yourself craving something else because your body cannot live on energy alone—it needs a whole bunch of micronutrients to function and without them, it starts to break down very quickly.

> Sugar is one of the most dangerous ingredients on the market. It's addictive, added to almost every processed food, and will make you overweight, depressed and sick if you eat too much. [59]

Sugar doesn't necessarily make you fat on its own (although it does rot your teeth) but it does play havoc with the systems that regulate our nutrition—and there's where the problems start; very soon your craving for proteins, fats and trace elements will have you heading for the pantry/fridge/supermarket and devouring even more calories just to get at the essential nutrients you're missing.

The biggest problem with table sugar is that it's a mixture of two simpler sugars (called a disaccharide), glucose and fructose.

---

58 http://opinionator.blogs.nytimes.com/2013/02/27/its-the-sugar-folks/
59 http://foodbabe.com/2013/04/25/stevia-good-or-bad/

Food Babe has an alternative—coconut palm sugar:

> One of the big pluses of coconut palm sugar—it's completely
> unrefined and not bleached like typical refined white sugar,
> helping to preserve all of its teeming vitamins and minerals. [60]

Bleached? Bleached! You run a food blog and you think that white sugar is bleached? Pure sucrose (fructose/glucose) is a white crystal; much like pure sodium salt is. We think she's probably confusing sugar with white flour.

Suggesting coconut palm sugar (CPS) is "teeming" with vitamins and minerals is well wide of the mark. It actually contains calcium, iron, potassium and zinc with some short-chain fatty acids, polyphenols and antioxidants and additionally a soluble fiber called inulin. Inulin is chemically a sugar but we can't taste it or break it down so it passes right through us, acting as a fiber.

It's technically better for you than sugar in the same way that 1,000 is larger than 999 but it's still sugar, it's still going to rot your teeth, and you can't get a realistic amount of nutrients from it. CPS is about 80% sucrose (table sugar) with most of the remaining 20% split to varying degrees between fructose, glucose, inulin and trace elements. As far as your body is concerned you're still eating sugar, with the potential problems that fructose can cause.

> Now is a good time to tell you that much of the added sugar
> on the market has been filtered through bone char. Often
> called natural carbon, bone char comes from the bones of
> cattle (and sometimes dogs). The bones are heated to very high
> temperatures, powdered, dehydrated, and turned into a charcoal
> filter to whiten cane sugar and remove impurities. [61]

Given that water boils at just 212°F (100°C) and bone char is created by heating recovered animal bones from abattoirs at temperatures as high as 1,300°F (700°C), no appreciable water is left to require dehydration. Although referred to as bone char, the end result is primarily carbon since the heating is done in the absence of sufficient oxygen for the carbon to decompose into carbon dioxide.

---

60   http://foodbabe.com/2011/12/19/ditch-refined-sugar/
61   The Food Babe Way, p. 156

Wait—did someone just say dog bones? Surely wouldn't they all go up with one big "woof?" (*Get your coat—Ed.*)

We've been unable to discover any reliable source that could verify this claim—but the reality is, since dogs are not used as food in the west (and only in very isolated places elsewhere), the supply of canine skeletal remains is likely as high as the demand for canine meat. Further, since the variant-CJD scare (mad cow disease) the supply of even skeletal animal remains is very tightly controlled. Prions (the agents responsible for CJD) are proteins, and therefore destroyed by moderately high temperatures, no reasonable agency would be willing to take the risk.

The reason bone char is so popular, apart from its relative cheapness and simple chemistry, is its efficacy at removing impurities (including heavy metals) from cane-derived sugars by a process called adsorption. Sugar beets store sugar in their root tuber and don't require this form of processing.

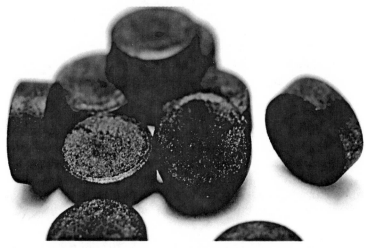

Figure 2.6: After processing, bone char looks like little black tablets of carbon—because that's all it is. (Honza Groh/wikipedia.com)

Adsorption sounds like absorption but the processes are entirely different. When something absorbs something else—say a sponge absorbing water—one material fills tiny spaces in the other by displacing something else: air in this case. This is great if you need to mop up a large amount of water but not very useful if you want to remove a tiny amount of impurity from a large volume of something.

Activated carbon (bone char is almost entirely pure carbon) is one of the most popular chemicals used for this task because it's cheap and easy to produce.

Perhaps the easier way to understand adsorption is to imagine an old-fashioned chalkboard (or even the pavement outside). When you scrape a piece of chalk over the surface, little bits of chalk dust get stuck to the surface and at an atomic level, this is what happens on the surface of the carbon.

Larger molecules of the product we want to keep (sucrose in this case) flow past the carbon but heavy metals and other impurities which are smaller, get lodged in the surface, and are unable to escape. Activated carbon has a vast surface area of up to 1200m² per gram (about 6½ football fields per ounce of the stuff).

Like a sponge, activated carbon has a limit before it's used up; but like a sponge you can wring it out and start again. Rather than wringing, it has to be heated so the impurities it's collected are burned off, but the idea is similar. Chemists will tell you that it's a lot more complicated than that (it is) but this should give you the basic idea.

Strict vegetarians and vegans may wish to avoid sugars processed this way. Although the char itself can't really get into the sugar (you'd see little black bits) it is derived from an animal source. The better vegan websites keep track of how manufacturers are sourcing their sugars and are the best source for this information. [62]

Food Babe herself claims to be allergic to sugar—but not just any sugar—only refined sugar.

> I found out I was incredibly allergic to refined sugar. About 3 months ago I was treated for this—it doesn't mean I can eat all the refined sugar I want now, rather it means that my body can tolerate it better. [63]

---

62 http://veganproducts.org/sugar.html
63 http://foodbabe.com/2011/09/22/seize-your-sugar-cravings/

She claims to have achieved this using acupuncture but there are two things that strike us. First, acupuncture is bunk. It has been tried and tested and never found to have any therapeutic effect at all. It does work as a placebo however and therein lies the trick. Food Babe fooled herself into believing she was cured of an allergy that was all in her mind in the first place. Second, make no mistake, psychosomatic illnesses are very real to the sufferer—and this is an admirable demonstration of that since sugar (i.e. sucrose) is the same compound be it from a sugar beet, sugar cane or corn syrup. Your body can't tell the difference.

On HFCS

> High Fructose Corn Syrup—This chemically refined sugar has been shown to cause more weight gain than regular sugar. Even when eaten in moderation, it's said to be a major cause of heart disease, cancer, dementia and liver failure. Some high fructose corn syrup is even contaminated with mercury. [64]

HFCS is a popular sweetener simply because it's cheap and, as it's roughly ¼ water, it's easily blended. US government subsidies on corn make this stuff really cost effective for the manufacturers, and it's available in three main concentrations: HFCS 90, 55 and 42. The number represents the percentage ratio of fructose to glucose. So HFCS 90, for instance, contains 90% fructose to 10% glucose.

Is it dangerous? The evidence says no. Regular table sugar (sucrose) is a mixture of 50% glucose/fructose so anything using HFCS 55 is roughly using table sugar (HFCS90 and HFCS55 are sweeter, so less is required). HFCS42 is less sweet than traditional sugar and contains a greater proportion of glucose.

Once HFCS gets into our guts, the effect is little different from eating regular sugar because sucrose is broken into its component glucose and fructose by our digestive system. Since the most common form is HFCS55, that's as good as saying it's the same as sugar.

It was widely reported in 2009 that a study had found measurable levels of mercury in roughly 50% of samples of HFCS. This PR disaster prompted

---

64   http://foodbabe.com/2014/07/29/fig-newtons-100-whole-grain/

the food industry to begin to switch from a chemical to an enzymatic process that does not require the use of strong acids.

It's worth pointing out that just a 4oz steak of bigeye tuna is enough to push a 180 lb adult well over their weekly limit for mercury exposure! Fish is a major source of mercury poisoning with the larger fish presenting much larger risks.

The mercury content of HFCS pales against the very real risk of too much sugar in our diet—sucrose, glucose or fructose—which is a major cause of obesity. Fructose, which our bodies are unable to use without considerable effort, is potentially indicated in non-alcoholic fatty liver disease. [65] It's not the HFCS that's a problem—it's our addiction to sweet things.

On Stevia

> That's why it's exciting to know there are alternative sweeteners made in nature, like "stevia," that don't wreak havoc on your health—or do they? Is Stevia safe? [66]

Stevia, from the *Stevia Rebaudiana* plant, is one of the newest non-sugar (non-carbohydrate) sweeteners on the market, although the plant's properties have been known to locals for centuries.

Rebaudioside A (a diterpenoid steviol glycoside) is the sweetest of glycosides and the one with the least unpleasant aftertaste. Glycosides are formed by bonding a simple sugar with another compound by replacing the hydroxyl (OH) group and account for many of the toxins and drugs extracted from plants.

Try saying that last lot while you're drunk—which is what might happen if you try this extraction at home. The bit we're interested in is rebaudioside A; that's the one that the food companies need to get from their stevia because the other compounds are far less pleasant tasting.

Rebaudioside A is easily purified to around 80% pure with other impurities comprising dulcoside A, stevioside, steviolbioside, rebaudioside B, C, D and F, and other steviol glycosides. Separating the A compound from the

---

65   http://www.ncbi.nlm.nih.gov/pmc/articles/PMC3577529/
66   http://foodbabe.com/2013/04/25/stevia-good-or-bad/

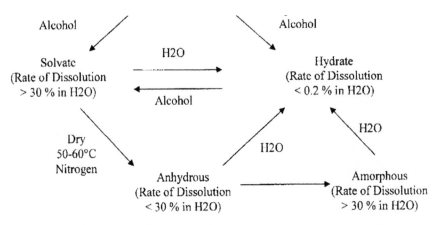

Figure 2.7: Image from the original patent application. (US Patents/Google)

others is difficult because they all have similar solubilities. But leave them in and the sweetness diminishes. A 2007 US patent (US20070292582 A1) reveals a process by which:

> *"In particular, this invention relates to a method for purifying crude rebaudioside A compositions comprising purities from approximately 40% to approximately 95% rebaudioside A to obtain a substantially pure rebaudioside A product with a single crystallization step."* [67]

In other words, it's fast and effective—and in business, efficiency equals profit and a development that would allow this alternative sweetener to enter the US market at a much lower price. Problem was, the FDA had already decided it didn't like Stevia and effectively banned the product from sale; despite having been used in Japan since the 1970s, and accounting for some 50% of the country's artificial sweetener market.

By the 1980s, aspartame was riding high in the billion dollar artificial sweetener market (the patent did not expire until 1992) and there are allegations that some wanted to keep it that way.

Jim May, owner of *Wisdom of the Ancients,* told the Sonoma County Independent that Nutrasweet had filed a complaint with the FDA. Nutrasweet's VP of public affairs, speaking in a 1997 issue of *Self* magazine, claimed the stories were an urban myth—but for whatever the real reason, Stevia remained a niche product until, according to Food Babe:

---

67   http://www.google.com/patents/US20070292582

Not until a major food company got involved did stevia become legal, and only after it had been highly processed using a patentable chemical-laden process...so processed that Truvia (Coca-Cola's branded product) goes through about 40 steps to process the extract from the leaf, relying on chemicals like acetone, methanol, ethanol, acetonitrile, and isopropanol. Some of these chemicals are known carcinogens (substances that cause cancer), and none of those ingredients sound like real food, do they? [68]

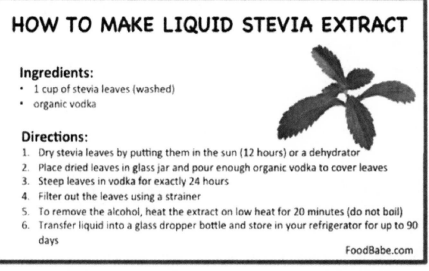

HOW TO MAKE LIQUID STEVIA EXTRACT

Ingredients:
- 1 cup of stevia leaves (washed)
- organic vodka

Directions:
1. Dry stevia leaves by putting them in the sun (12 hours) or a dehydrator
2. Place dried leaves in glass jar and pour enough organic vodka to cover leaves
3. Steep leaves in vodka for exactly 24 hours
4. Filter out the leaves using a strainer
5. To remove the alcohol, heat the extract on low heat for 20 minutes (do not boil)
6. Transfer liquid into a glass dropper bottle and store in your refrigerator for up to 90 days

FoodBabe.com

Figure 2.8: Food Babe's home-made Stevia extract uses a known carcinogen. (Food Babe LLC)

Ethanol is a carcinogen found in alcoholic drinks. It's a Class 1 IARC substance known to cause cancer in humans. But like all the other scary substances here, it's being used as a solvent. Food Babe comes to the rescue with her own recipe for liquid Stevia. This one uses ethanol diluted with oxidane; otherwise known as vodka. Wait—didn't she just say that method was bad?

Just don't use ethanol near an open flame as the evaporating fumes are extremely flammable.

---

68   http://foodbabe.com/2013/04/25/stevia-good-or-bad/

Much of Food Babe's sloppy research leads her to these ludicrous declarations—and this one is a fine example. She claims (see above) that Truvia *"goes through about 40 steps."* She gleans this fact from the patent by reading the "Claims" section, which we've reproduced in the appendix. Some familiarity with the arcane language of patents is an enormous help to understand this, but claims are generalizations to protect the inventors from ne'er do wells stealing their invention by changing some small detail and claiming it as their own. There aren't 40 steps at all, as this example process shows:

> *Crude rebaudioside A (77.4% purity) mixture was obtained from a commercial source. The impurities (6.2% stevioside, 5.6% rebaudioside C, 0.6% rebaudioside F, 1.0% other steviol glycosides, 3.0% rebaudioside D, 4.9% rebaudioside B, 0.3% steviolbioside) were identified and quantified using HPLC on a dry basis (moisture content 4.7%).*

> *Crude rebaudioside A (400 g), ethanol (95%, 1200 mL), methanol (99% 400 mL) and water (320 mL) were combined and heated to 50°C for 10 minutes. The clear solution was cooled to 22°C. for 16 hours. The white crystals were filtered and washed twice with ethanol (2×200 mL, 95%) and dried in a vacuum oven at 50°C. for 16-24 hours under reduced pressure (20 mm).*

> *The final composition of substantially pure rebaudioside A (130 g) comprised 98.91% rebaudioside A, 0.06% stevioside, 0.03% rebaudioside C, 0.12% rebaudioside F, 0.13% other steviol glycosides, 0.1% rebaudioside D, 0.49% rebaudioside B and 0.03% steviolbioside, all by weight.*

That might look a little arcane too, so let's look at it as a recipe (bearing in mind these are industrial grade chemicals that you can't buy in the shops—largely because they are dangerous intoxicants and need careful handling).

Diluted ethanol makes vodka. The best vodka in the world abides the Russian standard, which requires it to be colorless, odorless and tasteless, so the recipe we've reproduced here is little more than vodka and methylated spirits. It's probably worth noting that 95% ethanol is a standard industrial grade distillate—the other 5% comprises primarily water.

Are these carcinogenic? Sure. Are they toxic in the right doses? Absolutely. Would you want to consume them in this form? Hell no, but they are only part of the process, and are removed during steps 4-6 in our recipe. If you've ever let a pan of vegetable water boil dry or left your coffee pot on the heater too long, you'll notice that there is always some dry powder left behind. These are the soluble solids that remain when the solvent is removed. In these cases, the solvent is water—but it could just as easily be alcohol or even fat.

If you never did this in chemistry, you can prove it by mixing a tablespoon of salt in about two cups of cool water, bring the mixture to boiling, and stir until the salt dissolves. Now pour away most of the water and carefully simmer the remaining water until the salt crystals start to appear. The remaining water can be placed in an oven-proof container and placed in a medium oven (gas 4, 180°C, 350°F) until all the water has evaporated. What's left is relatively pure salt—but you'll notice that most of it has gone.

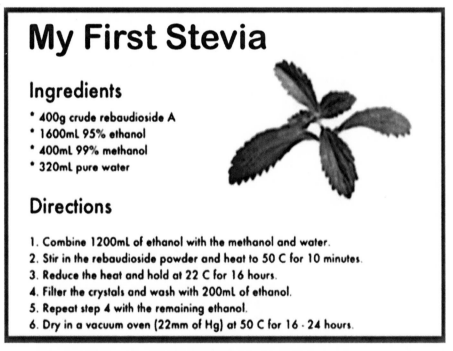

My First Stevia

Ingredients

* 400g crude rebaudioside A
* 1600mL 95% ethanol
* 400mL 99% methanol
* 320mL pure water

Directions

1. Combine 1200mL of ethanol with the methanol and water.
2. Stir in the rebaudioside powder and heat to 50 C for 10 minutes.
3. Reduce the heat and hold at 22 C for 16 hours.
4. Filter the crystals and wash with 200mL of ethanol.
5. Repeat step 4 with the remaining ethanol.
6. Dry in a vacuum oven (22mm of Hg) at 50 C for 16 - 24 hours.

Figure 2.9: Translating the industrial (patented) process, it's easy to see how few steps are really involved. Unfortunately, it's not the sort of equipment we have in our kitchens!

Precisely the same thing happens to the impurities in processes like the one described for rebaudioside here. They get washed away with the solvent and what little of the solvent remains is evaporated.

Sea salt you can buy at the store can be processed from sea water in much the same way. Imagine how much fish poo was in that!

Your dried salt no more contains water than the dried rebaudioside (stevia) crystals contain traces of methanol, ethanol, or whatever solvent was used to process it. White sugar can be purified in much the same way, by dissolving the product in a solvent (usually water) and recrystallizing the pure crystals, which tend to drop out of solution as it cools.

Looking at our translated recipe, it's fairly clear that Coca-Cola's process uses only a few, fairly innocuous steps, to remove the sweetener from the crudely processed leaves—nowhere near the complexity Food Babe implies. Although this is a chemical process, it's little different than growing some root vegetables in your backyard and washing the soil off before cooking them.

Food Babe objects to other additives in some stevia products, such as the natural sugar alcohol (polyol) erythritol. (If you've noticed that a lot of these words end in "ol" you'd be right. In chemistry, common names of alcohols end in "ol" so you can tell that xylitol, erythritol, sorbitol, methanol, ethanol, propanol and isopropanol and even cholesterol are all technically alcohols—but this list is far from exhaustive.)

We've been making alcohols for centuries by a process called fermentation, where natural yeasts (*saccharomyces cerevisiae*) are added to sugars and water and allowed to synthesize alcohol, which we consume in beers and wine. There's nothing spooky about that.

Moniliella pollinis is another natural yeast that can be used on an industrial scale to ferment glucose (sugar) to produce the sugar alcohol (erythritol), which can be purified and crystallized into a form most of us would recognize as sugar. Although it's not as sweet as sugar, erythritol cannot be processed by oral bacteria, so it doesn't rot your teeth.

The likely reason erythritol is added to stevia products is to reduce the bitter aftertaste. Unlike aspartame, rebaudioside A is not completely sweet, so this just gives the product that extra kick. On its own, erythritol has a cooling effect found in some chewing gums.

Our editor tried some pure processed stevia on his family. Apart from being underwhelmed, all but one of them reported an unpleasant (if mild) aftertaste.

On Pasteurized Milk

Cancer is something we all fear. Food Babe alludes to the disease and carcinogens many times through her blogs and in her book, *The Food Babe Way*. This next quote is one of the more disturbing demonstrations of just how a little bit of knowledge is dangerous:

> A Nutrition and Cancer study reported in 2011 that cow's milk stimulated the growth of prostate cancer cells in lab dishes, while almond milk suppressed the growth of these cells. Interesting isn't it? [69]

We might as easily say that toilet bleach suppressed the growth of cancer cells for what difference this makes. If this almond milk was made with bitter almonds it would contain a large amount of cyanide. Everyday sweet almonds contain a tiny amount of this deadly poison. Nowhere near enough to make us ill, but dunking unprotected cells in such a substance… who knows? Certainly not Food Babe.

This is the problem—we don't know, yet Food Babe takes such abstract remarks and touts them as relevant.

Do you know how much milk (almond or cows) gets into a prostate cancer cell?

None.

It's fair to say that when we drink milk, some of the products produced by our digestive enzymes get into our own system, and some of that complex mix of proteins and other substances will certainly reach a well-vascularized tumor. But that's a whole lot different from cooking a few cells in a petri dish.

---

69   The Food Babe Way, p. 40

On Caramel Colors

> Are you upset that the caramel coloring industry is going down the tubes. Is that why you like to spread lies about me? [70]

Moving on from the sweetener Stevia, we go from other people's misread science to Food Babe's misreading of it. Is the caramel coloring industry even a bona-fide industry? Is it really going down the tubes? Are people spreading lies about the Food Babe? Why are we about to use a lot more big words?

This is one of those histrionic comments Food Babe spouts when she detects negative sentiment heading in her direction. In this case she's pulled the "spreading lies about me" card from *Vani's Deck of Deflection*. Her stance against Caramel Class IV is well known, specifically because it contains minute traces of 4-methylimidazole (the 4-MeI bogeyman).

Caramelization is a normal part of cooking. We often refer to it as browning (technically, the Maillard reaction [71]). The food industry needs colors with predictable behaviors and since the early days, caramel has been divided into four classes depending on how it's formulated, with each class serving a specific need.

Class I: E150a (plain, caustic and spirit caramels) is produced by heating carbohydrates in the presence of an alkali or an acid. Primarily used to color spirits with a high alcohol content.

Class II: E150b (caustic sulfites process caramels) replaces the acid/ alkali with sulfites. Added to vegetable extracts and cognac.

Class III: E150c (ammonia, ammonia process, closed-pan ammonia process, open-pan ammonia process, bakers', confectioners' and beer caramels) uses heat in the presence of ammonium compounds. Used in beer, sauces, gravies and other goods. May contain traces of 4-MeI.

Class IV: E150d (ammonia sulfite process, sulfite ammonia, sulfite ammonia process, acid-proof, beverage, and soft-drink caramels).

---

70   https://twitter.com/thefoodbabe/status/559548770463924226 (tweet removed)
71   https://en.wikipedia.org/wiki/Maillard_reaction

Used in soft drinks and artificial colors. May contain trace amounts of 4-MeI.

But is it dangerous? Food Babe believes that it is, despite the multiple panels of expert opinion from across the world. More on this later.

> A 2-year government funded feeding study found that 4-Mel caused lung cancer in mice. [72]

Technically this is correct, but it's only part of the story because as per usual, Food Babe conveniently missed the fundamental tenet of toxicology, "the dose makes the poison." In this study the dose was equivalent to consuming 1,000 cans (about 87 US gallons) of a typically colored soft drink every day, which is patently ludicrous. The two-year study encompassed a typical rat's lifespan.

Of course, interest groups like the CSPI (one of Food Babe's quoted resources) sound like valid sources, but there is more to science and research than a clever name and flashy website.

> When The Center for Science in the Public Interest studied two different brands of soda earlier this year, they found that both had dangerous levels of caramel coloring and could be contributing to thousands of cancers in the US. [73]

Quoting from the International Program on Chemical Safety (emphasis ours):

"In the carcinogenicity portion of the study, the observations were generally similar to those in the chronic portion. Survival at 24 months ranged from 64-68% for males and 82-92% for females. Random variations in both benign and malignant neoplasms typical of the F344 strain and this age of animal were observed; however, there were no treatment-related differences. **The authors concluded that the feeding of caramel color IV at doses up to 10 g/kg b.w. for 24 months did not induce neoplastic changes or non-**

---

72   http://foodbabe.com/2014/09/02/drink-starbucks-wake-up-and-smell-the-chemicals/
73   http://foodbabe.com/2012/07/18/sabotaged-at-starbucks/

neoplastic changes of toxicological importance (*MacKenzie, 1985a* [74])."

Jim Coughlin, Ph.D.—a food scientist with over 35 years of experience in the field has this to say of 4-MeI:

"Foods and supplements have become major targets of regulatory enforcement and litigation activities in the past several years. Unfortunately, [California's Proposition 65] and its regulations focus only on the presence of trace levels of individual, listed chemicals in products, but not on the safety or benefits of the whole food or supplement product, nor about real harm to California consumers."

Food Babe isn't a food scientist, she even admits as much. Yet, rather than listening to the very clear message from a raft of qualified people, she chooses to focus on scare-mongering, presumably because fear sells books and affiliated products from her page.

Would Newcastle Brown Ale have to carry a warning under Proposition 65? We don't know, and neither does Food Babe. That doesn't stop her from using the weasel phrase "…would likely have to have a cancer warning label…" which is enough to scare the heck out of the casual reader and elicit eye-rolling from skeptics far and wide.

Newcastle, a UK brand, confessed to using what I would consider one of the most controversial food additives. Toasted barley is usually what gives beer its golden or deep brown color, however in this case, Newcastle beer is also colored artificially with caramel color. This caramel coloring is manufactured by heating ammonia and sulfites under high pressure, which creating carcinogenic compounds. If beer companies were required by law to list the ingredients, Newcastle would likely have to have a cancer warning label under California law because it is a carcinogen proven to cause liver tumors, lung tumors, and thyroid tumors in rats and mice. [75]

Another interesting choice of words here is "confessed," a weasel phrase used to imply the hiding of some guilty secret. "Confirmed" would be a less loaded choice, but this is a purposeful tactic to make things look darker

74   http://www.inchem.org/documents/jecfa/jecmono/v20je11.htm
75   http://foodbabe.com/2015/01/26/breaking-news-major-beer-brand-removes-caramel-coloring/

than they really are. Did someone really cajole the brewery into admitting this or did the put it out as part of their product development literature?

Although efforts to have 4-MeI removed from Prop. 65 (citing poor quality science) have so far failed, in 2012, the Office of Environmental Health Hazard Assessment (OEHA) raised the "safe harbor" limit 16µg to 29µg exposure per day.

This is where the legislation gets confusing. If a single bottle of Newcastle Brown contains 20µg of 4-MeI, that puts the bottle below the limit. But a California consumer drinking just two bottles would easily exceed the current limit. Just to confuse matters further, manufacturers are now producing Caramel Class IV with almost no 4-MeI at all. What's in yours?

Perhaps most revealing of all is that while 4-MeI is not definitively carcinogenic, ethanol (alcohol) most certainly is and Newcastle, like all alcoholic drinks has that in abundance.

On Coffee

Food Babe prides herself on reading those ingredients—and this one is a shocker:

> After reading the ingredients in a Pumpkin Spice Latte, I can tell you that there's absolutely no pumpkin. [76]

The clue is in the name—it's a Pumpkin Spice Latte. Pumpkin Spice Latte isn't supposed to have any pumpkin in it. It's not supposed to taste like pumpkin (which by all accounts isn't really tasty on its own.)

> Non-organic coffee is considered one of the heaviest chemically treated crops in the world, especially when it's imported from developing nations that allow pesticides that are restricted in the US due to health concerns such as Chlorpyrifos. [77]

Check that wording again.

---

76   http://foodbabe.com/2014/08/25/starbucks-pumpkin-spice-latte/
77   http://foodbabe.com/2014/09/02/drink-starbucks-wake-up-and-smell-the-chemicals/

Did Food Babe say considered? Considered by whom? See how those weasel phrases sneak in everywhere? Hiding in plain sight like this, the deliberate implication is that:

There are pesticide residues there and…

There's enough to cause harm.

Offering no actual evidence that Starbucks coffee has anything other than, well, coffee in it, doesn't stop the self-appointed Grand Inquisitor from leaping to a conclusion so far-fetched it would make Brian Williams blush. In an interview with *Fox News*, [78] Food Babe quite categorically stated that the coffee is "ridden with pesticides"—using the word "pesticides" no fewer than three times in under 30 seconds.

She doesn't even specify pesticide residue (which would be bad enough, if it were true) but claims that the final products contain actual pesticides.

Chlorpyrifos (also sold as Dursban, Piridane, Eradex and others) is moderately toxic to humans but the effects are primarily from acute toxicity caused by accidental or deliberate ingestion of the raw product. Farmers and their families using the product (children and pregnant women are most vulnerable) may also suffer from chronic exposure through inhalation of the aerosol. However, the amount remaining on products we buy and use is well below safe limits.

Pesticides used on these crops are sprayed on the berries and the plants. The beans are well protected inside the fleshy fruit. Any chance of detectable amounts of pesticides reaching the final stages (pre-roast) is fairly unlikely; and after that, they have to survive the roasting process.

Being a roasted product, courtesy of that infernal Maillard reaction, coffee may contain trace amounts of 4-MeI and acrylamide (both IARC 2b carcinogens), but pesticides? Well, there is one in there, but it's in pretty much all coffee: it's the caffeine! The coffee plant evolved caffeine to protect itself from insects. We just happen to use it as a stimulant.

---

78   http://video.foxnews.com/v/3344545093001/is-starbucks-organic-coffee-as-advertised/

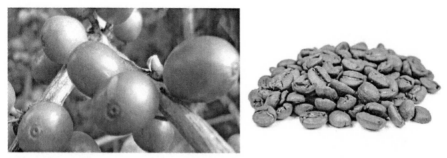

Figure 2.10: Coffee berries ripen on the plant (left) and go through a number of processes before being finally sold as usable beans (right). (George Hoaden/Lucy Toner)

Coffee is highly processed long before it reaches the shop. It's picked, washed, sorted and squashed, fermented, dehydrated, hulled, polished and then stored in an air-conditioned room for up to 18 months, then re-dried at 329°F before being roasted at temperatures from 374°F to 473°F (depending on taste), and finally ground into a powder before being doused in very hot water to extract the flavorings.

As expected with something as virally visible as this meme was, it rapidly appeared on the generally reliable Snopes.com website, which specializes in debunking urban myths and legends by testing the story against known facts. Snopes' researchers came to the same conclusions we did; completely independently and using different sources. Still, that didn't stop the Food Babe PR machine from admitting it was all a huge misunderstanding and poorly sourced material; because the best defense is offense, right?

> There's a bogus "Snopes" article that is circulating trying to disprove my research into the ingredients in the Pumpkin Spice Latte. [79]

Food Babe reiterates her so-called research (which Snopes and others have solidly refuted) but still fails to accept that the FDA and EFSA haven't found any reason to outlaw 4-MeI in quantities that we're exposed to in everyday life, continuing the assault by concluding:

> Millions of people continue to drink Starbucks flavored coffee drinks laced with this substance and could be harming

---

79   https://www.facebook.com/thefoodbabe/photos/a.208386335862752.56063.132535093447877/830361756998537/

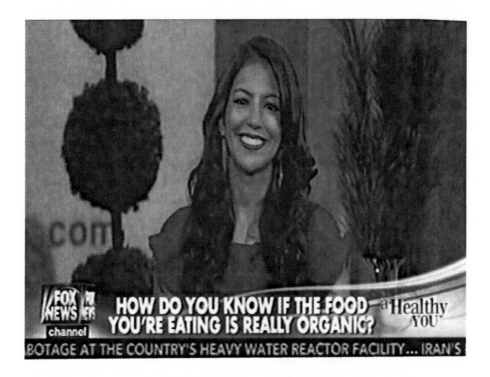

Figure 2.11: The beaming smile is well-rehearsed. But Vani is about to tell viewers that Starbucks coffee is "ridden with pesticides." Bon appétit! (Fox News—Mar. 15, 2014)
themselves. [80]

In The Food Babe Way, she goes even further, stating quite categorically:

> At most locations Starbucks doesn't serve organic coffee or organic milk; they serve nonorganic coffee made from beans doused with pesticides, and milk from cows fed GMOs and given antibiotics. If you drink Starbucks on a daily basis, you're exposing yourself to pesticides, GMOs, and antibiotics every day. [81]

So let's pause for a moment and pick apart these three very specific claims raised against conventional farming.

Remember from earlier that coffee plants don't produce beans, they produce a fruit that contains the seed we refer to as a bean. There is no evi-

80   https://www.facebook.com/thefoodbabe/photos/a.208386335862752.56063.132535093447877/830361756998537/
81   Food Babe Way, p. 83

dence the beans are ever "doused" in pesticides—there is simply no logic in doing so. The word doused means to: "soak, saturate, and pour over" and coffee beans simply are not processed like that. The closest they come is when the berries are sprayed and the bean, not unlike the seeds in an apple core or the stone in a peach, is protected deep inside the fruit.

What about GMOs? Aside from the fact that no reputable study has ever found any causative link between GM crops and adverse human health (not so much as a sniffle), let's assume there was a concern. Milk is a complex of fats, water, proteins, minerals and trace elements produced in the breast tissue of mammals. Any GM foodstuff fed to the cows is broken down into its constituent parts long before it even enters the animal's bloodstream. Any transgenic ("man-made") DNA sequence present before it entered the cow has been annihilated long before it could get to the animal's milk.

Finally, antibiotics. Antibiotics are known to get into the animal's milk as they are delivered into the blood. However, they are only given to dairy

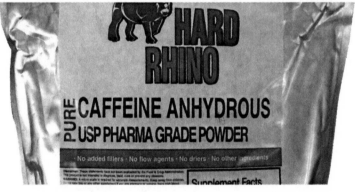

Figure 2.12: Hard Rhino pure caffeine—similar to that implicated in the death of Logan Steiner. (Jeanie Jaramillo, Texas Panhandle Poison Center)

(milk) herds as a treatment when the animals are sick and in need of treatment. During and after cessation of treatment, the affected animals are removed from production—the withdrawal period—until all traces of the medication have passed.

Not a single one of these claims are true. Your coffee is safe—you're just being conned into buying organic and spending more money than you have to.

As we mentioned, there's an interesting little addition to this story. Coffee contains measurable amounts of 1,3,7-Trimethylpurine-2,6-dion. Considerable quantities of this psychoactive drug remain in the final product and we consume it every time we drink coffee regardless of the purity of the source. It's an effective herbicide and insecticide, paralyzing and killing the insects that consume it and destroying plants that come into contact with it.

It's also known as caffeine

Although rare, even something as apparently innocuous as caffeine can kill a healthy adult in the right dose. Prom King Logan Stiner of Ohio died tragically on May 27, 2014 after ingesting pharmaceutical grade caffeine—a white crystalline powder widely available on the Internet. The coroner recorded the level of caffeine in Logan's blood to be 23 times that of a typical coffee drinker and his death was due to cardiac arrhythmia (abnormal heart rhythm) caused by acute caffeine toxicity.

Logan's death was preventable; the supplement, known as *Hard Rhino*, was sold in such a way as to bypass the FDA's laws. A website in his honor was set up at *LoganStiner.org*.

Caffeine is the active ingredient in energy drinks such as Red Bull. These have also been implicated in a number of deaths [82, 83] , particularly among young people who may treat it more like a soft drink or mix it with alcohol. A typical can contains about the same amount of caffeine as a 12oz Starbucks coffee but can be consumed at a far greater rate and may affect people who are genetically predisposed to caffeine sensitivity.

Chronic caffeine poisoning (caffeinism) may also present with many or all of the following symptoms: headache, light-headedness, anxiety, agitation, tremulousness, tingling in the mouth, fingers and toes, confusion, psychosis, seizures, chest pain, irregular heartbeat or palpitations, nau-

---

82   http://guardianlv.com/2014/06/teenage-girl-is-dead-after-consuming-red-bull-energy-drink/
83   http://www.caffeineinformer.com/death-by-red-bull

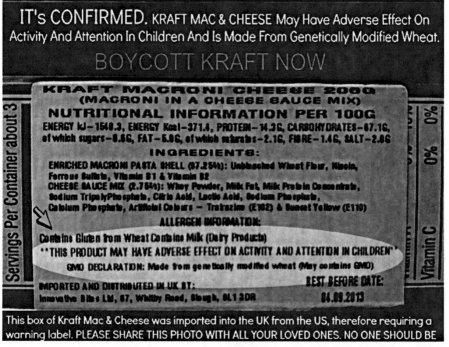

Figure 2.13: Based on the evidence of a sticky label alone, Food Babe "confirms" Mac N Cheese is made from GM Wheat based on a sticker! (Flo Wrightson/Food Babe LLC)

sea, vomiting, diarrhea & bowel incontinence, and even anorexia. [84] Food Babe's selective demonization of safe ingredients is arbitrary but effective at mobilizing an army of armchair warriors.

On Artificial Colors

Warning #1: This Product May Cause Adverse Effects On Activity And Attention In Children (This warning label is required because The US version of Kraft Mac & Cheese has artificial food dyes yellow #5 and yellow #6 which are proven to be linked to hyperactivity in children.)![85]

European readers will be more familiar with the E-numbers E102 (tartrazine) and E104 (quinoline yellow), which belong to a family of artificial azo dyes. This warning label, found by a Food Babe reader, was applied by a UK importer (*Innovative Bites Ltd.*) and is a requirement of EU law.

---

84   http://orthomolecular.org/library/jom/2004/pdf/2004-v19n02-p092.pdf

85   http://foodbabe.com/2013/05/30/illegal-gmo-wheat-in-kraft-mac-cheese/

This caution is due to another set of European directives. There is neither suggestion nor evidence that the importer, Innovative Bites, had the slightest inkling where the wheat was sourced from. Putting this on the label saves them from future litigation should it later transpire GM products were found in this food. It's simply lazy and unjustified. Further, take a guess how many varieties of GMO wheat exist on the market? If you guessed zero, you were right. As of publication, there are no available wheat varieties made using recombinant DNA or genetic engineering technologies considered genetic modification. [86]

However, there are wheat varieties created using "atomic gardening" in which a plant or seed is bombarded with mutagenic radiation with the intention of scrambling its DNA to induce new traits. Notably, these varieties can be sold as organic. However, Food Babe's claim that Yellow #5 and #6 have been proven to cause hyperactivity in children is another example of the tabloid level fear-mongering she is so frequently accused of.

Before we address Food Babe's fear-mongering and bad science, let us pause briefly and consider her hypocrisy and double standards. If Yellow #5 and #6 are as bad as she claims, why are these dyes found in so many of the products that Ms. Hari sells via FoodBabe.com? Her Tarte [87] and Josie Maran lip stains [88] contain not only these two yellows, but the villainous Blue #1 (from her campaign against Jello) and Red #40 (from her McDonald's wars).

Read Food Babe's article, *Holistic Health Care*, [89] in which she warns the reader that toxic chemicals will be absorbed into their bodies through their hair. Then put on your Food Babe Investigator Hat and read the labels on the Giovanni Hair Care [90] products that you purchased from Food Babe. com: Yes, there's Yellow #5, Red #40, Red #3...

Food Babe's hypocrisy aside, these additives and a possible link to ADD and ADHD were originally part of a UK study by Southampton University (the Southampton Six) which we'll examine in more detail in Chapter 13.

---

86 http://www.bloomberg.com/news/articles/2013-11-13/mutant-crops-drive-basf-sales-where-monsanto-denied-commodities

87 http://tartecosmetics.com/tarte-item-lipsurgence-natural-matte-lip-tint

88 http://www.josiemarancosmetics.com/coconut-watercolor-lip-stain-shine.html

89 http://foodbabe.com/2011/11/06/holistic-hair-care-how-why/

90 http://www.giovannicosmetics.com/GIOVANNI-INGREDIENT-LIST.PDF

Despite numerous attempts and meta-analyses by panels of experts, there remains no convincing scientific evidence these additives cause hyperactivity in the general population.

There is *limited* evidence these colors **may** affect *susceptible* children. However, it relies considerably on anecdotal evidence from parents, caregivers and teachers—often of children with pre-diagnosed ADD and related behavioral disorders. The link is not proven. Even if it was, it only appears to affect a small number of children, possibly due to uncommon genetic variants, in much the same way that aspartame must be avoided by people with PKU.

> Warning #2: GMO Declaration: Made from genetically modified wheat. (May contain GMO)(This warning label is required because the US version of Kraft Mac & Cheese contains GMOs.) [91]

Kraft spokesperson *Lynne Galia* told the New York Times:

> *Anyone implying that G.E. wheat is in Kraft Mac and Cheese or any of our products is wrong.* [92]

So, despite Kraft Foods categorically and unequivocally stating it does not use GMO wheat in its products, Food Babe doesn't care and stirs the pot even more. This story has been updated twice and not corrected despite the new information.

> If Kraft is using genetically modified (GMO) wheat in their Mac & Cheese, it is SERIOUSLY ALARMING for a number of reasons.

1. **GMO Wheat is not approved by the USDA for U.S. Farming. So where the heck is Kraft getting this wheat to put in their Mac & Cheese?**

2. **Last night in breaking news, it was discovered that GMO wheat had been illegally growing in Oregon. [93] So this begs the question—is there illegal GMO wheat in Kraft Mac & Cheese?**

3. **The USDA is investigating the illegal crop in Oregon—**

---

91   http://foodbabe.com/2013/05/30/illegal-gmo-wheat-in-kraft-mac-cheese/

92   http://www.nytimes.com/2013/06/06/business/gmo-label-on-kraft-mac-cheese-box-raises-alarm.html

93   http://www.huffingtonpost.com/2013/05/29/non-approved-genetically-modified-wheat-usda_n_3354275.html

> Don't you think they should investigate companies that are
> using GM wheat like Kraft too?

4. If Kraft is not using GMO wheat grown in the United
    States, they could be getting genetically engineered wheat
    from other countries that allow the production, and are
    importing it into the US. It is crazy to think that a company
    could be importing a crop that is not approved for use in
    the US and putting it our products without labeling!

5. There is only one other likely scenario for the GMO
    Declaration on Kraft's Mac & Cheese. The farm land that
    wheat is grown on in the US is so contaminated [94] from
    GMO crops like corn and soy, they have no choice but to
    declare our wheat genetically modified on the warning
    label when exported to other countries. This fact is very
    concerning if true and has dire implications for the entire
    farmland here in America.

6. The labeler could have mistaken GMO corn for GMO wheat,
    but if that is the case, Kraft needs to confirm either way.

Tin foil hats at the ready people! Call Alex Jones—where others see a lazy label on a gray import, we sense a huge conspiracy!

If we apply Occam's Razor—the idea the simplest explanation is usually the right one—it's easy to see this is a storm in a very small teacup, brought about by some lazy labelling of an imported product. Food Babe isn't interested in that. It doesn't serve her agenda. Instead, she spends six whole points explaining other rather extravagant scenarios.

You may note that at Point 5 here, Food Babe refers the reader to *Natural News,* specifically a piece by Mike Adams, perhaps the number one source of pernicious lies and misinformation on food. [95]

The story doesn't end there. Urban legends specialists Snopes.com got in on the act and strongly implied the label wasn't even real, stating in the 18 March 2015 revision:

---

94 http://www.naturalnews.com/040541_GMO_genetic_pollution_GE_wheat.html

95 http://www.geneticliteracyproject.org/2014/07/28/fbi-turns-up-heat-on-mike-adams-as-health-ranger-fiasco-widens-plus-adams-archive/

"Additionally, even if the label shown here were genuine, the commonly suggested interpretation of it would still be inaccurate." [96]

So we sent our Scottish mole on a mission. Although we received the same response as everyone else from Innovative Bites Ltd., i.e. not even an acknowledgement, we did manage to track down a bunch of labels placed on candy, imported into the UK by the company and several others.

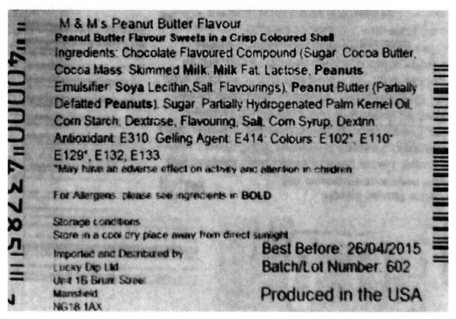

M & M s Peanut Butter Flavour
Peanut Butter Flavour Sweets in a Crisp Coloured Shell
Ingredients: Chocolate Flavoured Compound (Sugar. Cocoa Butter.
Cocoa Mass. Skimmed Milk. Milk Fat. Lactose. **Peanuts**
Emulsifier **Soya** Lecithin,Salt. Flavourings). **Peanut** Butter (Partially
Defatted **Peanuts**). Sugar. Partially Hydrogenated Palm Kernel Oil.
Corn Starch. Dextrose. Flavouring. Salt. Corn Syrup. Dextrin.
Antioxidant. E310. Gelling Agent: E414. Colours: E102*, E110*
E129*, E132, E133.
*May have an adverse effect on activity and attention in children

For Allergens please see ingredients in **BOLD**

Storage conditions
Store in a cool dry place away from direct sunlight

Imported and Distributed by
Lucky Dip Ltd
Unit 16 Brunt Street
Mansfield
NG18 1AX

Best Before: 26/04/2015
Batch/Lot Number: 602
Produced in the USA

Figure 2.14: Yellow 5, Yellow 6 and Red 40—shown here with their European designations– carry a warning label as required by European legislation. This pack of M&Ms was imported by Lucky Dip ltd. in Mansfield.

In most cases, the labels shared similar dire warnings. We did speak to an anonymous source who has previously dealt with Innovative Bites. He confirmed the labels are produced in house. We were also able to locate some candy imported by Innovative Bites and several other "grey" importers.

Snopes could not be reached for comment despite being offered hard evidence of the actual labels.

Yellow 5 and Yellow 6 can be contaminated with known

---

96   www.snopes.com/food/warnings/kraftgmo.asp

carcinogens (a.k.a. an agent directly involved in causing cancer). [97]

As with many of Food Babe's so-called investigations, this one cites the Center For Science in the Public Interest, a non-governmental organization with a mission to act as a consumer advocate. As grand as it sounds, the CSPI is not an academic institution and, while it produces detailed reports, those reports are not subject to peer review. As such we view it with a healthy dash of skepticism.

The offending chemicals listed are used in the production of azo dyes (including Yellow #6) and there is a chance a microscopic (if measurable) amount of contaminant may remain in the final product–but only a chance. Of these two, 4-amino-biphenyl has been discontinued since at least 2000 [98] leaving just benzidine to account for. It's true that exposure to benzidine in an industrial setting may be a hazard to health as detailed by the National Toxicity Program. [99] However, it is foolhardy (and bad science) to automatically transpose that finding onto the barely measurable amount ending up in the dye coloring our food.

Even the CSPI admits [100] (however vaguely) that the studies were unable to find conclusive proof Yellow 5/6 were responsible for neoplasms (cancer) in either mice or rats—let alone humans.

More detail on additives, their effects and the science appears in "E for Ingredients" on page 316.

On Artificial Flavorings

> Artificial flavor that could be made from anything—most likely petroleum [101]

Ah there are those weasel words getting into everything: "most likely petroleum [crude oil]"

Here's the list of flavorings made with petroleum:

---

97   http://foodbabe.com/2015/04/20/kraft-dumps-artificial-food-dyes-after-massive-petition/
98   http://www.epa.gov/airtoxics/hlthef/aminobip.html
99   https://ntp.niehs.nih.gov/ntp/roc/content/profiles/dimethoxybenzidineanddyes.pdf
100 http://cspinet.org/new/pdf/dyes-problem-table.pdf
101 http://foodbabe.com/2011/12/01/chemical-warfare-with-natural-flavor/

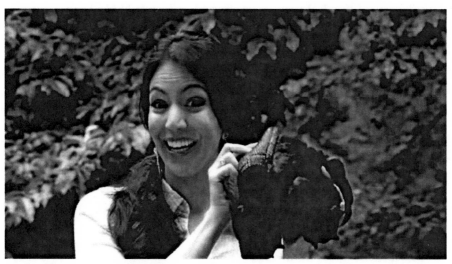

Figure 2.15: Look! This beaver's butt tastes like strawberry. Yummy! Beaver posed by model. (Food Babe LLC/YouTube)

...

Yeah, that's it. None as far as we can tell, although there are over 6000 products known to be made from crude oil, including some preservatives. Perhaps that's the source of the confusion?

It's worth pointing out that a founding principle of chemistry is that nearly anything can be made from anything if you have the right skills and equipment. Everything in the universe was, at some time, just a bunch of hydrogen atoms, including us; we're just nuclear waste!

Humans may never harness the power of stars to create heavy elements in large amounts, but we're pretty good at combining chemical elements and their isotopes into compounds; then combining those compounds into newer and more exciting ones. Carbon, the element of life, is probably the most versatile of all the elements and crude oil is a wonderful source of (relatively) simple carbon compounds that are just begging to be formulated into something more complex and diverse.

A simple piece of kitchen chemistry may serve as a demonstration. Crack an egg into a cold pan and you can see the clear albumen (there are several parts to it, but for now, just think of it as one) and the yellow yolk sac. If you were to heat the pan, in a short time you'd see the proteins in the albumen start to break down (denature) and the substance change from yellowish-tinted slippery jelly into a firm white mass. The cooked egg is chemically entirely different from the raw one (and a lot safer to eat!)

If that had been a fertile egg (farmed eggs are not fertile) and you'd popped it under a broody hen, you'd have a fluffy little chick in 21 days.

This natural process is entirely chemical in nature and so amazingly complex that we're only just beginning to understand it. Nature builds an entire chick from the proteins in the albumen. The yolk is used to feed the growing chick.

Making one thing from another thing often changes it entirely. So just because something is made from crude oil, it's no longer crude oil any more than the stuff that comes out of us is the same healthy stuff we shovelled in.

Some flavors come from beaver butts (according to Food Babe):

> Castoreum (or beaver butt) is just one of the ingredients that could be called a "natural flavor." But there are many other things called "natural flavors" that could be lurking in your food. [102]

You can't beat a good gross-out moment for igniting fear and solidifying righteous indignation in your uncritical army of followers. Even Food Babe has to admit that whatever comes out of dead beavers isn't the beaver's anal sphincter.

Castoreum is a broad term to describe both the exudate (gloop) that is formed in the beaver's castor sacs and the sacs themselves. Beavers use small amounts of the aromatic castoreum combined with urine to scent mark their territories, and therein lies the clue to the real usage of this rather unusual animal product.

According to Fenaroli's handbook, castoreum extract can be used for a broad range of vanilla flavorings. Food Babe claims it's used as a strawberry flavor but crucially, even IF (and it's a fairly dubious claim) it's used as a vanilla flavor, a person's average daily exposure is 81 nanograms/Kg—which is:

0.000000081 of a gram, which is 0.00000000324 of an ounce.

---

102 http://foodbabe.com/2013/09/09/food-babe-tv-do-you-eat-beaver-butt/

… and that's assuming the stuff even gets into your food in the first place. Based on Food Babe logic, we should avoid swimming at the beach to avoid swallowing fish poo.

Using these figures, castoreum must be extraordinarily potent. But wait -there's more—Food Babe thinks it's in everything!

> They [beavers] also flavor a ton of foods at the grocery store. [103]

The origin of this little dollop of drivel seems to have come from British Chef, and TV personality, *Jamie Oliver* when he appeared on the *Late Show with David Letterman* and claimed [104] castoreum is used to flavor vanilla ice cream. This prompted a concerned viewer to write to the *Vegetarian Resource Group* which did a more thorough investigation [105] and could find no evidence from the manufacturers that castoreum was being used to flavor… well, anything.

> It's far cheaper to use castoreum, or beaver's butt, to flavor strawberry oatmeal, than to use actual strawberries. [106]

When was the last time you tasted a vanilla flavored strawberry? Castoreum is supposed to be a vanilla flavor isn't it? That's some pretty strange voodoo going on right there. As for vanilla—industrial consumption (almost certainly all of which goes into food) is 8,700 times greater than castoreum. Fenaroli's usage estimate for both products appears to lie in the production rather than consumed quantities.

Castoreum does have a fairly pungent odor and because of this finds a use in high-end perfumery. So rather than eating beaver butt, you're more likely to be dabbing it behind your ears, girls—if it's in your budget!

Mmmmm! Hon, you smell like strawberries and vanilla! Have you been licking the beaver's butt again! Delish!

---

103 https://www.youtube.com/watch?v=nweK6VRM8a8

104 http://metro.co.uk/2011/04/06/jamie-oliver-vanilla-ice-cream-contains-beaver-anal-gland-649693/

105 http://www.vrg.org/blog/2011/06/17/beaver-gland-castoreum-not-used-in-vanilla-flavorings-according-to-manufacturers/

106 https://www.youtube.com/watch?v=nweK6VRM8a8

On Silly Putty

Dimethylpolysiloxane is commonly used in vinegary-smelling silicone caulks, adhesives, and aquarium sealants, a component in silicone grease and other silicone based lubricants, as well as in defoaming agents, mold release agents, damping fluids, heat transfer fluids, polishes, cosmetics, hair conditioners AND IN OUR FOOD! [107]

Dimethylpolysiloxane (also called dimethicone) is about as non-toxic as they come. Though it's a component used in the manufacture of Silly Putty, referring to dimethicone as Silly Putty is about as accurate as referring to vodka as nail polish remover. Still, that doesn't stop Food Babe from claiming that everything from McDonald's French fries to Domino's breadsticks contains the childhood playtime favorite.

Even if Silly Putty was used in large enough quantities to be noticeable in food (and we think it's fair to say you'd file a complaint if you found a lump of it in your fries) it could not do us any harm: millions of children have played with Silly Putty since it was first created and not a single incident of Silly Putty poisoning has ever been reported. Anywhere. Ever.

Now consider this stuff (dimethicone) is used as an adhesive and sealer in the production of fish tanks. Does that sound like the sort of thing that requires preserving? What with all those hungry fish and billions of bacteria, if there was a mere morsel of tasty nourishment in there, tanks would start self-destructing in a matter of weeks. Yet, despite this rather obvious reality, Food Babe says:

The FDA allows dimethylpolysiloxane to be preserved by several different chemicals that don't have to be listed on the label either, including formaldehyde! Formaldehyde is one of the most highly toxic substances on earth. It is linked to allergies, brain damage, cancer, and auto-immune disorders. [108]

Sounds scary doesn't it? This comes from misinterpreting the wording of the FDA's Code of Federal Regulations, Title 21 on formaldehyde:

---

107 http://foodbabe.com/2013/10/22/sillyputty/
108 http://foodbabe.com/2013/10/22/sillyputty/

"…a preservative in defoaming agents containing dimethylpolysiloxane, in an amount not exceeding 1.0 percent of the dimethylpolysiloxane content."

Preservatives are compounds that prevent growth of things like molds and bacteria in our food but it's pretty clear from the aquarium example that di methylpolysiloxane/dimethicone needs artificial preserving like trout need motorcycles.

This small amount of formaldehyde is allowed to preserve the defoamer as a whole. For simplicity, imagine the dimethicone made up 1% of the defoaming agent. That would make the total formaldehyde content 0.001%. This figure also has to be further divided by the proportion of defoamer added to the product. At these dilutions, any formaldehyde we are exposed to (our bodies even make the stuff) is completely harmless.

On Alcohol

Your liver is your main fat-burning organ. If you are trying to lose weight or even maintain your ideal weight, drinking alcohol is one of your worst enemies. [109]

That a medical professional wrote the foreword to The Food Babe Way and the above claim appears in the book (p. 128) is a pretty damning indictment of how much people trust Vani Hari.

Whatever the reason, the liver is not a fat burning organ. We don't burn fat; at least, not directly, because it has to be converted into something our cells can use for energy: glucose (which can be metabolized in our liver from a number of more complex molecules, including fats).

Most of the direct burn (oxidation) happens in the muscles. And the bigger the muscle, the bigger the burn.

The team felt this issue was so important, we've devoted an entire chapter to it later in the book. But Food Babe pushes enough misinformation on alcohol to fill more than a chapter:

Is beer really healthy? Why are the ingredients not listed on the label? Which brands can we trust? Which brands are trying to

---

109 http://foodbabe.com/2013/07/17/the-shocking-ingredients-in-beer/

slowly poison us with cheap and harmful ingredients? [110]

Phrasing like this isn't just misleading, it's plain wrong. Beer producers aren't trying to *slowly poison us*. We're quite capable of doing that to the entire biosphere without any help from them. Most cars create more potentially carcinogenic compounds just driving to the mall than you'll ever find in your six pack of ale.

Unsurprisingly, she brings up the tried and true beaver butt in her discussion of beer as well, this time in the Food Babe Way:

> Natural flavors that could come from anything, including a beaver's anal gland. [111]

A gross allusion with no basis in reality. Sure, they might use flavorings, but castoreum is far too rare (and therefore, expensive) to dump into beer willy nilly. Artificial colors, though, are a different story:

> Caramel coloring, classified as III or IV, made from ammonia, and considered a carcinogen. [112]

We've already covered 4-MeI and the rather overblown claim that it causes cancer. This error is worth pointing out again: caramel coloring is not "made from ammonia" it's made in the presence of it. Even the source of the confusion, California's Proposition 65, [113] has admitted it poses "*no significant risk.*" Naturally, Food Babe isn't about to admit to that. It's a ready-made stick to beat the producers with, and admitting she's wrong would require huge public U-turns.

On GMO

> GMO stands for "genetically modified organism" and is a plant or animal that has been genetically engineered with DNA from bacteria, viruses, or other plants or animals. [114]

---

110 http://foodbabe.com/2013/07/17/the-shocking-ingredients-in-beer/
111 The Food Babe Way, p. 129
112 The Food Babe Way, p. 129
113 http://oehha.ca.gov/public_info/facts/4MEIfacts_021012.html
114 http://foodbabe.com/faq/

Food Babe doesn't seem to understand GMOs; she just wants to create an unnecessary climate of fear surrounding them. Time after time she uses the same weasel phrases like "may be GMO." The technology is referenced over 90 times in The Food Babe Way: GMO sugars, GMO corn (and corn products), GMO yeast, GMO soybean... and so on. On her website (as of February 2015) she lists over 90 different ingredients that "...*could be GMO or genetically engineered.*" [115]

The phrase "Genetically Modified Organism" is a vague and misleading term that refers to a specific set of breeding techniques; not to an ingredient or product that can be scooped into a bowl. GMOs include organisms with new genes from the same or different organisms, with genes whose activity has been down-regulated (reduced), or with genes that have been "edited" in some way.

But what most people don't know is that many "conventional", so-called "non-GMO" breeding techniques involve radically modifying the plant in a laboratory, such as altering a plant's genome using chemical or radiation mutagenesis, or "wide cross" hybridizations, in which large numbers of genes are moved across organisms of different species to create plant varieties that couldn't be produced in nature. Notably, these genetic manipulations, among others, can be certified and sold as organic and "non-GMO."

Indeed, the vast majority of foods we consume, outside of certain wild herbs and mushrooms, berries, and game have been manipulated to states unrecognizable from their indigenous ancestors, and with considerable genomic changes though they aren't considered "GMOs" in the modern vernacular. Some varieties created in these ways result in offspring being unable to reproduce. In certain cases, it leads to a technique known as grafting for plants such as fruit trees, and it's something we'll examine in detail later.

A GMO has to be a living thing, otherwise it's not an organism. Something that is derived from a GMO might or might not contain genes modified with molecular genetic engineering (and if it's been cooked or processed even that likelihood is severely diminished.)

---

115 http://foodbabe.com/possible-gmo-ingredients-a-z/

I am not sure if this is the correct place post these photos. If not please accept my apologies and remove them. I bought these bananas two days ago. I don't remember seeing these fiber looking strings before. Are these things normal or am I seeing something more in this ?

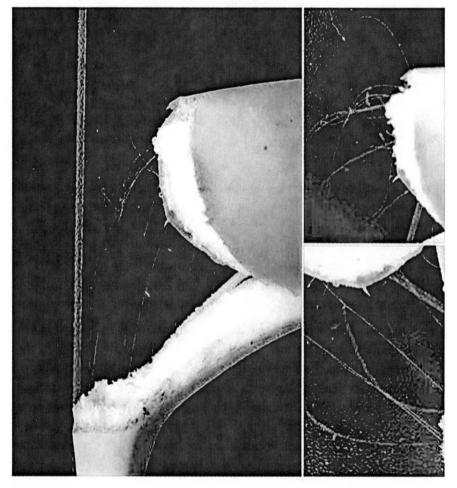

Like · Share

Figure 2.16: The banana in the picture is perfectly normal—what you can see here are part of the fibrous structure the skin is composed of. Without the fibers, the skin would be unable to protect the soft fruit and seeds inside. Ignorance is a breeding ground for fear, and in the US, fear of GM is a new form of McCarthyism fuelled by people like Food Babe who are laughing all the way to the bank. (Facebook/Kevin Folta)

So, from that list, things like corn and corn products (corn flour, corn oil) may have been derived from GM corn, and soy products from GM soy. Food Babe also demonizes things like milk powder. We think she means GM cows, such as the strain produced in New Zealand by AG Research in 2012 to produce milk without the whey protein, beta-lactoglobulin. This is essential for the 3% of children born with an intolerance. But to date this particular breed remains experimental.

From the sublime to the ludicrous… Food Babe claims the following are genetically modified: sucrose, glucose and fructose (sugars), erythritol, sorbitol, glycerol, maltitol (sugar alcohols), MSG, aspartame, and even phenylalanine (the substance created when we metabolise aspartame). Every one of these are chemicals, and fairly simple ones at that.

So what is a GMO anyway?

The acronym stands for "Genetically Modified Organism." An organism is loosely defined as any living thing, including plants, animals, and microbes. So what makes an organism "genetically modified?" Essentially genes are portions of genomes, which are identical copies of all of the genetic material in any organism. In multicellular organisms, there is an identical copy of the genome in every cell of the body. Like a book in English is written in 26 letters of the alphabet, the genome of any organism is written in four nucleotides, denoted as A,T, C, and G. Genes code for proteins, which are the most basic functional components of living things. Proteins serve all functions of life, from structure, immunity, metabolic, enzymatic functions, and more.

Proteins are large molecules composed of amino acid chains. The sequence of amino acids in any protein determines its 3D structure. Like the 3D structure of a cooking utensil or car part determines its function, so does the structure of a protein. Varied sequences of the four nucleotides code for different permutations of amino acids, changing the resultant protein. This is similar to binary code, in which variations of just two "characters" (0s and 1s) encode complex computer functions.

Proteins dictate almost everything a living thing is and does. Your bones are weak or strong? Proteins. Your bestie's enviable blue eyes? Lack of certain proteins. Your son always wins his swim meets? A complex interaction of proteins and environment. Likewise, the characteristics of plants (tall, short, sweet, pest-resistant, fibrous, etc.) depend on the types and expression levels of its proteins, determined by DNA sequence.When it comes to genetically modified crops, there is no injecting of vegetables with syringes, no cackling scientist sneaking toxins into franken-fruit, and no covert plot to harm consumers despite what biotechnology opponents would have us think.

Foods considered genetically modified (GM) are engineered using molecular transgenic technologies. Remember, proteins are encoded by only four nucleotide bases present in all life on earth: A, T, C, G. Nothing is altered in a GMO except for the sequence of a few of these nucleotides, often just a handful out of a billion or more "characters." Nothing is added that doesn't already exist in nature. And our friend Mother Nature alters these sequences on her own, achieving change slower than molasses in January—AKA evolution. Genetic modification does this in a targeted, efficient manner, moving or enhancing traits that already exist in nature. Benefits range from helping farmers' crops resist pests or survive drought, to reducing harmful compounds, to increasing vitamin content of staple foods.

No matter where this laundry list of chemicals came from in the first place they don't contain DNA… not now, not ever. It's almost as ridiculous as a Non-GMO Project verified salt. There is no "organism" in salt to modify. Yet it's no surprise that the state of the market allows for just that, a "GMO-free" salt known as HimalaSalt.

GE yeast is another interesting one. Yeast is a simple, single-celled organism brewers use to convert sugars into alcohol. As the alcohol content rises, the yeasts are killed off. At the end of the process all that remains is a brew which has to be clarified, either by standing, or using a compound such as isinglass (another one of Food Babe's gross-out culprits because it's made from fish's swim bladders).

GE yeasts are just more efficient at taking more complex carbohydrates and converting them to glucose, which is then converted to alcohol. In other words, it's just more efficient.

The National Centre for Biotechnology Education at the University of Reading (England) had this to say:

> *"It is now over 20 years since the first research on the genetic modification of brewing yeasts, and many modified strains have been developed. However, no brewers in the world currently use genetically-modified yeasts."* [116]

Even if you want to avoid GMOs created in labs using advanced biological techniques, avoiding products like refined sugars and oils is pointless. Genetic modification affects the plant's DNA. By the time the plant has been harvested and processed into sugar or oil, there's no DNA left.

DNA is a very fragile molecule held together with a sugar (not the stuff we eat) and it's destroyed (in humans) by the enzymes in the mouth and degrades to less complex molecules within seconds of being exposed to the acid environment in our stomach. With the exception of specifically evolved bacteria, it's irrevocably altered (denatured) by temperatures no warmer than a cup of coffee (about 70°C/160°F).

> What GMO crops are proven to do is produce novel proteins that have never before existed, with which we did not evolve, and which are not required to be tested for safety before being put into the food supply. [117]

Genetic engineering expert Dr. Kevin Folta's pithy response says it all:

> *"Except in nature where they came from."*

...and...

> *"we didn't evolve with 99% of the stuff we eat today."*

The next two quotations, although sourced from Food Babe's website, actually belong to a young farmer, author and speaker, Birke Baehr. Now Birke is a bright kid; but he doesn't grasp the science behind genetically engineered crops and listening to him speak is telling—almost a sock puppet for someone equally ignorant but an awful lot more invested in tradition. As such, his passion isn't matched by his knowledge, and that's dangerous.

---

116 http://www.ncbe.reading.ac.uk/ncbe/gmfood/yeasts.html
117 http://foodbabe.com/an-open-letter-to-food-babe/

> GMO food that is fed to animals has been linked to sickening them with diseases, like kidney & liver toxicity, cancer, infertility, birth defects, and death. Scientists have found genetically engineered D.N.A. in animal tissue, that we end up consuming in the end. [118]

Birke doesn't provide a source for this claim so we can only guess where it came from. The hard fact is, GM food hasn't been linked to any such thing, although there are a bunch of other things that could cause this laundry list of maladies. Birke appears to be regurgitating what he was primed with.

Being ruminants, cattle have different stomachs. It's a nasty place down there and DNA is going to have a skeptic's chance at a natural food expo of getting out intact. Assuming some did survive, it has to pass into the bloodstream, where it's facing an army of defense mechanisms designed to target and destroy foreign DNA.

The bovine digestive system is completely different than ours. A cow's stomach has four chambers (sometime referred to as four stomachs):

- The *reticulum* and *rumen*: the first and second chambers start to break down the complex cell membranes—cellulose—using a combination of enzymes, bacteria and viruses. Ruminant animals belch some of this material (called cud) back into their mouths and continue to chew it. (Chewing the cud.) This portion of the stomach, along with the omasum, has a honeycombed appearance and is consumed in many cultures as tripe.
- The *omasum*: following the reticulum/rumen, the omasum absorbs much of the ingested water.
- The *abomasum*: the final "chamber" is where food is finally digested by a complex of enzymes called rennet. This is where nutrients are absorbed.

It's fair to say we don't know if any of this DNA can horizontally transfer into the bacteria populating the gut. But if they are doing this anyway, so what's a little extra DNA on your plate? If the GM opponents are so convinced they'll transfer all that DNA into our genome, shouldn't we all be

---

118 http://foodbabe.com/2013/05/13/birke-reports-gmos-in-meat/

turning into hideous plant-animal-bacterial-fungal hybrids? After all, non-GE food contains just as much DNA as GE varieties.

As is usually the case with these claims, they don't stand up to even a little scrutiny. They are scary so some people—even you—might be tempted to believe them. It's easy to accept what others are telling us if they seem to sincerely believe it themselves. Just like Birke, who also wrote of GM fish:

> It was discovered by a study done by Purdue University that when only 60 "frankenfish" were released into a habitat of about 60,000 wild fish that in only 40 fish generations there was a complete extinction! [119]

This is a fairly typical example of blissful ignorance because the argument doesn't hold any water. Let's say the Atlantic salmon matured from egg to adult in just one year (they don't, but let's assume they do.) That would take 40 years to complete—and the technology itself is barely 40 years old as of 2013, when this post was written.

Calling any GM organism Franken-something isn't just an insult to a great piece of 19th century literature, it's an insult to the intelligence of the people who know a little about genetic engineering.

This is such a fascinating subject, we've provided a chapter explaining just why this is both ignorant and offensive (if effective as a PR stunt). Head over to Chapter 5 to see where "Frankenfood" really is in our food supply—the answer might shock you.

So how did Purdue manage to study the GM salmon?

It cheated. It used a computer model to simulate the introduction of the more competitive fish into a traditional eco-system and, like all models, made a lot of assumptions.

Could it happen and does it matter? A number of strategies are in place to ensure this sort of thing can't occur—such as farming the fish in special tanks, miles away from any waterway; and making infertile offspring incapable of breeding. Even if they did escape into the wild, they could not reproduce.

---

119 http://foodbabe.com/2013/01/31/birke-reports-why-we-shouldnt-trust-gmo-salmon/

Extinction is a natural process—not a pleasant one if you happen to care enough about your species to worry about it. It's a fact of nature. Our own species is systematically destroying our entire biosphere. We've already driven a number of species to extinction, with many others threatened or teetering on the brink.

Our own species is heading for the same fate. If we don't pull our fingers out soon, this beautiful planet could be devoid of human life in just a few centuries. This is a factor that drives people like Birke Baehr and it's a noble cause. But it's like sticking your finger in a hole in the bottom of the boat while water is pouring in from the sides, and worse, convincing everyone else that your contribution is going to save the day.

On Seafood

In fact, scientists have found that the inflammatory potential of tilapia is far greater than that of a hamburger or bacon. [120]

This little nugget of misinformation derives from the simplistic idea that omega 6 fatty acids are found in large quantities in "dry" fish such as catfish and tilapia. As University of Minnesota researcher on human lipid and lipoprotein metabolism Dr. William Harris is keen to point out, not all fatty acids are created equal. That includes omega 3, 6 polyunsaturated fatty acids (PUFAs) and omega 9 monounsaturated fatty acids (MUFAs).

Omega 3, the family thought most beneficial to heart health, comes in several forms: docosahexaenoic (DHA) and eicosapentaenoic (EPA) are found in temperate, oily sea-fishes such as albacore tuna, mackerel and oysters (not so much in other shellfish though). Most of us only receive about 150mg of these essential fatty acids per day despite experts recommending around 500mg!

If we don't get sufficient omega 3, our bodies use arachidonic acid, a member of the omega 6 group. Harris says that provided we have sufficient omega 3 in our diet, the amount of omega 6 is easily balanced out because our bodies use the omega 3 compounds first. Were you to get enough omega 3 from tilapia, the omega 6 content is irrelevant because your system will just

---

120 The Food Babe Way, p. 172

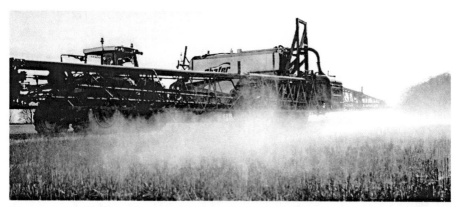

Figure 2.17: A Chafer Sentry applies glyphosate to stubble on a field in England. Herbi-cide application is a vital part of modern agriculture. (Chafer Machinery/flickr.com)

throw it away. As Dr. Harris mentions in his interview with foodinsight. org:

> *"Some people think omega-6 fatty acids should be avoided because they are purported to promote an inflammatory response in the body, which actually is not true. Some metabolites of omega-6's are inflammatory and some are anti-inflammatory."* [121]

So what about salmon? Food Babe has a fair bit of unpleasant news for aficionados of the fishy feast, so beloved of banquets and buffets:

> Farmed salmon are often fed a mixture of highly contaminated fish meal and fish oil mixed with corn and soy products, because it is cheap and helps fatten them up. This practice leads to horrible side effects. It turns the salmon gray, because they are not eating the creatures that make their flesh naturally pink. [122]

Salmon farms use dyes to color the fish's flesh to match customer expecta-tions, but that's where it ends. Wild-caught salmon's flesh color is a product of the carotenoids (the same compounds that make carrots orange) present in their diet of krill and other marine crustaceans. (Eat enough carotenoids and you too can look like a spray tan gone wrong.)

Interestingly, about 5% of Chinook (King) Salmon have a genetic trait that prevents them from absorbing carotenoids, making their flesh white. Over

---

121 http://www.foodinsight.org/newsletters/food-insight-interviews-dr-bill-harris-omega-3-and-omega-6-fatty-acids
122 The Food Babe Way, p. 171

the years this variety has become sought after, and therefore, rather expensive.

Food Babe tells us farmed fish are contaminated with PCBs—polychlorinated biphenyls—a type of industrial waste. A 2004 study [123] in Science revealed the discovery of PCBs in both farmed and wild caught fish, but the toxins were present in much larger quantities (up to eight times as much) in the farmed animals.

So there is some truth in this, but it's a case of exaggeration of evidence (neglecting to mention both forms contain PCBs). The levels discovered, while detectable, were fairly low: 37 parts per billion for farmed fish (0.0000037%) compared with 5 parts per billion for the wild caught. The current limit for safe human consumption is 2000 parts per billion.

PCBs (and potentially other toxins) get into salmon through their diet of processed fish such as herring, which is more economical to feed than growing billions of krill. US-farmed fish stocks are said to be lower in PCBs than those originating from Europe. The European Salmon industry was fairly upset at the results, particularly as there is no demonstrable risk to human health.

We know omega 3 fatty acids are good for us—in particular for cardiovascular health—so it's important to balance the tiny (and disputed) risk from PCBs against the very real risk of a heart attack or stroke. Scientists found that the PCBs tended to bioaccumulate in the fish's skin and outer fatty layers. If you are concerned about consuming even minute amounts of these toxins, those are the areas to avoid. Bear in mind you'll also be missing out on some omega 3s.

Wild caught salmon have lower concentrations of PCBs simply because their primary food source (krill, shrimp and other tiny crustaceans) is closer to the bottom of the food chain, so less is absorbed over time.

So what about "chicken of the sea"—the larger shrimp and prawns aficionados relish on seafood platters?

> Ninety percent of the shrimp we eat is imported. This farmed shrimp is tainted with antibiotics, residues from chemicals used

---

123 http://www.sciencemag.org/content/303/5655/226.short

to clean pens, and filth like mouse hair, rat hair and pieces of insects. Even E. coli has been detected in imported shrimp. [124]

That sounds pretty nasty—just as well she doesn't know what wild shrimp eat! The antibiotics she mentions aren't actually in the seafood. What she means by tainted (those weasel words again), is that *metabolites* of antibiotic can be detected. [125] This is no more being tainted with antibiotics than Subway's bread was tainted by yoga mats because azodicarbonomide was used in the manufacturing process. The real question is this: are these creatures reaching our plates or is Food Babe (who is really just parroting research from other organizations) making a mountain out of a molehill, or no hill at all?

Despite Food Babe's criticism of the FDA, its import restrictions are designed to protect public safety, particularly following some nasty findings dating back to 1979, where unpleasant things were found lurking in imports from Bangladesh, Hong Kong, India, Indonesia, Taiwan, and Thailand.

For this reason, just because a plant producing farmed shrimp in, say, Indonesia sends a batch of shrimp to the USA, there's no guarantee it's ever going to get into the food supply.

The FDA's guidance notes read as follows:

> *"Districts may detain fresh (raw) and fresh frozen shrimp from Bangladesh, Hong Kong, Indonesia, Taiwan, and Thailand, without physical examination for filth, decomposition and Salmonella, except those firms listed in the Green List whose shrimp should not be detained under this guidance. To overcome the appearance of a violation for detained shrimp, any importer/owner may have the shrimp sampled and analyzed by a private laboratory and submit documentation to FDA for review."* [126]

The question here then, is not so much if "filth, adulterants or contaminants" were detected, but when. Detection at the checkpoint is one thing—

---

124 The Food Babe Way, p. 172

125 http://www.fda.gov/Food/FoodScienceResearch/LaboratoryMethods/ ucm239765.htm

126 http://www.accessdata.fda.gov/cms_ia/importalert_35.html

finding these impurities in the store is quite a different story, and the FDA takes its responsibility very seriously.

On Pesticides

> Avoiding neurotoxic, endocrine disrupting, carcinogenic and teratogenic (birth defect) chemicals is of course more protective of people's health, not to mention the health of other species including the microorganisms both human and soil health depend on. [127]

Food Babe is very pro-organic (and that's her choice) but she seems unaware that organic farmers use pesticides too (at least, they do if they want to stay in business). The only difference between an organic pesticide and a traditional one is the organic one must have a "natural" origin:

> One thing that totally baffles me is that the word "conventional" is used to describe produce that is grown with pesticides. There's nothing conventional about using toxic chemicals to grow food. [128]

US organic regulations stipulate that natural substances (except where prohibited) can be used in organic farming. Indeed, some organic pesticides are so nasty they've been widely restricted in the USA. Rotenone is just such a product, but by no means the only one. Conventional farming has to use chemicals to protect crops from pests and disease and those chemicals are toxic (to something) by definition. The idea that organic farmers don't use toxic chemicals is understandable. But ultimately, the joke is on those who literally buy into the hype.

Food Babe hates glyphosate with a vengeance. Perhaps because Monsanto developed it (and sold it as Roundup) or perhaps because its method of action is biological—and plants can be modified (cue Monstanto rants again) to make them immune to the effect.

Glyphosate is not organic. Ironically, one of its biggest opponents is a Ph.D. qualified computer language specialist, Dr. Stephanie Seneff. Dr. Seneff, insofar as horticultural experts are concerned, is nothing more than a layperson with a grudge. Her papers have titles like this:

127 http://foodbabe.com/an-open-letter-to-food-babe/
128 The Food Babe Way, p. 43

"Aluminum and Glyphosate Can Synergistically Induce Pineal Gland Pathology: Connection to Gut Dysbiosis and Neurological Disease," "Glyphosate, pathways to modern diseases II: Celiac sprue and gluten intolerance" and even "Empirical Data Confirm Autism Symptoms Related to Aluminum and Acetaminophen Exposure."

Not one of these three sample papers are in her doctoral area of expertise. For example, the correlation between the rise of autism and the switch from aspirin to Tylenol/paracetamol (acetaminophen) occurred primarily in the USA. Countries that did not make the switch (preferring to stay with aspirin) saw precisely the same rate of increase in autism diagnosis. The best evidence we have to date suggests the condition is primarily (and probably entirely) genetic, resulting from a complex interaction of specific variations across genetic loci.

Another of Seneff's diatribes against glyphosate (the active herbicide in Roundup) relies on similarly specious correlations (read, worthless). We'll cover those in Chapter 2.

> We now know from research that glyphosate found in genetically modified foods is a toxin that can accumulate in your body the more you are exposed to it. It has been linked to kidney disease, breast cancer and some birth defects. It compromises your immunity. And it slows down your metabolism. This is bad, bad, stuff. [129]

There is no credible current research to support this assertion (any of it) when glyphosate is used as a pesticide and at normal exposures through food.

Glyphosate herbicides are known to have an acute toxicity in humans (>85mL orally of the concentrated solution with elderly patients suffering the worst). However, the toxic effect is from the polyoxyethyleneamine surfactant. Surfactants are chemicals that help the product spread itself across the plant's leaves, enabling a smaller amount to be used per acre, reducing costs and human exposure; soap is an everyday surfactant. Indeed, the dose makes the poison. We ingest minute amounts of things like soap,

---

129 The Food Babe Way, p. 43

toothpaste, vodka, and vinegar; but we certainly wouldn't drink them by the glass or the gallon.

On Preservatives

It's fair to say that there may be some element of risk in adding chemicals to our food. However, contrary to the rather ludicrous claim they're there to increase profits, they exist to prevent spoilage. Food-borne pathogens can cause illness and even death.

> TBHQ is one scary chemical. It's created from butane (a very toxic gas) and can only be used at a rate of 0.002 percent of the total oil in a product. [130]

If butane is such a toxic gas, why is it used in throw-away gas lighters, camping stoves, camp lights and movable heaters? It's about the most commonly used portable gas there is. Butane is mildly toxic but most injuries are by deliberate inhalation, causing asphyxiation. TBHQ (tert-butylhydroquinone) isn't all that scary in reality, because we're exposed to minute amounts of it, and only in a very limited number of foods. [131]

> Among the worst of these preservatives are the nitrates, used in meats to prevent bacteria growth and maintain color. Toxic to the brain, nitrates are linked to Alzheimer's disease and many types of cancer. [132]

The most common salting methods involve common table salt (sodium chloride) or a mixture of salt and a nitrate/nitrite mixture as follows:

Prague Powder #1: 6.25% sodium nitrite to 93.75% table salt.

Prague Powder #2: 6.25% sodium nitrite and 4% sodium nitrate & 89.75% salt.

Commercially available Prague powders are slightly pinkish from an added dye as the raw salts are all white crystalline powders.

---

130 The Food Babe Way, p. 23
131 http://www.inchem.org/documents/jecfa/jecmono/v042je26.htm
132 The Food Babe Way, p. 48

Saltpeter (*potassium nitrate*), a component of gunpowder no less, was in common use in the middle ages but has fallen into disuse. It is still found in a specialized branch of French pork cuisine, called charcuterie.

The big shocker here though is if you want to avoid nitrates, you'll have to give up veggies. Most aquarists will tell you that they keep live plants in their tanks because the fish excrete ammonia. That is broken down into nitrites and then nitrates by bacteria in the water. Gardeners similarly use piles of rotted horse and chicken manure for the same reason. This is part of what biologists refer to as the nitrogen cycle.

These forms of dietary nitrites and nitrates aren't dangerous. Our own bodies make them! Doctors have used a variation in the form of glycerol trinitrate (GTN) spray or tablets for the treatment of angina pectoris for many decades. Nutritionists and medics have long recognized the link between the consumption of nitrate rich foods (fresh fruits and vegetables) as essential to good cardiovascular health. [133] But as always, remember one primary tenet of toxicology: the dose makes the poison. Kavin remembers her family doctor advising her not to prepare homemade carrot purees for her infants (or in this case, advising her husband. Kavin can't cook!). Parents should avoid homemade green beans, carrots, squash, beets or spinach, though store bought purees of the same are okay, as they've been tested for safe nitrate levels. [134]

The chemicals responsible for gut cancers and implicated in Alzheimer's disease are *nitrosamines*. They form when nitrites are heated in the presence of amino acids. In everyday language, if you like your bacon extra crispy, you're consuming large amounts of the stuff. Ironically, some of this early fear has translated into greatly lowered amounts of nitrogen-based preservatives in meat, which means lower nitrosamine production during harsh cooking.

Periodically, there are outraged allegations on social media claiming that fast food is brimming with preservatives, such as this one by *Live Well Centers*:

> *"Our fast "food" display is now 2 years old. The word food is question-able, since the bread-like and meat-like substances have not molded or*

133 Lundberg J.O., Carlström M., Larsen F.J., Weitzberg, E. Roles of dietary inorganic nitrate in cardiovascular health and disease. Cardiovascular Research Feb 2011, 89 (3) 525-532; DOI: 10.1093/cvr/cvq325

134 http://www.marchofdimes.org/baby/choosing-baby-food.aspx

spoiled in any way. Bugs won't even bother with it. Please think twice about giving this to your kids. You have a choice, but they don't. We truly are what we eat." [135]

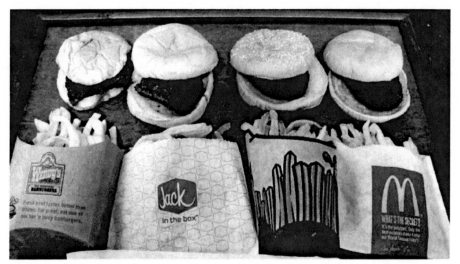

Figure 2.18: This fast food display isn't what is claimed. (Live Well Centres/Facebook)

The picture contains burgers and fries from four different fast-food eateries, including McDonald's and Wendy's, apparently untouched by any living thing.

You put what in your mouth? Yuck!

This experiment is easy to replicate with fresh food or meats in your own kitchen by cooking fried potatoes, freshly ground meat, or freshly baked and toasted bread. Leave the food undisturbed where the air can get to it and amazingly, even months later, you'll see that, like the Live Well Centers' display, it's still "fresh."

To illustrate, the authors did this with bread (Figure 2.19). A slice was cut in two, with one piece (on the right) being left to dry out in free air and the one on the left remaining in a sealed bag to make sure moisture couldn't escape.

---

135 https://www.facebook.com/117036525022242/photos/a.294460993946460.69795.117036525022242/350927234966502/

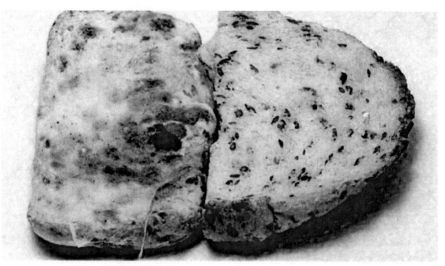

Figure 2.19: A slice of supermarket bread; cut into two. The one on the right, allowed to dry naturally, the one on the left, kept in a bag of moist air. Note that mold "preferred" the store-bought whole grain, seeded bread over the McDonalds. (Brian Jobson/ Brian Jobson Photography)

Ah, but that's not McDonald's bread, so to be as thorough as possible in an admittedly poorly-controlled experiment, we did it with a McDonald's cheeseburger too. (Figures 2.20—2.21)

This viral demonstration proves desiccation works. The bread dries out quite rapidly, the potato fries/chips are protected by the oil absorbed during cooking, and the meat is sealed and dried with any remaining bacteria killed during the cooking process. These products aren't meat-like or bread-like– they're just dried out bread and meat. Nutritionally speaking, they may have questionable value, but to suggest that they're not real food is bordering on ludicrous. It also shows the lengths some interested parties will go to in order to instill unfounded fear and disgust.

The same goes for other products such as eggs and meat, where bacteria may be present at point of sale. Great Britain famously had the 1988 "Egg-wina" incident where junior health minister Edwina Currie slightly misquoted a scientific advisory, saying:

> *"Most of the egg production in this country, sadly, is now affected with salmonella"—Edwina Currie MP, December 1988*

Fresh egg sales plummeted around 60% and four million laying hens were slaughtered as a result. Although the Public Health Laboratory Service, the source of the original report, stood by its findings, Currie's position proved untenable and she was forced to resign.

As The Telegraph reported [136] in 2001, Mrs. Currie wasn't so far off the mark after all. A strain of salmonella, PT4, was sufficiently resistant to heat to survive the light cooking found in soft-boiled and lightly fried eggs, and eggs used in custards and mayonnaise. With the clarity of hindsight, it's highly likely deaths were prevented despite Ms. Currie being forced to fall on her sword.

We've been cooking our food for thousands of years. Although cooking releases flavors and makes some nutrients more bioavailable, this example shows that it can also protect us from live food-borne pathogens.

Consuming raw foods is dangerous if they are not prepared correctly, particularly for young children, pregnant women, the elderly, and the immunocompromised (such as people living with HIV or undergoing certain cancer therapies).

The CDC has identified eight common pathogens responsible for 128,000 hospitalizations and around 3,000 deaths each year. Bacteria live and reproduce very quickly, from a single organism to trillions in just 24 hours. Each generation can replicate in just 20 minutes—that's 72 generations in a day. Assuming ideal conditions, this is how the numbers stack up:

Generation	Hours:Mins	Bacterial Count
1	0:20	1
2	0:40	2
4	1.00	4
…	…	…
71	23:40	2,361,183,241,434,820,000,000
72	24:00	4,722,366,482,869,650,000,000

136 http://www.telegraph.co.uk/news/uknews/1366276/Currie-was-right-on-salmonella.html

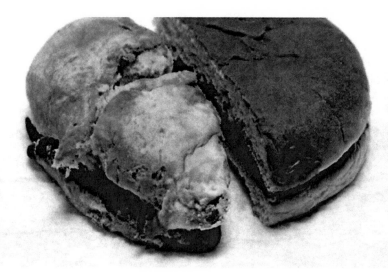

Figure 2.20: Do try this at home—if you can stomach it. Two halves of the same McDonald's cheeseburger. The one on the right remained in open air to dry naturally while the other was kept in a sealed bag to retain moisture. (Brian Jobson/Brian Jobson Photography)

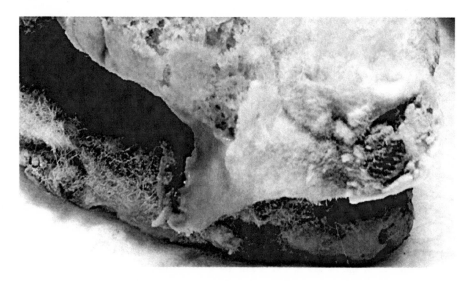

Figure 2.21: Close up: although the McDonald's bun contains a smaller amount of nutrition for the mold, the decay does take place all the same. (Brian Jobson/Brian Jobson Photography)

A Rogue's Gallery of Common Foodborne Pathogens

- *Salmonella*: found in raw milks and raw milk products, on meat and some fruit and vegetables like sprouts and melon. Salmonella is also spread through poor food handling techniques where someone has contaminated their hands with fecal matter and failed to wash before handling food. Such a person may by asymptomatic and unaware they are carrying the bacteria.
- *Listeria monocytogenes* and *E. coli*: found in unpasteurized dairy, ready-to-eat foods, under-cooked meat, poultry and seafood.
- *Norovirus*: in addition to raw milk, this nasty bug can spread on most fresh foods via unwashed hands and from surfaces contaminated with other foods.
- *Clostridium perfringens* (aka. *C. perfringens*) also known as the "buffet bug." Illness is primarily a result of the toxins produced by the bacteria, which can multiply extremely rapidly in the correct environment.
- *Campylobacter*: found in many meat and dairy products but also present in untreated water. This bug can survive freezing temperatures so it's important to cook all food to the correct temperature.
- *Staphylococcus aureus*: a bug most of us carry without suffering any ill health, but that can be a different story if it contaminates our food. Most prepared foods subject to manual handling (salads and cold cuts, for instance) are a prime source of this nasty.
- *Toxoplasma gondii*: a parasitic organism somewhat larger than a bacterium but still extremely dangerous to susceptible individuals. Cat litter trays (cat poop in general) are the major vector for this. Pregnant women are at the greatest risk as toxoplasmosis can cross the placental barrier and infect the unborn child. Ladies with cats, you're off litter duty during pregnancy, though that barely compensates for the aches and pains, right?

All of those bacteria are living, eating, pooping and dying on, or in, your food. Feel queasy yet? Well ladies, you may want to pop a leftover morning sickness pill.

Like us, bacteria have ideal temperatures at which they thrive, although some can survive at extremes. The so-called danger zone for most pathogens –where they begin to reproduce up to the point where they are destroyed– ranges from 40°F/4°C (refrigerator temperatures) up to 160°F/71°C. Even at 160°F, some bacteria will survive for many minutes, and very few are required to re-establish a new colony. Products intended for long-term storage without the addition of chemical preservatives may be heated (under pressure) to temperatures of up to 240°F/115°C. A few of the more common pathogens we would face were it not for preservatives appear on page 94.

> Then there are the preservatives BHA and BHT, both banned all over the globe but still allowed in the United States. [137]

The simple answer to this is: BHA and BHT are *not banned* in the EU, which refers to them as E320 [138] and E321. [139] They may not be in common use, but aren't banned as yet and may never be. E320 (butylated hydroxyanisole) may be banned in the future as it is on the IARC list of possible carcinogens like 4-MeI. That's a selective precaution when you consider that ethanol is a known carcinogen, and even Food Babe doesn't eschew her wine and tequila.

Humans have been preserving food for centuries with various methods depending on the type of food. The oldest are smoking, salting and desiccation (drying) and in some cases, even sweetening. All of these methods were created long before the invention of the refrigerator or freezer, and in many cases allow food to remain edible for many months or longer.

Desiccation (drying), the chemical-free method of preservation, isn't suited to everything but can be applied to foods as diverse as milk, eggs, coffee, potatoes, tomatoes, beans, mushrooms, fish and meats too, with some considered great delicacies. Many fruits such as apples, bananas and grapes

---

137 The Food Babe Way, p. 48
138 http://www.ukfoodguide.net/e320.htm
139 http://www.ukfoodguide.net/e321.htm

are preserved this way. It's claimed, for instance, that freeze dried eggs are edible after a quarter of a century. We'll pass, thanks.

On Heavy Metals

> How would you like a nice big helping of aluminum, lead, mercury or arsenic for dinner? Sounds crazy, I know but you could be filling your body with heavy metals without knowing it. So how do they turn up in our bodies? The answer is through pesticide-sprayed food, farmed fish and food packaging material. [140]

Now that's a pretty scary claim! And, like much of what Food Babe says, it's broadly wrong with a sprinkling of truth– just nowhere near enough to make an informed choice.

Arsenic is used in North America as an adjunct in some feed additives for swine and turkeys. *Nitrosone, Roxarsone, Carbarsone,* and *arsanilic* acid all contain arsenic, although it's reported that after 2013 all but Roxarsone will be phased out. Roxarsone is prohibited in the EU and it seems probable the FDA will follow suit in time.

Despite this being the likely primary vector for arsenic in humans (not necessarily to toxic levels) it's both concerning and telling that Food Babe has never once mentioned it (so far as we are able to tell) in either her blog or book. Rather ironically, it's widely thought that low levels of arsenic might also protect against bladder cancer—yet another example of the dose determining the poison.

Most of the lead we ingest comes from lead compounds floating around in the environment. Lead is a very common metal in the earth and was used for years in primers (lead oxide), as an anti-knocking agent in gasoline, and even as a material for water pipes. Its use has been phased out in most of the industrialized world, where copper and advanced plastics have replaced it.

That said, there's still a lot of it around and since it doesn't biodegrade, it tends to hang around in soil until it gets taken up by a plant. From there it may pass into an animal and ultimately to us. Lead (and mercury) may

---

140 The Food Babe Way, p. 54

bioaccumulate in fatty tissues for years and only become a problem when we lose weight!

Although aluminum toxicity has been suspected for years, the 1988 Camelford incident in which a van accidentally dumped tons of the stuff into the town's drinking water supply [141] really threw it into sharp focus. The dose (which was astronomical in that case) made the poison.

Comparatively little aluminum gets into our systems. Most goes straight through without being absorbed and most of what's left leaves via our urine. The tiny amount remaining can bioaccumulate in our brain, bones, lungs, liver and thyroid but the the scientific consensus is *clear*: this has no detrimental effect on our health.

Fatakdi Powder, used in Indian cuisine as a pickling spice, is pure alum and a major source of aluminum. It has also been used for centuries to seal minor cuts and as an antiseptic. We wrap our food in aluminium foil. Though Food Babe may wear a figurative foil hat, she is very particular about avoiding the stuff. Exclusively wrapping her food in parchment paper. If aluminum really were as toxic as Food Babe claims, we could expect to see endemic levels of these diseases among users and yet we don't. In normal use, aluminum is safe.

Since most free aluminum in blood plasma is evacuated via the kidneys, people with impaired kidney function may feel happier using steel or cast iron cookware and utensils, as highly acidic foods such as tomatoes can cause significant amounts of the metal to leech into the meal. Affected persons may also wish to avoid aluminum foil whenever possible and practical.

Another aluminium source is antacids: *Gaviscon*, *Maalox* and Alka-Seltzer contain aluminum hydroxide to counteract the laxative properties of the magnesium hydroxide. Also, many anti-perspirants contain various aluminum salts (and they're not always obvious).

We should stress, most people are quite able to deal with these levels of environmental aluminum without effort and only people with poor renal

---

141 http://www.dailymail.co.uk/news/article-2608449/Village-damned-Mysterious-suicides-Agonising-illness-And-25-years-UKs-worst-case-mass-poisoning-evidence-dirty-water-KILLED-people.html

(kidney) function [142] such as those on dialysis need to take extra precautions.

Which leaves us with perhaps the most toxic of the bunch, mercury. Like the other metals, mercury bioaccumulates in animal tissue.

Farmed fish are fed very strict diets so the likelihood of them containing appreciable amounts of mercury is low. Wild caught fish, however, are a different story. The bigger the fish, the bigger the mercury exposure.

Mercury (from industrial use of methylmercury) gets into seawater where it is rapidly absorbed by single-celled algae. The algae are eaten by simple crustaceans such as krill and shrimp, which are eaten by larger fish, and some filter feeders such as oysters. In this way the mercury moves up the food chain, bioaccumulating in the tissues of ever larger fish: a process called bioamplification or biomagnification.

From a human perspective (and according to the EPA), smaller fish and seafood such as Atlantic salmon, oysters and pollock are safe to eat every day whereas trout, albacore and bluefin tuna should be restricted to a few times a week. Big fish like shark, king mackerel, and bigeye tuna are restricted to a few times a month at most.

On Detoxing

You probably feel pretty wretched as you crawl out of bed the morning after a fun night on the town and a few too many, or after a delicious but over-indulgent holiday feast. Time for detox?

Well your doctor will tell you: detoxing doesn't work.

Detoxing is a con, pure and simple. It's marketing to sell you all sorts of "healthy" potions at inflated prices. Now, Food Babe will tell you time and again that detoxing works. She's touted everything from parsley to so-called "supergreens" as detoxifying agents.

It's all unsubstantiated misdirection. Your body does all the detoxing for you—it's been doing it from the day you were born (your mother did it

---

142 http://www.ncbi.nlm.nih.gov/pmc/articles/PMC2664589/

while she carried you) and it will keep on detoxifying until you kick the proverbial bucket.

The only thing you can do to help your body detox is to drink enough water to make sure your urine is clear to very pale yellow (dark yellow is a sure sign you're dehydrated). All those phytochemicals and other sciencey sounding stuff you sometimes see touted? If you're already getting a balanced diet, your body has those in abundance anyway.

It's true that these various concoctions make you feel better but that's due to something called the placebo effect. Indeed, many people grudgingly complain that placebos are "just in your mind."

Since "you" exist in your mind, everything you perceive is under that direct control: pain, hunger, pleasure, thirst, excitement—everything. Placebos might not have any active ingredients as such, but they can still be shown to create measurable physiological effects. If you believe something is doing you good (provided it's not actually bad for you) then for minor ailments at least, it very well might be.

This is the best case scenario with "detox" juices. The very ritual of preparing your chosen detox (and the more complicated the better) is sufficient to convince yourself you're about to feel better. Practically speaking though, a glass of tap water will have the same effect of flushing the toxins out of your body. It works just as quickly and in some cases, even faster than these potions because it's the water that does the work. Everything else is just window dressing.

This is why we can't survive for long without water—it's the universal solvent. As your liver breaks down the toxic chemicals your body produces, it dumps them back into your bloodstream, where they are filtered out through your kidneys and into your urine. (This is what doctors mean when they refer to the renal pathway.)

Some "detoxifying" potions contain mild diuretics (things that make you pee more) but they are actually acting against your body's systems, making the kidneys work harder by producing larger volumes of urine. Because your liver can only break down toxic chemicals so fast, these drinks force you to drink more or risk dehydration, which will actually make you feel worse.

> Most people think dandelion is just a weed that grows beautiful
> yellow and white flowers but they actually are one of the most
> healing greens you can buy. [143]

This particular piece of Food Babe nonsense is made worse because dandelion contains a substance called caffeic acid. What's the big deal? Why, it's a group 2B carcinogen!

Another 2B carcinogen is 4-MeI, the compound over which Food Babe bullied Starbucks—eventually creating a viral meme that accused the company of using cancer-causing substances in its Pumpkin Spice Latte .

Remember: even though probable carcinogens have the ability to cause cancer, we can't assume they will. One of the most potent carcinogens in daily life is alcohol and yet, few people think twice about imbibing large amounts in quantities orders of magnitude larger than the trivial amount of 4-MeI in a cup of coffee.

Food Babe created such terror over this substance, the Office of Environmental Health Hazard Assessment (California's Proposition 65) makes the following note [144] about 4-MeI.

> *"Because of the significant public interest in this chemical, a Notice
> of Proposed Rulemaking identifying a proposed No Significant Risk
> Level (NSRL) is being published concurrently with this listing notice."*

So you either believe that 4-MeI does give you cancer (and therefore so does Food Babe's dandelion detox):

– OR –

You accept the science and enjoy your dandelion juice, your Starbucks Pumpkin Spice Latte, and your chardonnay. Bottoms up!

On Cooking Oils

> What they don't tell you in this video is that the "solvent" that is
> most often used to extract the oil is the neurotoxin hexane—and
> as you can see it's literally bathed in it. ...it surely isn't healthy. [145]

---

143 http://foodbabe.com/2012/03/17/super-detox-juice/
144 http://oehha.ca.gov/prop65/prop65_list/010711list.html
145 http://foodbabe.com/2015/02/04/cooking-oils/

Want to avoid n-Hexane? You're going to have to wear a breathing apparatus—particularly when you fill your car.

Calling it a neurotoxin is willful ignorance of the science! Scientists measured levels in Chicago [146] at two parts per billion (2ppb). You're exposed to it every time you visit the gas station. Inhalation of n-Hexane is far more toxic than ingestion, and the "detectable" amount in cooking oil is testament to the sensitivity of modern instruments.

In the 1970s some Japanese workers suffered neurological symptoms by inhaling n-Hexane at 500-2,500ppm (that's over a million times more concentrated) for up to 14 hours a day over periods from six months to many years. Every one of them subsequently recovered.

Something smells, but it's not n-Hexane!

> Before it [Canola Oil] was bred this way, it was called Rapeseed Oil and used for industrial purposes because the erucic acid in it caused heart damage in animal studies. [147]

Erucic acid is one of the large number of "fatty acids" found in nature. Food Babe's quote appears to derive information from schoolboy Birke Baehr's misreading of the available data, from which he concludes:

> Rapeseed oil is toxic because it contains significant amounts of a poisonous substance called erucic acid. [148]

Birke goes looking for the scary and hype-worthy while ignoring everything else (*confirmation bias*). In establishing a safe limit for erucic acid, scientists in New Zealand found:

> *"A tolerable level of human exposure has been established on the basis of the animal studies. There is a 120-fold safety margin between this level and the level that is associated with increased myocardial lipidosis in nursling pigs."* [149]

They go on to say that the rat is not a suitable candidate for establishing toxicity of erucic acid—in particular because the digestion of fatty acids

---

146 http://www.atsdr.cdc.gov/toxprofiles/tp113.pdf
147 http://foodbabe.com/2015/02/04/cooking-oils/
148 http://foodbabe.com/2012/12/28/birke-reports-dont-let-organic-cooking-oils-fool-you
149 http://www.foodstandards.gov.au/publications/documents/Erucic%20acid%20monograph.pdf

differs between primates (and us) and rats—invalidating the original toxicological data.

It's in the reports. They just don't read them thoroughly or interpret them correctly.

On Writing

> Next time maybe you should get an interview or practice some journalism. [150]

Remember at the start of this chapter, we pointed out that we have asked for an interview, multiple times, but have been repeatedly ignored. This snappy little tweet was in response to discussion surrounding a blog reply written by someone using the name Nicky Castillo, in reply to an open letter to the Food Babe from a group of food science students:

"I applaud the authors' efforts here. Yet as a former Food Babe staff member, I can guarantee that she won't respond or engage. I often wonder if people think she believes all of her cockamamie information. Answer: she does not. She's not an idiot, she's just a liar. She sells these lies to pay the bills and the only manner in which to maintain this web of lies is to protect her airtight bubble of ignorance by never engaging experts. She has been so successful with her lies that her husband even quit his banking job to run the site full time. The point is, it's all just a facade for a business. In fact, we used to debate with her about how ridiculous some of her claims were, but she would respond in a flippant manner and state that her crazy advice will bring more eyeballs to the site and more money. In the end, I resigned as I was disgusted by the entire business. So that being said, and back to my original point, you're not going to receive a response."

Which seems on the face of things to be a pretty damning indictment (not to mention, remarkably brave). Only the next day, greeted by a flurry of interest from the blogging and science community, Castillo drops a bombshell:

---

150 https://twitter.com/thefoodbabe/status/559748839607762944 (tweet deteled)

"I wish I could share more, but I've already been contacted by attorneys."

But, as was confirmed just a day later, the post was simply an elaborate "Poe" (a satirical comment or remark that is indistinguishable from the real thing) as Castillo owned up.

"Alright. I didn't expect what I had intended to be a satirical comment to get so many responses as the goal was to elicit a response from Food Babe, not others. Of course, I am not using my real name so how could I have been contacted by attorneys so quickly? I thought that comment would make it clear that I was writing in jest and would not be taken seriously. In any case, I never worked for Food Babe. Again, I just wanted to push her to engage. I'm glad so many people are interested in dialog with Food Babe such that she can embrace science. My actions indicate just how frustrated I am as well about this topic. My apologies for misleading anyone."

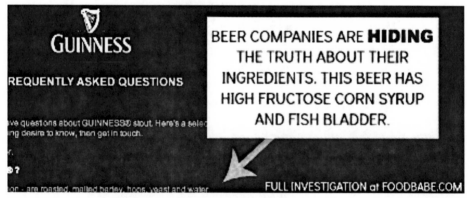

Figure 2.22: There's *what* in my beer! (Food Babe LLC)

What make this Poe so effective was that it spoke to what many in the science community felt was really going on. It's a form of confirmation bias: our natural tendency to believe things that agree with our current thinking.

One thing we know for sure is that Food Babe refuses to grant interviews to anyone she suspects of being on the other side of the argument. A number of writers and journalists have contacted her and been ignored.

The suggestion from this angry tweet that we all "practice some journalism" is completely at odds with her own form of journalism, which is limited entirely to her largely baseless views and actively silencing dissenters. Although Castillo has probably never even met her in person, his/her observations ring true.

Stoking fear like this serves a purpose—frightened people spend money. And, of course, Food Babe has the products and services to calm those fears– often sold through affiliate programs but now branching out into book sales. All the while she creates a fog of confusion around the real problems big food poses. As food scientist John Coupland told NPR reporter Maria Godoy for *The Salt*, these distractions are diverting attention from issues such as food-waste, hunger, and childhood obesity through poorly regulated advertising.

> Dear Future Science Students In Training[151]

This is the patronizing opening line of Food Babe's response to the open letter from Matt Teegarden, John Frelka, Diane Schmitt, Stephanie Diamond, Jacob Farr and Diana Maricruz Pérez-Santos (on which "Nicky Castillo" commented). The difference between the letter's authors and Food Babe is that they already know way more about food science than she has managed to glean since she began her research in 2009.

Professor Folta brilliantly analyzed the reply; the full text is available online, [152] but, for easy reference, we've expanded a few points:

> First, synthetic ingredients in our food should be proven safe before they are put into our bodies. [153]

How do you prove something is safe? That's like trying to prove the existence of the invisible, fire-breathing dragon under your kid's bed. You can prove something is dangerous , in much the same way that you can prove that fire is hot, but proving something unequivocally safe is an impossible target.

---

151 http://foodbabe.com/an-open-letter-to-food-babe/
152 http://www.geneticliteracyproject.org/2015/01/28/kevin-folta-deconstructs-food-babes-response-to-students-in-scathing-fashion/
153 http://foodbabe.com/an-open-letter-to-food-babe/

Is organic food "safe?"

We can't just assume natural ingredients (including colorings) are safe either. The entirely natural color carmine/cochineal has been shown to cause severe allergic reactions in susceptible people.

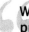 When there is significant evidence, short of certainty, we should protect the public from unnecessary risk. [154]

What evidence? Aspartame, MSG, gluten, 4-MeI... all have been tested to destruction by real scientists working in their own field. The best and most widely respected studies have never demonstrated one iota of risk when these additives are consumed at everyday levels. Even at much higher intakes, there remains no solid evidence of toxicity. And remember, this comes from a writer who openly and strongly promotes the use of unpasteurized milk as key to a healthy lifestyle.

But this last quote is perhaps the most telling of all, considering Food Babe has a policy of ignoring or brushing aside any actual science that disagrees with her own Google University findings.

As is traditional in print journalism, I am going to start a Corrections/Editor's Note feature on my web site. I want to be sure that if there are any mistakes, we admit and correct them immediately. [155]

Some articles have received minor corrections but the main thrust of the mantra is repeated at every step, sometimes diluted with weasel phrases such as "*I believe to be...*" which leaves the ball firmly in the reader's court. This is a clever and dangerous tactic because Food Babe has already established a brand of trust based on a foundation of fear, half-truths and misunderstanding. Also, while traditional print journals are discarded over time, the Internet never forgets.

One example of what might loosely be called a correction can be found in her discussion of beer and the use of high-fructose corn syrup and GMO ingredients in beers.

---

154 http://foodbabe.com/an-open-letter-to-food-babe/
155 http://foodbabe.com/category/most-controversial/

Food Babe posted a so-called "correction" explaining that the company "reached out" to her and explained that they didn't use HFCS. Nevertheless she has continued to prattle on about isinglass (which is *produced* from swim bladders). Despite this, the scary image remains (Feb 2015).

To get this into context, water is produced by an explosive, exothermic reaction between hydrogen and oxygen; but we can all agree that water is neither hydrogen nor oxygen any more.

It's just water.

On Her Critics

> Instead of focusing on the issues at hand I've raised about the food industry, their go-to criticisms are ad hominem personal attacks: they've attacked me, as a woman, in ways they'd never attack my male colleagues. I am personally being subjected to hate speech, harassment and cyber-bullying on a daily basis. [156]

The worst part of this statement is that it's probably partly true. But playing the sexism card is a crafty move because, while there are some vicious childish trolls out in the largely lawless land of the Internet, they are heavily outnumbered by people who have a legitimate bone to pick with Food Babe. Not that she cares, apparently; if you're not part of her solution then you're automatically part of the problem.

Even scientists? Especially scientists!

We should not forget this is a lady who was, at one time, "a nationally-ranked debater." [157] who "placed at Harvard's prestigious debate tournament."[158] Yet rather than engage with critics, most of whom have nowhere near her competitive debating experience, she seeks to silence them at every junction.

> Apparently, science that people don't like-that conflicts with their paid positions or sources of funding—can just be written off as pseudo-science (or an ad hominem attack). Given where we are today, where 1 in 3 women will get cancer, and 1 in 2 men will, I think we need to look for answers on how to live healthier lives

---

156 http://foodbabe.com/2014/12/06/food-babe-critics
157 The Food Babe Way, p. 9
158 The Food Babe Way, p. 9

and break free from the downward spiral of disease our country is facing. True health starts with the quality of our food supply. [159]

Oh the irony! At very best, Food Babe is an engineer who lays the blame for the world's ills firmly where it will play to her monetary advantage. She funds a lavish lifestyle by cherry-picking pseudo-science and refuted papers that agree with her position. This is surely the height of hypocrisy.

> I've never claimed to be a scientist or nutritionist, but a high percentage of the "expert" scientists, doctors, registered dieticians and nutritionists in this field have a financial relationship with the entities I investigate. [160]

While it's true that good food is key to living a long and healthy life, it's only part of an almost infinitely larger puzzle. Food Babe derides science that doesn't agree with her non-GMO, organic agenda.

Moreover, she unwittingly falls into the trap of researcher bias that plagues even the best of scientists. This is a form of research one might also call "cherry-picking," where we (sometimes unconsciously) select the research that agrees with the point we're making.

This isn't pseudo-science, it's **bad** science. But in order to deflect this criticism, she claims to cite experts:

> On a regular basis, I seek the counsel of many credentialed (sic) experts in this field and present my data which often includes access to published, peer-reviewed research. [161]

Unfortunately, there's more to consulting an expert than sticking a metaphorical pin in a Google search. Published, peer-reviewed literature is no longer the gold standard it once was. *Dr Stephanie Seneff, Ph.D* is an expert—in artificial intelligence. That hasn't stopped her from publishing several seemingly scientific diatribes about the "connection" between glyphosate (aka Roundup) and the rise in a whole host of diseases. Scientists are not infallible nor are they always free from bias. The key is differentiating between the weight of empirical, reproducible scientific consensus, and

---

159 http://foodbabe.com/2014/12/06/food-babe-critics
160 http://foodbabe.com/2014/12/06/food-babe-critics
161 http://foodbabe.com/2014/12/06/food-babe-critics

one-off studies with outlier results. Food Babe tends to cherry-pick these one-off studies to support her advice, though the advice flies in the face of the majority of scientific research.

> There was controversy surrounding a talk I gave at a University recently when a professor—who publicly supports and argues for Monsanto and other biotech companies by writing for their industry funded websites—claimed that I refused to answer questions following my talk. Yeah, okay. [162]

That would be Kevin Folta (again) who writes of the visit:

> *"There's something that dies inside when you are a faculty member that works hard to teach about food, farming and science, and your own university brings in a crackpot to unravel all of the information you have brought to students."* [163]

… and more recently observed:

> *"This Facebook post frames the problem we face as educators. So much of the public is clueless, paranoid, and knows nothing about basic biology. This is why folks like US-RTK [US Right to Know] must silence and intimidate scientists. If anyone learns, they lose their power to influence them."* [164]

Food Babe is one of the progenitors of this sort of paranoia. When she started, her heart was probably in the right place, but money, fame and ignorance have misplaced her intentions. She's not interested in revising her opinion—and why should she be? It's brought her wealth, fame, and even cult-like worship.

> What they say: I ban anyone that disagrees with me on social media.
>
> The truth: I give my moderators full authority to delete comments and ban insulting, harassing, or cyberbullying commenters. [165]

---

162 http://foodbabe.com/2014/12/06/food-babe-critics

163 http://kfolta.blogspot.co.uk/2014/10/food-babe-visits-my-university.html

164 http://kfolta.blogspot.co.uk/2015/02/this-is-what-we-are-up-against.html

165 http://foodbabe.com/2014/12/06/food-babe-critics

No one wants to read offensive, misogynistic or threatening comments on blog posts. A moderator's job is to seek out and remove these before they cause harm or offense. If it stopped there, books like this and blogs discussing Food Babe's antics would have probably never reached critical mass.

Yet, the tipping point has already come, and her glass house has already fallen and shattered. This is purely testament to the way that almost all comments left standing on her social media pages by moderators are sycophantic and adoring. Anyone challenging the status quo is almost immediately banned and there is evidence some people have been banned in advance, without ever having left any comment on any thread or post.

This is impossible to prove conclusively without access to records from Facebook and Twitter, but thousands of people have related this experience. Many more have started to see it as a badge of honor—seeing just how far they can push the envelope of truth (that is, post scientifically validated fact) before they find the door slammed and locked.

> What they say: I'm not an expert because I am not a scientist or doctor or nutritionist.
>
> Truth: There is an old saying, "these issues are too important to leave up to the experts." [166]

We're not aware of that saying– old or otherwise. Food Babe doesn't cite where these words come from. While it's true that important issues need not necessarily be complex in nature, they invariably are, and science in all its myriad forms tends to be complex.

> What They Say: Our findings are based on pseudoscience or we hate science and we are "fear mongering."
>
> Truth: If our findings didn't have any concerns, do not have a solid basis in fact, why are companies willing to drop these controversial chemicals? [167]

To answer this question with a (rhetorical) question:

---

166 http://foodbabe.com/2014/12/06/food-babe-critics
167 http://foodbabe.com/2014/12/06/food-babe-critics

"Why do you think the weedy kid would give up his lunch money when the bully towering over him threatened to break his nose?"

Every day the bully comes back demanding more—and Food Babe likewise encourages her army of followers to keep the pressure up until something gives.

> Continue to ask Starbucks to drop caramel coloring level IV immediately (I hear the detractors on Facebook (sic) pages are getting paid 60 cents per post by BIG FOOD or BIG AG PR firms to talk back to the #FoodBabeArmy! Their bullying won't keep us from seeking the truth and demanding safer ingredients!) [168]

Food Babe's "army" has been a massive thorn in the side of these companies. Even when other activists or just normal product development may be the reason for removing specific additives, Food Babe is quick to claim the credit.

To see how this works in practice, imagine being in a theatre where a single patron throws a tomato at the stage. That person will be removed and the show can carry on as if nothing had happened. Now imagine 50 people all stood up and started throwing vegetables at the stage. That small group would easily bring the show to a grinding halt; at least until they were dealt with. But that takes time and resources, while the rest of the audience is inconvenienced.

Much the same remains common on the Internet where single "hackers" command huge armies of zombie PCs to attack sites they want to take down using something called a DDOS (distributed denial of service) attack. Such attacks employ a simple technique where each zombie node calls the target server at the same time. Just like a telephone exchange, a server can only handle a finite number of simultaneous requests and eventually it will break down under the stress, making it unavailable to legitimate callers.

In the 7th Century BCE, Marc's namesake, the Athenian lawmaker Draco, was killed by a crowd in the Aeginetan theatre. It was customary at the time to show affection by gifting clothes. So much clothing was piled upon the unfortunate lawyer he was suffocated to death—literally killed by kind-

---

168 https://www.facebook.com/thefoodbabe/photos/a.208386335862752.56063.132535093447877/829564730411573/

ness. An alternative (and more likely) interpretation is that the people of Aegina simply wanted him dead. It's entirely possible this act of selfless love was planned in advance and perpetrated by his enemies, who would reasonably claim "He tripped, officer."

Food additives only become controversial if someone in authority says they are harmful. But that authority need not be an expert, it just has to be someone who can leverage enough people to create a panic—perhaps a celebrity or a blogger with a large following. If enough people are convinced, a small mass of true believers is created and the genie is out of the bottle.

Food Babe need not be the one to identify the additive in question. In fact, we have been unable find a single instance where she has done the research herself. But such is the size of the Food Babe Army that at the single press of a button, she can command her followers to overload the switchboards and PR offices of large companies until they buckle under the pressure. Worst of all, with every success they claim, they become ever more powerful. They stand girded by their successes, undaunted by their failures.

Fortunately, the tide has turned for the Food Babe Army. In the wake of Yvette d'Entremont's viral take-down, [169] Food Babe still has a large following, but has been largely discredited in the eyes of mainstream media. We hope that companies will take Food Babe's fallen credibility into account, and will choose not to give in to her army's pressure any longer.

> In order to create social change, all you need is passion. To think you need a degree in food science or whatever else in order to share your personal journey to inspire people to eat real food or encourage companies to do the right thing is small minded. [170]

Sharing a personal journey is one thing –misrepresentation of harmless chemicals and using celebrity to harangue companies into submission is quite another. Food Babe's lack of relevant qualifications– and convenient interpretation of the science she does occasionally cite– are precisely demonstrative of why one needs either advanced degrees in these subjects, or access to experts and a grasp of the scientific method to maintain credibility. Case in point:

---

169 http://gawker.com/the-food-babe-blogger-is-full-of-shit-1694902226
170 http://foodbabe.com/2014/12/06/food-babe-critics/

> What They Say: The dose makes the poison and food additives are safe.
>
> The Truth: That food industry orthodoxy is outdated and dangerous. [171]

Some forms of caramelization, for instance, naturally produce minute amounts of presumed carcinogens such as 4-MeI and furan. The amounts are so small they pose no practical risk against a background of uncertainty, such as diesel fumes and strong alcoholic drinks. Food scientists know this, as do those who grasp the meaning of empirical evidence.

Suggesting otherwise isn't just dangerous; it's arrogant and irresponsible.

On Chlorophyll

> Wheatgrass, however, is one of the best source of living chlorophyll available. In the 1970s, Ann Wigmore popularized the use of fresh-squeezed wheatgrass juice to treat cancer patients who had been written off an "incurable" after conventional cancer treatment. In a miraculous turn of events, Wigmore saved her own gangrenous legs from amputation with her own wheatgrass treatments and eventually competed in the Boston Marathon. [172]

The problem with this statement is that it's entirely anecdotal and without corroboration. Internet searches, perhaps predictably, suggest this story relies considerably upon interpretation. Occasionally referred to as "Dr.," her claimed doctorate was not in medicine and may have even been awarded honorifically—that is, without doing any actual academic studies.

This is confirmed by a 1988 article in the *Boston Globe* which states that Wigmore was permitted to claim a treatment for HIV/AIDS (under the 1st Amendment) by Judge Robert A. Mulligan. Judge Mulligan ruled that, under the law, Wigmore was not permitted to represent herself as a doctor even though she could claim miraculous treatments without evidence of their efficacy.

---

171 http://foodbabe.com/2014/12/06/food-babe-critics/
172 The Food Babe Way, p. 88

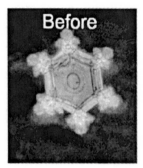

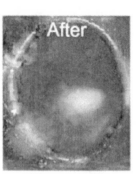

Microwave oven

Harmful Effects of Electromatic Waves As Illustrated by Dr. Masaru Emoto in book "The Hidden Messages in Water"

The distilled water heated in the microwave resulted in a crystal similar to that created by the word "Satan "

More Info at FoodBabe.com

Last by not least, Dr. Masaru Emoto, who is famous for taking pictures of various types of waters and the crystals that they formed in the book called "Hidden Messages in Water," found water that was microwaved did not form beautiful crystals—but instead formed crystals similar to those formed when exposed to negative thoughts or beliefs. If this is happening to just water—I can only imagine what a microwave is doing to the nutrients, energy of our food and to our bodies when we consume microwaved food. For the experiment pictured above, microwaved water produced a similar physical structure to when the words "satan" and "hitler" were repeatedly exposed to the water. This fact is probably too hokey for most people—but I wanted to include it because sometimes the things we can't see with the naked eye or even fully comprehend could be the most powerful way to unlock spontaneous healing.

Figure: Emoto's book, **The Hidden Messages of Water,** *was a bestseller, like* **The Food Babe Way.** *Critic* **Dwight Garner,** *writing in the* **New York Times Book Review,** *described it as a head scratcher that had him questioning the very sanity of the reading public.* [1]

---

1   https://en.wikipedia.org/wiki/Masaru_Emoto

Dr. William T. Jarvis (Ph.D.) writing for *The National Council Against Health Fraud* [173] sums up the chlorophyll hypothesis:

> *"The fact that grass-eating animals are not spared from cancer, despite their large intake of fresh chlorophyll, seems to have been lost on Wigmore."* [174]

Claims for a miraculous recovery from her post-trauma gangrene are similarly dubious. As laymen, we often think of gangrene as being fatal or at least, life changing. The implication laid out here by Food Babe is that the gangrene had travelled into Wigmore's legs although the evidence seems to suggest that only her feet were affected. It's not clear, as of this writing, the extent of the damage although we might assume it was the dry form—the least dangerous.

Gangrene is a result of loss of blood flow to an affected limb (typically in the extremities) and does not always require amputation if the blood flow can be restored (revascularization) before permanent damage occurs—leading to surgical intervention or autoamputation. (Autoamputation is a process where an affected digit—such as a finger or toe—dies and falls off.)

When most of us think of gangrene, it's the wet or gaseous variety which are both far more serious. In any event, had Wigmore suffered severe ischemia to her entire legs, it's unlikely she would have been able to walk again had she even survived.

On Microwaves

One of Food Babe's more catastrophically obvious mistakes was her "research" into microwaves. This post (originally dated July 30, 2012) has long since been deleted and systematically removed from the normal archives, but can be found on the web if you know where to look. [175]

> Microwaves create carcinogenic compounds in your food

---

173 http://www.ncahf.org/

174 http://www.ncahf.org/articles/s-z/wheatgrass.html

175 https://skeptic78240.wordpress.com/2014/11/11/food-babe/

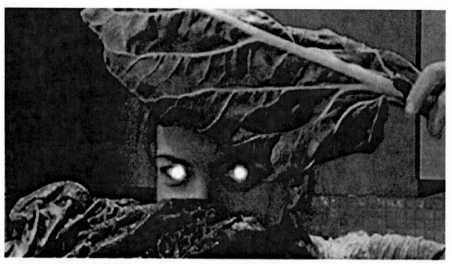

Figure 2.24: Jeepers, creepers, where d' you get those peepers? Vani Hari plays with Rainbow Chard in the kitchen. Image modified for comedic effect. (Original: Food Babe LLC.)

While it's true that cooking can (and does) create tiny amounts of potentially carcinogenic chemicals, this is a function of heat, not of the means by which the heat is imparted. It has absolutely nothing to do with the microwave radiation which is, rather ironically, quite weak as radiation goes.

Amazingly (or not) Food Babe is still regurgitating this utter baloney in her (first) book—word for word! She is correct to advise that foods should be removed from their packaging and cooked on conventional dishes. Beyond this, her claim simply isn't supported by evidence.

> Microwaves destroy the nutrient value of your food.

No more than any other form of cooking. In fact, scientists have discovered that although raw food contains more nutrients, the act of cooking makes some nutrients more bioavailable. It's difficult to get sufficient nutrition from raw food, and humans and their ancestors have been cooking for at least 250,000 years (probably a lot longer). This same argument also appears in her first book—it was wrong then and it's just as wrong now.

> Microwaves were never thoroughly researched before adoption in the United States.

Percy Spencer discovered the microwave cooking technique shortly after World War II; he developed the idea from early radar. Early commercial microwave ovens were produced before 1950 and the first kitchen top units didn't appear until around 1967. Food Babe's claim about WW2 personnel:

> ... studies produced indicated that several of the German soldiers developed cancers of the blood and that microwaves voided nutritional content of the food.

... should really speak for itself, given that the war was already over.

> Microwaves provide unnecessary daily exposure to radiation

A working microwave oven is protected by a Faraday cage. There's no way that radiation should leak out unless the cage is damaged– at least, not microwave radiation. Radiation is everywhere—from the light we see to the heat that keeps us warm—even TV signals. The radiation we need to worry about is a whole different animal. The most common form, one that really does cause cancer, is something many of us perceive as healthy: ultra-violet from the sun and tanning beds.

> Microwaves can create severe health issues

The only way a microwave oven can cause harm is if the numerous safety features are deliberately disabled, or you are sufficiently small and limber enough to get inside while simultaneously operating the complex controls. Let's be realistic, it's not going to happen.

The idea that some magic happens inside the oven that turns food against us is patently ludicrous, as millions of people prove every day.

> Microwaves have been associated with the increase in obesity

This little gem appears to stem from author Michael Pollan's book, *Cooked*, which Food Babe quotes:

> *"The microwave oven, which stands at the precise opposite end of the culinary (and imaginative) spectrum from the cook fire, exerts a kind of anti-gravity, its flameless, smokeless, anti-sensory, cold heat giving*

us a mild case of the willies. The microwave is as antisocial as the cook fire is communal."

This suggests that Mr. Pollan, apparently a first-order Luddite, would be happier if we all returned to Palaeolithic times. There is some sense in this argument, but in reality we can enjoy much the same familial bonding by sitting down at a table to enjoy the meal that one or more of us has prepared.

Food Babe develops her argument like this: since microwaves have made it easy to cook processed food, we eat more junk and end up fat. This is really a non-sequitur. The reality is far more complex and nuanced.

Obesity is more clearly associated with access to unhealthy food and sedentary lifestyle than it ever has been with microwaves. Far fewer children than ever before engage in imaginative and physical activities due in part to cheaper television, video games, and other modern lifestyle factors.

(This page was intentionally microwaved in pressurized oxygen and stored in a disentangled quantum state until you opened it.)

On Night Vision

> Rainbow Chard is one of my favorite plants to juice! The leaves are huge! My favorite benefit of eating this member of the beet family—is NIGHT VISION. Yes—everyone can get rid of their night vision goggles if they just add rainbow chard to their diet. [176]

There are so many reasons why this is wrong that it's hard to know where to start. The error stems from the fact that people in countries where vitamin A resources are sparse tend to suffer from night blindness. Across the developed world, we all get more than enough vitamin A complex from our diets. This comes primarily from meat and fortified products. Fat-soluble vitamins (A, D, E and K) are found in foods rich in fats, such as full-fat milk. Only strict vegans need to worry about this limitation.

A side effect of this discovery strongly suggests that not only is Vani completely mistaken about the effect of vitamin A (our bodies take what they

---

176 http://foodbabe.com/2011/10/22/rainbow-bite-juice/

need and no more) but that even vegetables rich in vitamin A are relatively poor sources of it. You'd be better off eating a steak.

Food scientists have known this for a long time, and someone should tell the Food Babe. This sort of overconfidence in her abilities (Dunning-Kruger syndrome) is what leads the Babe into making either idiotic or disingenuous pronouncements such as this:

> I'm grateful for the advances made by generations of tireless independent scientists, doctors, and nutritionists. Without their work, we would not be able to have conversations like the ones we are having here about what goes in our food and why. But just because you have a degree, doesn't make you right. [177]

While it's true that having a degree doesn't make you right—scientists like Stephanie Seneff have proven that beyond doubt—it does make you much more likely to be right when you're in your own field. If you're a writer without a degree in the field in which you opine? That's fine; indeed not all science writers have science degrees. These non-expert writers do best disseminating expertise, consulting with scientists, and communicating the clout of scientific consensus. Science isn't rigid or black and white, it's constantly being refined. That's why it's better than the firmly rooted dogma that Food Babe and those like her are so happy to repeat

On Air Travel

> When your body is in the air, at a seriously high altitude, your body under goes some serious pressure. Just think about it—Airplanes thrive in places we don't. You are traveling in a pressurized cabin, and when your body is pressurized, it gets really compressed!

Poor Food Babe, this blog of hers is now infamous. She's since realized you can't pull such drivel and get away without ridicule, and did her best to scrub it out of existance. Alas, the Internet is forever. Her adversaries saved this misinformation trove for posterity using a web archiving service.

Food Babe's first mistake is to assume that the cabin air is pressurized beyond one atmosphere. This is the pressure we experience at the beach,

---

177 http://foodbabe.com/2014/12/06/food-babe-critics/

and pretty much what we feel most of the time unless we're at very high altitude, where the air pressure drops. The cabin of a modern airliner is pressurized for passengers' comfort. We feel pressure as a discomfort in our ears when we experience a sudden change (you hear a pop when they do—that's your eardrum snapping back into position). Some airlines give you candy to suck on, as the action of swallowing aids the pressure correction. A pilot confirms this:

> "I fly the Airbus A330. 8000 ft is correct (straight from the Airbus Flight Crew Operating Manual). Cabin pressure is maintained after takeoff in accordance with a preprogrammed pressure schedule which is obviously somewhat less than the rate of climb of the aircraft, until it reaches cruise altitude. At maximum cruise altitude the cabin pressure in an A330 cannot exceed 8000ft [equivalent altitude] and this is a typical figure (plus or minus a bit) for most big jets. This equates to a pressure differential of around 8 psi. If the differential goes above 8.85 psi, safety valves open to dump excess cabin pressure." [178]

By way of saving the best for last, perhaps the most hilarious quote from Food Babe's blog is this one:

> The air you are breathing on an airplane is recycled from directly outside of your window. That means you are breathing everything that the airplanes gives off and is flying through. The air that is pumped in isn't pure oxygen either, it's mixed with nitrogen, sometimes almost at 50%. To pump a greater amount of oxygen in costs money in terms of fuel and the airlines know this! The nitrogen may affect the times and dosages of medications, make you feel bloated and cause your ankles and joints swell.

Most people should know that the air we breathe is mostly nitrogen anyway—around 78% in fact. Oxygen makes up around 20% and the rest is just trace gases such as argon and carbon dioxide. Even if you didn't—what sort of sense does this statement really make? Simply grabbing fresh air from outside the plane is far more efficient than having to carry lbs of extra weight of nitrogen in weighty, pressure-safe containers!

---

178 https://skeptic78240.wordpress.com/2014/11/11/food-babe/

> Compression leads to all sorts of issues. First off your body's digestive organs start to shrink, taxing your ability to digest large quantities of food. Secondly, this compression reduces the ability for your body to normally circulate blood through your blood vessels. Sitting down for long hours while this is happening, exacerbates these issues, leading to what they call "Economy Class Syndrome." Economy Class Syndrome results the action of sitting in a cramped space for a long period of time, thus resulting in blood flow loss to the legs. A unhealthy person or someone who eats a poor diet, smokes, has heart disease, diabetes or an auto-immune disorder has a larger risk of developing DVT, which basically causes a blood clot in your one of your large veins in your leg and you risk death. [179]

Economy Class Syndrome is a real thing but it has nothing to do with the cabin pressure. DVT (a deep vein thrombosis)—is a classic symptom of sitting in one place for too long and can happen to anyone. The thrombus (clot) itself is not always evident until it dislodges, moves through the bloodstream and lodges elsewhere causing a complete blockage. One of the the more poignant examples in recent history relates to 20-year old Chris Stainforth, who died after developing the condition during a 12 hour stint on his XBox. [180] Sitting for long periods puts us all at increased risk of this condition, which is another reason why everyone needs to be aware of this silent killer.

> Additionally, the pressurized cabin reduces the humidity by 40% of what humans typically thrive at. The Sahara Desert has more humidity at ~25% than your airplane does at ~10%. Remember your body is made up of 50% water, if the humidity is reduced by 40%, your body becomes very dehydrated, very quickly and usually without you feeling the effects until after you get off the plane. Dehydration causes all sorts of issues from fatigue, headaches, constipation, light headedness and even death in extreme cases.

Humidity can be measured in two ways: absolute—the actual amount of water present in the atmosphere; and relative—the amount of water vapor the air could hold vs. the amount it's actually holding right here and now. Food Babe and weather reports use the relative measurement because that's

---

179 https://skeptic78240.wordpress.com/2014/11/11/food-babe/
180 http://www.dailymail.co.uk/news/article-2020462/Xbox-addict-20-killed-blood-clot-12-hour-gaming-sessions.html

what affects us and it's directly related to the temperature we're experiencing. The warmer the air is, the more gaseous water it can hold.

This is crucial for humans (all land and air dwelling life in fact) because it affects our liquid cooling system (perspiration) directly. At 75°F with a relative humidity of 0% we feel like it's only 69° but at 100% relative, the same 75° feels like 80°. That's a big difference and it's all to do with how the air affects the surface of our skin.

On a very hot day, say 90° (32°C) dry air feels rather pleasantly warm; ramp up the humidity and we start to perspire, feeling clammy and uncomfortable as the sweat stands on our skin unable to evaporate away into the saturated air. For humans, a relative humidity of about 45% (between 40-60%) feels quite comfortable. Humidity is also thought to be the reason for the seasonal (winter) spike in influenza when the levels drop. [181] The flu virus is thought to prefer drier air. Ironically, when the temperature outside drops, turn up the heating and that creates drier air in our homes and at work—creating a haven for flu to thrive.

Dehydration on airplanes is largely due to the consumption of diuretics such as caffeinated drinks and alcohol. It's important to stay hydrated at all times—not just when you're flying. Modern aircraft have some of the best regulated atmospheres we can enjoy.

Long Live the King

We expect by now that you will be starting to understand why we quoted Erasmus at the head of this chapter. Food Babe's "army" (and you might even be one of them) are led by deception. Where knowledge is key, the one with the smallest shard of information can manipulate those with none; bend them to their will.

For all of her misunderstanding and misrepresentation of good science, Food Babe is an excellent manipulator. This was, by her own tacit admission, something she excelled at in college with her position in the debate team. Remember that in debating, all that matters is to defeat your opponent in the minds of the judges. To plead a better case, provided your opponent can't catch and expose your misdirection, you win.

---

181 http://www.nih.gov/researchmatters/march2010/03082010flu.htm

This technique has served her well. Even on the ropes—exposed in the popular media by experts such as Yvette d'Entremont, David Gorski, and John Coupland, Food Babe pulls no punches in undermining her opponent's position.

For the remainder of this book we're going to look at some of these facts in more detail, how Food Babe leverages fear of illness, tells us what we want to hear and exploits the very followers she claims to love for her own financial gain.

■

3

Ring a Ring O' Roses

"The fundamental cause of the trouble is that in the modern world the stupid are cocksure while the intelligent are full of doubt."—Bertrand Russell (1872-1970) British Philosopher

The famous children's rhyme dates back to the Victorians and perhaps before that. It's widely thought the words allude to the belief (widely held until the discovery of microbes) that nasty smells were the cause of illness. We have, in fact, developed a sense of disgust when we smell rotting odors because they are invariably a sign bacteria are present. By extension, those bacteria can make us ill. Countering the stench by using strongly scented flowers was thought to overcome the risk.

Average life expectancy was surprisingly short until the discovery and wide use of antibiotics—perhaps as little as 45 years in the latter part of the 19th century. This number is skewed largely by the huge death rate of the under 6s. In the 21st century people in the west are living longer, healthier lives. Although some parts of the developed West are now suffering a virtual epidemic of obesity, many people will live well into their 80s and beyond. Modern science and medicine keep us fitter for longer, with many deadly diseases now consigned to the history books.

Bogeymen (and Women)

There is an increasing body of evidence to suggest that diet is only one part of a much bigger picture. Modern living as a whole is more to blame than a poor diet, although very poor diet leading to morbid obesity is a problem of its own. For research purposes, there is very little evidence of a strong correlation between cancer in rodents and cancer in humans, where humans are subjected to tiny amounts of these chemicals, and only on occasion.

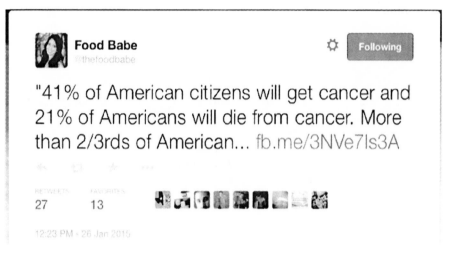

Food Babe
@thefoodbabe
Following

"41% of American citizens will get cancer and 21% of Americans will die from cancer. More than 2/3rds of American... fb.me/3NVe7ls3A

RETWEETS 27 FAVORITES 13

12:23 PM - 26 Jan 2015

Figure 3.1: Not that I want to put the fear of God into anyone but... (Food Babe/Twitter.) Tweet since deleted.

Cancer is the ultimate bogeyman and (probably) the most feared of all non-communicable diseases. It's an overriding term for a whole raft of illness and primarily a disease of older people when the machinery that helps our regulate cell growth goes awry.

Despite popular myths that cancer is a modern disease, it is as natural as scales on a fish, and 100% of them are caused by genetic mutations. [1] When the genomes in our cells function properly, they tell our cells when to multiply, when not to grow, and when to self-destruct. When they don't, cells grow out of control and voila, cancer.

The statistics suggest that (assuming rates remain static) roughly half of us will be diagnosed with some form of cancer and a fifth of us will die as a direct result.

That's a scary figure. Even if we are fortunate enough to not develop the condition, we're almost certain to see a friend or loved one go through it. Some cancers are common, some rare; some people are genetically predisposed to certain forms (breast cancer in particular), and some are strongly influenced by relevant environmental factors like pollution, alcohol consumption, obesity, and viral infection. We can't all escape cancer, but we can

---

[1] http://www.mayoclinic.org/diseases-conditions/cancer/basics/causes/con-20032378

do our best to reduce our risks by not smoking, drinking in moderation, getting vaccinated against HPV and keeping to a healthy weight.

McMillan cancer support, perhaps the UK's pre-eminent charity on cancer and its treatment, lists the risks in more detail:

> *Three-quarters (75%) of all newly diagnosed cancers occur in people aged 60 or over.*

> *Less than 1 in 100 (1%) of cancers are diagnosed in children under 15.*

About 1 in 10 (10%) cancers are diagnosed in people aged 25-49. There is no easy answer as to why cancer rates are climbing in the general population. The primary reason is age—the older we get, the more likely we are to receive a diagnosis of cancer because our bodies are starting to wear out. However, we're also spotting cancer much sooner than ever with improved screening, a more informed public and huge leaps in technology so doctors can see tumors earlier than ever before.

Rates of lung cancer remain troublingly high despite a fall in new smokers with around 80% of cases first diagnosed in people over 60 years of age. [2]

Further, the American Cancer Society has a highly detailed breakdown for North America on its site, providing detailed statistics on a state-by-state basis. [3]

Cancer rates have appeared to be on the increase since the early 20th century. The biggest rise occurred after calorie-dense foods become more available, access to work became easier, and work itself became less physical. In the Victorian Golden Era, from the middle to the late 19th century, we worked harder and longer, slept better, and ate a completely different diet. While these factors don't directly affect cancer risk, the related higher rates of obesity do. In addition, cigarettes are now well-known to be major factors affecting public health, closely followed by obesity. [4]

Breast cancer is the most commonly found cancer in women (though men are susceptible, especially with certain genetic mutations like BRCA 1 and 2). Age is the most likely determinant factor, with most diagnoses occurring

---

2   http://www.macmillan.org.uk/Cancerinformation/Cancertypes/Lung/Aboutlungcancer/Riskfactorscauses.aspx

3   http://www.cancer.org/acs/groups/content/@epidemiologysurveilance/documents/document/acspc-036845.pdf

4   Clayton P, Rowbotham J. How the Mid-Victorians Worked, Ate and Died. International Journal of Environmental Research and Public Health. 2009;6(3):1235-1253. doi:10.3390/ijerph6031235

in women over 50 years old, although it can and does strike earlier. Faulty genes aside, experts have identified some of the most common risk factors:

- *HRT—particularly using the combined form (progesterone and estrogen) increases the risk, although that has to be offset against the symptoms of not taking the treatments.*
- *Having your first children later in life (post 30) or not having them at all.*
- *Not breastfeeding at all, or less than a year in total for all of one's children.*
- *Early onset puberty (pre-12 years old) or late menopause—onset post 50 years old.*
- *Current use of birth control pills increases breast cancer risk very slightly, though the risk drops as soon as one stops taking them.*
- *Other factors include: smoking, being overweight (especially after menopause) and drinking alcohol, although it's not clear how much these factors add to the risk.*

Prostate cancer is the second most common cancer in American men, with skin cancer being the most common. Age is the greatest contributing factor, with an estimated 80% of males in the 80+ bracket thought to have some degree of the disease. [5]

> *"Food Babe conveniently missed out the doses administered—equivalent to consuming 1,000 cans (about 87 US gallons) of a typically colored soft drink—every day for the rest of your life..."*

Risk factors in prostate cancers are less well-understood than those for breast cancer, but what is known is that African-American or Afro-Caribbean men living in the West are at the highest risk, and Asian men in China and Japan at the lowest. So far, investigation into factors causing this discrepancy have had mixed results.

So many factors have changed over the last 150 years that it's hard to quantify and enough to drive the most dedicated researchers or critical thinkers to throw up their hands in frustration. When scientists perform experiments

---

5 http://www.cancerresearchuk.org/cancer-info/cancerstats/types/prostate/incidence/uk-prostate-cancer-incidence-statistics

they typically have a "control"—an identical scenario to whatever they are testing. They are careful to only change a single variable—that is, whatever they hypothesize is causing the effect in question.

A simple example would involve planting some identical seedlings in two boxes. One box remains open to the light; the other is sealed shut. After a specific amount of time, you can come back and see which seeds have grown and which have died. Children perform experiments like this to see how light affects plant growth, typically on rapidly germinating seeds like cress.

If you change more than one condition (watering one group and leaving the other dry, for example) you can't be sure if it was the water (or lack of it) that caused some effect, or the light, or the lack of it. Now imagine trying to study the effect of an unknown (but huge number) of changes.

Dietary obesity was extremely uncommon until just a few decades ago, which is likely one of the biggest contributing factors to modern cancer. Nevertheless, one wouldn't glean this by following the Food Babes and Mercolas of the world. The natural food and supplement industries continue to try to pin cancer risk to food choice despite a woeful lack of well-controlled studies supporting this.

They also all but ignore the role of true environmental risk factors. For example, in the mid-Victorian era, alcoholic drinks weren't common, salt intake was low and beer was weaker than what we typically drink today. Few could afford luxuries like wines or spirits, and the vast majority were within healthy weight ranges.

Powered transport was a thing they could only dream of and no one even thought about powered flight or nuclear war. The air was free from much of the environmental pollutants that we're faced with just by breathing.

While Food Babe is right to espouse a diet of healthy food and exercise, this is already an accepted mantra from medical experts and has been for decades. However, she creates a climate of fear by frequently referring to toxins and carcinogens, often where the effect has been demonstrated in animal models—typically rodents. In these experiments, the animals are given huge doses of experimental chemicals for extended periods, nowhere near the real-life exposure a human would encounter.

Carcinogenic compounds are grouped in a number of ways, but Food Babe's preferred reference is the International Agency for Research on Cancer (IARC), which classifies them into five broad groups. Note the delivery method and level of exposure are as important as the compound itself. A substance that might cause cancer when inhaled or applied directly to tissues may be rendered completely inert by our digestive system for instance.

- *Group 1: substances are known to cause cancer in humans.*
- *Group 2A: substances that probably cause cancer.*
- *Group 2B: substances that possibly cause cancer in humans.*
- *Group 3: substances that cannot be classified as carcinogenic.*
- *Group 4: substances that are probably not carcinogenic.*

(See"IARC Group 1" on page 364, "IARC Group 2a" on page 368 and "IARC Group 2b" on page 371.)

Even light to moderate alcohol consmption has now been implicated as a risk factor in breast cancer, [6] and according to the BMJ

> *"Heavy alcohol consumption has been linked to increased risk of several cancers, including cancer of the colorectum, female breast, oral cavity, pharynx, larynx, liver, and esophagus, and possibly to a higher risk of cancer of the stomach pancreas, lung and gallbladder."* [7]

The BMJ's findings for women is particularly stark.

> *"For women who have never smoked, risk of alcohol related cancers (mainly breast cancer) increases even within the range of up to one alcoholic drink a day."* [8]

Just A Spoonful of Sugar...

Any toxicologist will tell you: the dose makes the poison.

Everyone knows that, apart from food, we need air and water to survive. Lack of air will kill us faster (minutes) than lack of water (days). Lack of food comes in a poor third in that race because we've evolved to survive many weeks without food. This makes sense since air has always been avail-

---

6   http://www.bbc.co.uk/news/health-33975946

7   http://www.bmj.com/content/351/bmj.h4238

8   http://www.bmj.com/content/351/bmj.h4238

able (we've only started poisoning that in the last few centuries). Water is fairly available since it's the most common compound on the surface of our planet... but food? Well food supplies come and go with the seasons. All land-dwelling animals, and broadly speaking, all life on earth is subject to the same rules, although the times vary.

So by way of example, let's consider the effects of water and air, more specifically, oxygen on our bodies. Air is about 21% oxygen—but as the 70's rock song goes "Love is like oxygen, you get too much you get too high, not enough and you're gonna die."

Too much oxygen, a condition called hyperoxia, has various effects on our tissues depending on a number of factors, such as the length and type of exposure. Deepwater scuba divers are specially trained in the use of 100% oxygen and use special equipment to avoid this potentially dangerous condition.

Exposure at raised pressures (above atmospheric pressure) has a toxic effect on the central nervous system (spine, brain) [*Paul Bert Effect*]. [9] Exposure to 100% oxygen at lower pressures is more damaging to the lungs [*Lorrain Smith Effect*], [10] with short term effects such as blurred vision and confusion leading to seizures and damage to the sensitive tissues in the lungs (the alveoli). Studies have found that provided the person survives, the body repairs itself over time and makes a complete recovery.

Lack of oxygen or hypoxia (sometimes called hypoxemia, meaning low oxygen in the blood) is similarly survivable for very short periods. However, this is far more dangerous, as the liver and brain are likely to become irreparably damaged in just a few minutes; the heart and other tissues fail shortly after that.

The most common modern cause of hypoxia is asthma, which causes the airways in the lungs to narrow, making it difficult to breathe. Sufferers use steroids to reduce the inflammation and restore normal breathing, but even today, people still die from asthma-related hypoxia.

As you can see from this example, dose makes a considerable difference in how a substance is tolerated. We need oxygen to survive but if we don't get

9   http://medind.nic.in/jac/t03/i3/jact03i3p234.pdf
10   http://www.medscape.com/viewarticle/778505_3

enough we will die. Indeed, in the right amounts, otherwise toxic chemicals are no more harmful than sitting on your couch unwinding in front of the idiot box (less so, in fact).

Water is another one of life's essential nutrients—it's the most widely used solvent in nature and industry and arguably the most important naturally occurring compound on the planet. We drink gallons of the stuff every week, and everyone knows that without it we'd die.

But you don't want lungs full of the stuff, even though few people would consider that plain water is toxic. And yet the route matters. We have water in our lungs (not much, but it's there) and if you're ever unlucky enough to find yourself in very dry, hot air, you'll start to feel the effects fairly quickly. From this simple example, you can see that water isn't toxic if we ingest it, but inhaling it is a whole different ball game. We'll say it again: The route is important.

It might sound crazy, but plain old-fashioned water, right out of your RO (reverse osmosis) system if you have one, can be as just as toxic and just as deadly as the chemicals you keep under your sink.

> "All things are poison and nothing is without poison, only the dose permits something not to be poisonous."—Paracelsus 1493-1541

Water intoxication (dilutional hyponatremia) is what happens when you overdose on plain old water . While death is unusual, the effects of even mild hyponatremia can be highly unpleasant. Long-distance athletes are most vulnerable to this effect, which occurs when they drink too much water and lose valuable electrolytes (such as sodium and potassium).

In 2013, 17-year old endurance BMX rider Daniel "Sausage" Jamison collapsed from exhaustion and mild hyponatremia at the end of a gruelling 50-mile ride across North East England. Keeping his energy up with high-caffeine drinks proved to be too much, and Jamison collapsed and crashed his bicycle just a few tens of yards from the finish line in full view of the film crew. He made a full recovery.

Others have not been so lucky, such as 40-year-old Jacqueline Henson. Ms. Henson lost her life after drinking a full gallon (about four litres) of water over a short period. [11] Several people have died from water intoxication as a side effect of using MDMA (ecstasy). [12] The most well-known case is probably that of 28 year-old California mother Jennifer Strange, who lost her life trying to win a game console for her children during a radio competition entitled, *"Hold Your Wee for a Wii."* [13]

Pets and Poisons

The real problem with laboratory animals (typically mice and rats) is they are not humans (which might sound obvious) but it can lead to some very disturbing results, like the one that suggested the early artificial sweetener, saccharin, was carcinogenic. With subsequent studies confirming the findings, this warning was mandated in the US from the 1970s to late December 2000:

> *"Use of this product may be hazardous to your health. This product contains saccharin, which has been determined to cause cancer in laboratory animals."* [14]

After extended studies on humans, this statement was repealed because, while saccharin is carcinogenic in rodents, it has no effect on us.

If rodents aren't your thing, many of us has or has had either a cat or a dog. Food that's perfectly acceptable and even good for us, can either make them ill, or in some cases be fatal. Here are a few examples to be mindful of:

- *Caffeine in coffee and tea (and, in particular the related compound, theobromine in cocoa products such as chocolate) can be fatal to dogs and horses—even in surprisingly small quantities-because these animals are unable to process these compounds like we can.*
- *The small amounts of mercury in tuna won't do us much harm, but over time, can make a tuna-addicted kitty very sick indeed.*
- *Plants from the allium family, such as onion, garlic, and chives contain a compound that destroys a cat's red blood cells, leading to anemia and death*

11   http://news.bbc.co.uk/1/hi/england/bradford/7779079.stm
12   http://www.drugscope.org.uk/resources/faqs/faqpages/why-do-people-die-after-taking-ecstasy
13   http://articles.latimes.com/2007/jan/14/local/me-water14
14   http://www.cancer.gov/cancertopics/causes-prevention/risk/diet/artificial-sweeteners-fact-sheet

- *Xylitol, one of the sugar alcohols and a widely used sweetener, while harmless to us, interferes with a cat's insulin levels, leading to liver failure and death.*
- *Raw liver is loved by many cats, but too much can lead to vitamin A toxicity that affects their bone development and repair and may even be fatal.*
- *Avidin, a protein found in raw eggs, interferes with the absorption of biotin, an essential amino acid for cats.*
- *Raw fish contains an enzyme called thiaminase that destroys thiamine, a B vitamin your cat needs to keep its nervous system in good health.*
- *Dog food (when given to cats) is not nutritionally balanced and lacks the essential amino acid taurine that cats need to survive. The same amino acid is synthesized by dogs, so they don't need to consume it in their diets.*
- *Grapes (and their derivatives like raisins) may cause acute kidney failure in both dogs and cats.*

For Whom the Belle Tolls

As we were researching this book, news began to emerge of another charismatic (attractive) young woman, Australian author Belle Gibson, who had claimed to have various forms of cancer. She was exposed as a liar who could be suffering from Münchausen Syndrome: in her case, Münchausen by Internet. Sufferers concoct incredible stories of survival from terrible disease, often against all odds, and spread their protracted claims via social media where it can spread at alarming speeds.

At this juncture, it's unknown if Gibson is suffering from a true psychiatric condition or if she is just a fraud motivated by greed. Although her alleged health problems are considerably different from Food Babe's, the way she motivates her followers bears a striking resemblance to this "Hey, look at me, I should be sick, but I'm not because..." approach. Gibson produced a book, The Whole Pantry, and assisted in the creation of an app for Apple's iDevices including the Apple iWatch.

Her stories are emotive and deeply personal, as with this widely reported post on her @Healing_belle Instagram account from mid-2014:

> "With frustration and ache in my heart… it hurts me to find space tonight to let you all know with love and strength that I've been diagnosed with a third and forth (sic) cancer. One is secondary, and the other is primary. I have cancer in my blood, spleen, brain, uterus, and liver. I am hurting."

Following this she spoke to Stephen Fenech, editor of techguide.com.au:

> "Six weeks ago I was re-diagnosed with multiple cancers, but I'm feeling on top of the world. I get out of bed for what we do. We really believe that we're changing people's lives." [15]

That's a pretty remarkable recovery for someone with metastatic tumors affecting some of their major organs, and yet, no one had thought to question her claims.

Gibson's social media outpouring began in 2009, aged just 20, when she claimed to have been diagnosed with a malignant brain tumor but had eschewed conventional treatment, opting for a program of healthy diet and exercise instead.

Five-year survival rates for these, (thankfully rare) cancers are bleak, but Gibson seemed to make a miraculous recovery. With money pouring in and claims that sums of $300,000AUD had not been delivered to the various charities, things began to unravel. The Australian's journalist Richard Guillaitt unearthed evidence of her true age being 23, despite her 2009 "diagnosis" making her 26. Her self-diagnosed "stage two malignant tumor of the brain" turned out to be a lie.

The WHO describes a Grade II (note, not stage 2) tumor thus:

- *Relatively slow* growing
- *Sometimes spreads to nearby normal tissue and comes back (recurs)*
- *Cells look slightly abnormal under a microscope*

---

15   http://www.techguide.com.au/news/apps-news-feed/embattled-whole-pantry-developer-belle-gibson-told-tech-guide-she-was-diagnosed-with-cancer-twice/

- *Sometimes comes back as a higher grade tumor*

A malignant tumor would have been grade III or IV, and a grade II tumor is not considered malignant. [16, 17]

Staging is a system doctors use to describe the spread of a cancer—it metastasizes to neighboring (stage 2 and 3) or distant (at stage 4) parts of our bodies through our lymphatic system. With many cancers, it's the metastasics that kill you, as they are the hardest ones to treat because the tumor has invaded other parts of our body. [18]

That might be just an "accounting" error, but as the net began to close in, even the most dedicated of her followers began to ask questions, as Gibson shut down social media accounts, deleted incriminating posts, and allegedly fled her native Australia for the USA.

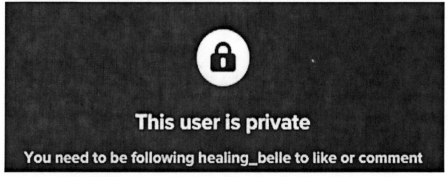

Figure 3.2: *Gibson's Instagram account was set to private as questions surrounding her numerous claims started to appear. (Belle Gibson/Instagram)*

As of March 2015, repercussions surrounding Gibson's claims were starting to echo around the world with her book and App being quietly pulled. Penguin Random House UK said in a statement:

> *"We are disappointed to have not received sufficient explanation or evidence from Ms Gibson in response to recent allegations. We have withdrawn The Whole Pantry recipe book from sale in Australia and*

---

16 http://www.hopkinsmedicine.org/neurology_neurosurgery/centers_clinics/brain_tumor/diagnosis/brain-tumor-grade.html

17 http://www.abta.org/brain-tumor-information/diagnosis/grading-staging.html

18 http://www.cancer.gov/cancertopics/diagnosis-staging/staging/staging-fact-sheet

do not have any plans to publish in the UK or elsewhere in light of this."

Paul Olsewski, publicity director for Simon & Schuster's Atria imprint, told the Sydney Morning Herald:

"In light of recent allegations we are seeking clarification from Belle Gibson and her representatives regarding details of her biography and charitable endeavors. Any and all decisions regarding publication of The Whole Pantry will be made when we have had the opportunity to evaluate all the available information." [19]

While we were still wondering if Gibson ever had cancer in the first place, the answer came in an interview she gave to The Australian Woman's Weekly.

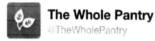

The Whole Pantry
@TheWholePantry

☼   +👤 Follow

@702sydney For the record, I haven't retreated to the United States. and didn't. Media, continue to "humiliate and condemn" - Belle.

↩   ⟲   ★   •••

RETWEETS   FAVORITES
4   2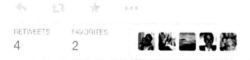

Figure 3.3: Gibson appeared to tweet from the Whole Pantry trying to shift blame from herself. (ABC Radio Sydney/Twitter)

"No. None of it is true," she said.

So the entire empire was built on lies, making it a fraud no different than any other.

---

19   ttp://www.smh.com.au/national/publisher-penguin-pulls-belle-gibson-cook-book-the-whole-pantry-20150316-1m0dsc.html

The Fear Babe

What is different though is people who followed Gibson's fallacious advice have died and will die as a direct result. Not only is that unconscionable, it's the ultimate reality we face when we take health or even dietary advice from Internet celebrities.

Who is left to pick up the pieces? The families of loved ones? The doctors now faced with treating patients left cheated, hopeless and alone? The law—something to stop such obviously outrageous claims from being courted by an uncritical media?

The truth is, we are all losers –except perhaps Belle Gibson herself, who continues to attempt to spin the situation to her own gain.

With that in mind, it's worth clarifying that Food Babe does not give direct health advice without disclaimers, and yet, it remains notable how little thought publishers give to remarkable claims. Surely therefore, they should shoulder some of the responsibility.

If Gibson leaves any lasting legacy for publishers everywhere it may be that they are more careful to validate their authors' claims. Even though Gibson has been exposed and has admitted her deception, people will continue to trust her… as we're about to show holds true with Food Babe herself.

Then I Saw Her Face! Now I'm A Believer!

Just as our minds are living things, the ideas they contain have lives of their own and are strengthened by challenges. When the resident ideas fend off an attack from within their walls, they are strengthened by the experience, learning from the mistakes in reasoning that prompted the attacks in the first place.

Perhaps the most extreme example of this is when a belief becomes so strong (the idea is so deeply entrenched) that no amount of contradictory evidence will unseat it. Psychic "medium," and admitted fraud, M. Lamar Keene, refers to this as "true believer syndrome," although the term was coined in the 1951 book, *The True Believer* by American author, Eric Hoffer. Keene notes:

> *"The true-believer syndrome merits study by science. What is it that compels a person, past all reason, to believe the unbelievable. How can an otherwise sane individual become so enamored of a fantasy,*

an imposture, that even after it's exposed in the bright light of day he still clings to it—indeed, clings to it all the harder?"

In his book, *The Psychic Mafia* [1976] Keene admitted that his "partner" Raoul was entirely fake. Despite that, his congregation continued to believe he was real.

Another notable example was created by stage magician and investigator James Randi (the guy who exposed Uri "spoon bender" Geller).

In 1988, Randi guided little-known stage performer José Alavarez in creating the appearance he was channeling a 2000-year-old spirit, "Carlos," and was able to commune with the dead. Part of the act involved a tennis ball placed into Alavarez's left armpit, which allowed him to temporarily reduce his radial (wrist) pulse so that even a qualified (but unsuspecting) nurse or audience member could be fooled into believing a physiological phenomenon was occurring. (This part is important because even intelligent or educated people are easy to fool– particularly when they are "primed" by the stage setting. Many stage magicians have attractive assistants, who wave and strike poses as the magician works in order to divert our attention from the trickster.)

For the stunt, Randi and Alavarez travelled to Australia where the media publicized his appearance without bothering to check his (deliberately faked) credentials. But the biggest clue was that Alavarez/Carlos didn't charge for his services. Even the "Atlantis Crystals" he offered for sale were only available on a promissory order. No money changed hands.

This is a remarkable contrast to every other guru and charlatan practising. It doesn't matter if they are in touch with spirits from the other side, claim to have evidence we're being invaded by reptilian overlords, or declare aspartame and MSG are bad for you: money is the only thing that will budge them; and they're not cheap.

When the Alavarez hoax was revealed on Australian television, most viewers were shocked and disappointed (as you might imagine), but a considerable number remained true believers: completely unshakable in the belief "Carlos" was real. The revelation the whole thing had been a carefully engineered hoax serves as a stark demonstration of our willingness to believe in the supernatural. These people vocally protested that the revelation was faked and that dark forces were afoot.

Such delusions are so strong they are unstoppable, and it's thought that some people are more susceptible than others. Anti-science fear mongering is more grounded than 2000-year-old spirits but it shares much of the same features, and triggers the same "true believer" effect in a sizable number of people. Just what percentage of a population is prone to this is difficult to quantify, but we know that it's large enough to cause serious diversions for those trying to solve very real problems.

Even if it's just 0.1% of the population (a fairly conservative estimate), and the adult population of the USA (18+) is 240,000,000 people, that suggests around 2.5M people are open to this sort of psychological manipulation. Often, this minority is very vocal, and has been known to influence policy.

We should point out that just because a person is susceptible, it doesn't mean they will automatically fall into the trap. A lot will though, and using these figures (aided by the myriad forums these people flock to), there is a strong implication that the problem is huge—no matter where we fall on this spectrum.

True believers become prophets of their own delusion—recruiting others by spreading the memes (by which we mean distorted facts, half-truths and blatant lies) because in their mind, everyone else is wrong and they're right. Weak believers, i.e. those not sufficiently skeptical to examine the ideas, are recruited along the way; swept along in a tide of follow-the-leader like the children followed the Pied Piper of Hamelin.

Food Babe's angry quote about being called the Jenny McCarthy of food demonstrates this: the allusion is one of equivocation, not sexism and it's not fallacious in this case because Ms. McCarthy—another attractive, telegenic personality—has taken an entirely fallacious stance against vaccinations based on the long disproved Wakefield paper, and ignores every piece of evidence to the contrary.

Like McCarthy, Food Babe shows every sign of being a true believer.

She is not alone. GMO technology has been attacked from a number of fronts—from playing God (*appeal to nature fallacy*) to complete misrepresentation of the science (*appeal to ignorance*) or outright lies. Because GMO technology is one of the cutting edge developments in modern biology, it is poorly understood by the public at large. This effect isn't new, but for the first time in our history, technologies and ideas under threat from ignorance may be vital to our very survival.

You won't hear a politician (publicly) express doubt for this very reason—it's career suicide. Yet, as Russell observes, it's the very essence of careful, reasoned, and intelligent thought. The surer we are of (particularly complex) facts, the more likely we are to be wrong! This is also the essence of the oft-observed Dunning-Kruger effect—particularly as people fall prey to the wrong end of it.

Belief is a powerful thing.

Combine the true believer with the truly ignorant and you have a deadly combination. Expose believers to a charismatic leader and you have a deadly epidemic.

An Apple a Day...

On October 5th, 2011, the world lost one of its most iconic and leading lights when Apple bid farewell to its co-founder Steve Jobs. People have a love/hate relationship with Apple's products but that has nothing to do with Jobs' death from pancreatic cancer, a disease that, in its intraductal papillary mucinous neoplasm form, claimed the life of actor Patrick Swayze two years earlier.

Pancreatic cancer is aggressive and invariably fatal due to the difficulty in early diagnosis and treatment—with one exception: islet cell neuroendocrine tumors—the very type Jobs was diagnosed with in 2003. As brilliant as he was, Jobs eschewed mainstream oncological (cancer) treatment that may have cured him and instead, followed a variety of alternative methods, one of which reportedly bears a striking resemblance to the so-called metabolic treatments including Gerson Therapy.

Gerson Therapy (a.k.a Gerson diet, Gerson method, Gerson treatment, Gerson program), probably the best known of the diet-based alternative treatments for cancer, was a regimen developed by German born Dr. Max Gerson, who began treating his tuberculosis patients using the Gerson-Sauerbruch-Hermannsdorfer diet. By 1928, Gerson had further developed the supposed therapy and began using it on cancer patients, reporting excellent results that were viewed with skepticism by his peers. Variations of Gerson's ideas include Kelley's treatment, Gonzalez treatment, and Issels whole body therapy.

Some of these "treatments"—such as Issels—recommend the removal of teeth that have mercury fillings (on the assumption that mercury is leaching from the teeth and entering the body). Others add vitamins and other supplements to the basic diet of raw, juiced fruit and vegetables. This idea may have derived from the observations of the Victorian golden age, when the American diet was already losing touch with the consumption of large amounts of fresh vegetarian fare.

Gerson's therapy in particular also advocates the use of coffee enemas with variations incorporating hydrogen peroxide.

There are lots of variations on the same ideas:

- *Increase the levels of phytonutrients in the diet.*
- *"Detox" the body using powerful enemas to clean the bowel.*

Water-based enemas have a long history, but their most popular proponent was one Dr. John Harvey Kellogg, the man best known for inventing corn flakes (the breakfast cereal) but lesser known for being thoroughly odd even by today's standards. [20, 21]

He believed that most maladies were caused by an imbalance of intestinal gut flora (bacteria) and to maintain that balance, strongly advocated the use of water and live yogurt enemas. This may seem laughable today, but we have to remember this was in the early part of the 20th century.

Enemas are still widely believed to be therapeutically valid in many forms of alternative anti-cancer treatment based around the idea that increased absorption of caffeine through the colon invigorates the liver and causes it to remove toxins from the bloodstream more effectively.

Evidence supporting this thesis does not exist; at least not in any respected form. In fact, people with tumors of the colon and rectum, diverticuli-

---

20   http://intactivists.blogspot.co.uk/2011/05/john-harvey-kellogg.html
21   https://www.psychologytoday.com/blog/sex-dawn/200902/time-boycott-kellogg

tis, Crohn's disease, and ulcerative colitis can (and have been) seriously harmed or killed by such practices because the bowel can be punctured by the equipment or the pressure, leading to conditions such as fecal peritonitis. Patients with impaired heart or kidney function may experience an overload of fluid leading to life-threatening electrolyte (sodium, potassium, calcium) imbalances. Besides that—it's just unpleasant.

Another possible "alternative" therapy includes large doses of "vitamin B17" (also known as Laetrile, or *amygdalin,* the naturally occurring form). B17 isn't a vitamin and is converted to cyanide in the body. Laetrile is not approved by the FDA in the US. Supporters claim (without proper evidence) that cancer cells take up the cyanide and die, leaving the healthy tissues untouched. Use of Laetrile may cause mild symptoms like nausea and headache, but in some cases, it can also lead to vomiting and potentially lethal cyanide poisoning.

The claim for amygdalin efficacy is derived from the Hunza and the Karakorum peoples living in an area near the border of Pakistan and China, who are "cancer-free." Since they have a diet rich in amygdalin, that must explain it.

What they don't tell you is that these isolated tribes have a diet rich in vegetables, don't drink, or smoke, and get lots of exercise, don't overeat, have very low rates of obesity, and are fairly removed from the air pollution most of us are exposed to in the industrialized West.

According to the American Cancer Society, in 1978 the National Cancer Institute conducted a *post hoc* (after the fact) study of an estimated 75,000 people who had used Laetrile. Of the 400,000 doctors queried, just 93 reported positive results and of those, only six showed any sign of improvement: a fact that could easily be attributed to any number of other factors. In percentages, that's a 0.12% reporting positive results and just 0.001% reporting shrinkage of the cancerous tissues. [22]

Several more deaths are recorded and linked with a practice known as cell therapy, where cells from live animals are either injected directly or consumed orally. Given the recorded cases of gangrene caused by cell therapy,

---

[22] http://www.cancer.org/treatment/treatmentsandsideeffects/complementaryandalternativemedicine/pharmacologicalandbiologicaltreatment/laetrile

[23] the practice seems positively barbaric, let alone stupid of 11 on a 10 point scale.

The Wellness Warrior's Passing

During our early research, on February 26, 2015, the world lost Jess Ainscough, another shining star and promoter of Gerson therapy. The news left doctors numbed, and followers stunned. Ms. Ainscough, a former online editor of Dolly magazine, began the "Wellness Warrior" blog shortly after being diagnosed with a rare form of cancer, epithelioid sarcoma, aged just 22. Such tumors appear in the soft tissue of the hand or arm and usually require complete removal of the affected limb.

In Ainscough's case, her best chance of survival meant losing her left arm, part of the collar bone and her left shoulder blade; a debilitating loss for any person, let alone an attractive young woman in the prime of life. Ainscough tried the alternative, perfusion therapy, which involves isolating the limb and delivering chemotherapy in huge doses.

It didn't work.

So Ainscough opted for Gerson therapy and her condition remained largely the same.

> "The therapy involves drinking 13 fresh organic veggie juices per day (yes that's one an hour, every hour of my waking day), five coffee enemas per day and a basic organic whole food plant-based diet with additional supplements." [24]

When her mother, Sharyn, was diagnosed with breast cancer she followed her daughter's lead, apparently eschewing conventional treatments. Sharyn lost her fight in 2013, almost exactly to the day predicted by the median survival rate for that particular cancer if left untreated. Her mother's death deeply affected Ms. Ainscough, as she reflects in this 2014 update:

> "This year absolutely brought me to my knees. I've been challenged, frightened, and cracked open in ways I never had before. After my mum died at the end of last year, my heart was shattered and it's still

---

23   http://www.quackwatch.org/01QuackeryRelatedTopics/Cancer/cellular.html

24   http://scienceblogs.com/insolence/2013/10/17/sharyn-ainscough-dies-tragically-because-she-followed-the-example-of-her-daughter-the-wellness-warrior/

in a million pieces. I had no idea how to function without her, and it turns out my body didn't either.

"For the first time in my almost seven year journey with cancer, this year I've been really unwell. I've lived with cancer since 2008 and for most of those years my condition was totally stable. When my mum became really ill, my cancer started to become aggressive again. After she died, things really started flaring up. For the past few months, I've been pretty much bedridden." [25]

In her five years or so of self-belief, and by setting an example, Ainscough convinced an unknown number of people to try Gerson therapy either with or as an alternative to conventional therapies. Her redoubtable charisma and fearless belief that she was healing herself spread like a virus before the unthinkable reality caught up with her... and many more will likely follow.

Gerson's outmoded, unscientific therapy was about to claim another victim. As cancer specialist Dr. David Gorski notes in this epitaph on his blog:

"One wonders if Jess Ainscough might have been persuaded not to do Gerson therapy if there had been a doctor caring for her who truly knew what the treatment involved, how it is based on an oversimplified understanding of cancer and the Warburg effect, and an understanding of human physiology that was becoming outdated a century ago." [26]

This is, we fear, the true price of tolerating "alternative" therapies for life-threatening diseases, and it's a price that's never worth paying. Science doesn't always get it right, but it's self-correcting—something you won't find the Gerson Institute or its followers openly advertising. It's deeply saddening and hard for those of us with scientific minds to accept. Food Babe makes a number of references to Gerson's treatment, like this one for a $2,500 juicer...

This juicer is highly recommended for the Gerson Therapy, a natural treatment to heal one's body through organic raw juices, a vegetarian diet and specific guidelines. [27]

25 http://scienceblogs.com/insolence/2013/10/17/sharyn-ainscough-dies-tragically-because-she-followed-the-example-of-her-daughter-the-wellness-warrior/

26 http://scienceblogs.com/insolence/2015/03/04/alternative-oncology-versus-oncology/

27 http://foodbabe.com/shop/the-best-juicers-and-blenders/

… and lists the outfit on both her website resources and in her book [28] and proudly name-drops Charlotte Gerson (daughter of Max Gerson) when bragging about her appearance on the Food Integrity podcast. [29]

Right now, an unknown number of people in Ainscough's native Australia are thought to be experimenting with metabolic treatments like Gerson therapy (one estimate put it as high as 66% of all cancer patients) and an unknown number are lowering their chance of survival in the same way across the developed world. Every life lost this way is lost without reason.

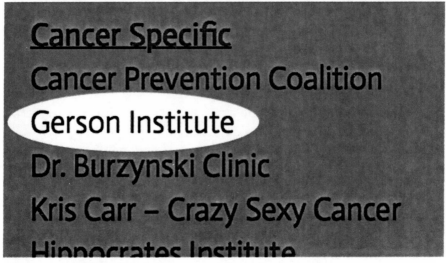

Figure 3.4: Food Babe lists the Gerson institute under cancer centers . (foodbabe.com/informativewebsites/)

Despite repeated failures and untold suffering as a direct result of following Gerson's methods, an institute set up in his name continues to claim (without supporting evidence):

Over the past 60 years, thousands of people have used the Gerson Therapy to recover from so-called "incurable" diseases, including:

- *Cancer (including melanoma, breast cancer, prostate cancer, colon cancer, lymphoma, pancreatic cancer and many others)*
- *Diabetes*

---

28 The Food Babe Way, p. 343

29 http://foodbabe.com/2013/06/13/listen-how-i-became-the-food-babe-on-food-integrity-now/

- *Heart disease*
- *Arthritis*
- *Auto-immune disorders, and many others.* [30]

A staggering and rather arrogant observation on the Gerson Institute's blog contains this passage:

> *"Some critics have taken her death as proof that alternative or holistic therapies don't work, but we disagree. There is no guarantee that any medical treatment, alternative or conventional, will work for every patient, every time–especially for patients like Jess, who have advanced or terminal cancer diagnoses. Cancer is a devastating and deadly disease, and the Gerson Therapy cannot save everyone."* [31]

This much is true of conventional medicine, but a bigger question remains: can the Gerson therapy save anyone? Such a dismissive attitude, rather typical of holistic practitioners, is like the chastised child who doesn't want to engage in discussion because she knows she will lose.

"La-la-la. I'm not listening."

The following quote by Stephen Barrett, M.D. comes from Quackwatch. [32]

> *"Charlotte Gerson claims that treatment at the clinic has produced high cure rates for many cancers. In 1986, however, investigators learned that patients were not monitored after they left the facility. [33] Although clinic personnel later said they would follow their patients systematically, there is no published evidence that they have done so. Three naturpaths (sic) who visited the Gerson Clinic in 1983 were able to track 18 patients over a 5-year period (or until death) through annual letters or phone calls. At the 5-year mark, only one was still alive (but not cancer-free); the rest had succumbed to their cancer."* [34]

So of 18 patients in that sample (statistically quite small) only one was still alive after five years and still sick with the disease, representing a failure rate

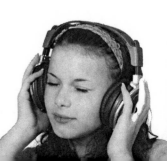

---

30 http://gerson.org/gerpress/

31 http://gerson.org/gerpress/in-memory-of-jess-ainscough-the-wellness-warrior/

32 http://www.quackwatch.org/01QuackeryRelatedTopics/cancer.html

33 Lowell J. The Gerson Clinic. Nutrition Forum 3:9-12, 1986

34 Austin S, Dale EB, DeKadt S. Long-term follow-up of cancer patients using Contreras, Hoxsey and Gerson therapies. Journal of Naturopathic Medicine 5(1):74-76, 1994

of 100% (or less than a 6% survival rate) after five years. Compare that to the current status of treatment in Great Britain where the ten year survival rate is at 50% overall and 78% for breast cancer. [35] In America, our odds are even better, with The Lancet's 2007 [36] appraisal claiming a 63% survival after five years. [37]

The team on this book sincerely hope, that should any of our readers be unfortunate enough to develop cancer, that they seek qualified medical attention from an oncologist. More people survive this terrible disease than ever before, but quack treatments from unqualified people put your health at risk.

American philosopher George Santayana wrote in his 1905 treatise, *Reason in Common Sense*:

"Those who cannot remember the past are condemned to repeat it."

The most popular reworking is widely attributed to Winston Churchill:

"Those who fail to learn from history are doomed to repeat it."

Although no record is made of this in the UK's official Hansard recordings, Churchill did make this rather lengthy statement in May 1935.

"When the situation was manageable it was neglected, and now that it is thoroughly out of hand we apply too late the remedies which then might have effected a cure. There is nothing new in the story. It is as old as the Sibylline books. It falls into that long, dismal catalogue of the fruitlessness of experience and the confirmed unteachability of mankind. Want of foresight, unwillingness to act when action would be simple and effective, lack of clear thinking, confusion of counsel until the emergency comes, until self-preservation strikes its jarring gong–these are the features which constitute the endless repetition of history." [38]

RIP Jessica. Here's hoping someone will learn from your terrible sacrifice.

■

---

35   http://www.cancerresearchuk.org/cancer-info/cancerstats/survival/england-and-wales-cancer-survival-statistics

36   Lancet Oncology, 2007. No. 9, p. 784-796

37   http://www.ncpa.org/pub/ba596

38   http://www.winstonchurchill.org/publications/finest-hour/finest-hour-156/wit-and-wisdom-2

4

Burn, Baby! Burn!

"Even though we all know the facts, it's hard to resist the lure of a tan"—Jane Krakowski, American Actress

It's not an exaggeration to say **skin cancer kills** [1] but Food Babe has other ideas. Although she correctly correlates sunlight with health (specifically, vitamin D production in our skin) this advice is dangerous. Sure the sun is good for us, but there's a caveat. Her complete lack of understanding (or plain lazy research) makes this advice potentially very dangerous indeed.

> Go outside without sunscreen! On vacation I got loads of Vitamin D from the Sun. There were several days I did not wear sunscreen, and in the winter, I NEVER wear sunscreen. You must get sunshine! The sun's rays are pure wonderful energy your body needs— spending a small amount of time in the sun without sunscreen will not give you skin cancer! [2]

What, specifically, is a small amount of time? What sort of sun exposure? What time of day? Where in the world? What is your skin type? Being of Indian descent, both our co-author Kavin Senapathy and Food Babe's skin contain more melanin than someone of European ancestry and less than someone of predominantly African ancestry. Poor Kavin regrets believing in her youth that she didn't need sunscreen because her caramel skin would protect her. Perhaps she's a bit vain (she readily admits it), but she attributes at least a few of her laugh lines to failure to use sunscreen in her teens and twenties!

Indeed, though Northern Europeans (many Americans are directly descended from these people) are most at risk, people of all hues should heed the "always wear sunscreen" mantra. These distinctions are why we have to listen to those with credible, evidence-based takes on the issues and should treat

---

1   http://www.cancerresearchuk.org/cancer-info/cancerstats/types/skin/mortality/uk-skin-cancer-mortality-statistics
2   http://foodbabe.com/2011/09/22/seize-your-sugar-cravings/

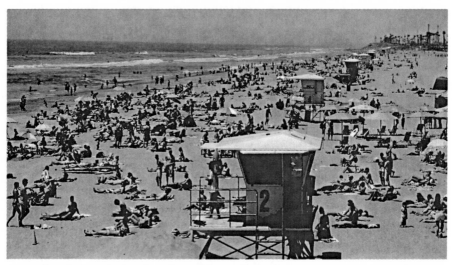

Many of us flock to the beach and spend hours in the sun trying to tan—without realising it's doing untold and lifelong damage to our skin. (Andrew Schmidt/PublicDomainPictures.net)

bloggers like Food Babe with skepticism and often derision. To do otherwise is dangerous, not only to our critical-thinking but to our health.

Ultra-violet radiation is a very powerful light from the sun that's invisible to our eyes but readily absorbed by our skin. Tanning is a production of melanin in response to the skin damage caused by exposure to too much UV radiation. Yes, we did say damage, and that's before you visibly burn.

There is no such thing as a healthy tan.

Doctors and scientists used to think that visible lines were a result of the aging process but we now know that they're also a direct result of exposure to UVA from sunlight.

During the Italian renaissance and the English Victorian era, dark skin was considered unattractive by the rich and well-to-do. The working class who, by and large, worked the land or on the sea were naturally exposed to huge amounts of sunlight and while that may have increased their vitamin D levels, their skin would become wrinkled and leathery with the advancing years. This can be seen in rare photographs from the era as the rich have clear, pale skin while the workers are swarthy and deeply lined. The Victorian obsession with staying out of the sun inspired the age's in-fashion accessories: rich women would wear delicate gloves and hold elaborate parasols to protect them from the sun.

Our hope is that before you reach the end of this section (which is large just because it's so important) you'll realize the best anti-aging cream you can buy is a good sunscreen and the best anti-aging treatment money can't buy is the knowledge of when to avoid the sun.

Sunlight is more dangerous than we thought just a few decades ago. Researchers are now identifying an increase in deadly melanomas in people with very dark skin. Rather than being completely immune to the effects of UV radiation, we now know that everyone should protect their skin—particularly during the summer months and while the sun is at its peak (from around 10am to around 3pm). Somewhat surprisingly, this even applies on overcast days, in the winter, and when you might be travelling by car or train.

Unsurprisingly perhaps, we're our own worst enemy. Because of advances in science and technology, our lifespans are vastly longer than they used to be. When we add our ability to travel to visit places on earth that we have not adapted to? Suddenly, those cheap flights to paradise are starting to look more expensive in terms of our health in our twilight years.

Melanin in our skin helps to protect us from some UV radiation—it's a many headed beast—and this is where the problems start. Dermatologists divide skin types into six categories (phototypes) from type 1 which burns very easily and produces very little melanin to type 6 which is very dark skin and does not burn easily.

Having sufficient melanin that comfortably tolerates high levels of sunlight can lure us into a false sense of security; damage is being done much deeper, lying in wait for decades before the effects become apparent, by which point, it's already too late. According to the American Cancer Society, over 3 million people are diagnosed in the US alone every year. [3] A 2006 study (currently the most recent data we have) says that there are more cases of skin cancer each year than the incidents of breast, prostate, lung and colon cancer combined. [4] Having a "nice healthy tan" (ironically, it's not healthy at all) only gives us the equivalent of SP4 which isn't even close to sufficient protection.

---

[3]   http://www.cancer.org/cancer/cancercauses/sunanduvexposure/sun-cancer-facts)
[4]   http://www.skincancer.org/skin-cancer-information/skin-cancer-facts

The Fear Babe

The *British Association of Dermatologists* estimates that 80% of cases of skin cancer (80,000 of the 100,000 new cases every year in the UK alone) are preventable. It's not clear how many of those cases are attributable to vacations abroad, the use of home and commercial tanning salons, or even climate change. The fact is, even in the relatively cool British climate, skin cancer is a serious issue that cannot be ignored.

Australians have perhaps the highest rates of skin cancer in the developed world with current estimates suggesting 80% of all types of cancer in the nation occurring on the skin and up to 99% of those being a direct result of exposure to the sun. [5]

We'll look at what ultra-violet does to our skin shortly, but let's take a few moments to understand what it actually is.

The name ultra-violet comes derives from "beyond violet"—if you were to look at a spectrum (on a rainbow for example) with red at the left and bluish/violet at the right, then UV is a little further to right. Over to the left—just left of red is infra-red. People can't see either of these extremes—although specially developed equipment can. Radio telescopes, for instance, are designed to see these extreme forms of light.

What isn't obvious, and something that wasn't even realized until around the turn of the 20th century, is that the color of visible light (the "color" of all light in fact) is directly related to the amount of energy that took to create it. What we see as red is relatively weak but violet is many times (up to 100,000x) more powerful.

Scientists sub-divide infra-red and ultra-violet into broad groups as follows: near, mid and far infra-red, and near (UVA) and extreme ultra-violet (UVB and UVC). We're really concerned with mid infra-red, which is responsible for much of the warmth we feel from the sun (and even a lover's touch on our skin) and UVA and UVB. The energy of each photon—packet of light—is measured in eVs (electron volts) but since this is rather difficult to follow, we've changed the figures into something rather less complicated.

Mid IR	*12—1500*
Visible light	*1500—3000*

---

5   http://www.cancer.org.au/about-cancer/types-of-cancer/skin-cancer.html

UVA	3,000—4,000
UVB	4,000—4,500
UVC	4,500—12,000

Notice how the lower numbers are responsible for that cozy feeling in front of a bonfire or fireplace. This warmth is due to the way the mid-IR (invisible electromagnetic radiation) from the fire makes the molecules in our skin vibrate.

If we get too close to the fire or turn it up too high however, we get a nasty burn or worse. Let's imagine you can warm yourself in front of a 1Kw electric fire. On a chilly day, that's the sort of pleasant balmy heat we would expect—although you would not want to touch it. Now imagine yourself sitting in front of a 250Kw furnace. How long could you stand the heat? Amazingly, when we go outside during the summer months (even when it's overcast and there's a cool breeze blowing) that's essentially what we are doing.

You might notice from the chart that visible light—the radiation we can see—is much more powerful—perhaps 10x as much. So why doesn't that cause discernable pain? Put simply, our skin reflects most of this light and what isn't reflected is absorbed by the melanin pigmentation. However, although melanin absorbs some UV, it can't absorb all of it. This is crucial to those of us with darker skin types—doubly so since a melanoma (the deadliest form of skin cancer) is naturally inky black-brown in appearance. They are far more difficult to spot on darker skin: putting those with darker skin at risk of simply not noticing a cancerous spot. Experts estimate that 95% of all melanomas are directly attributable to sun damage.

Of the three spectra of ultra-violet, our atmosphere protects us from UVC—which is only really a problem for astronauts—and also blocks a large amount of UVB. Precisely how much UVA or UVB reaches us depends on a number of factors—including altitude—making high-altitude climbers particularly susceptible. For another protective shield (thanks, atmosphere!) the ozone layer stops most of the sun's UVB rays from reaching us. Realistically, this is the most dangerous form for humans (and all life) but only around 5% hits the ground. Although UVB doesn't travel very deep into our skin, it's the one associated with delayed effects such as sunburn, skin damage (premature aging) and skin cancer. How delayed? Experts believe the "latent" period, that is the time between damage and actual cancer diagnosis, can be any-

Table 4.1: Common Ingredients in Modern Sunscreens

Ingredient	UVA (340-400nM)	UVA (320-340nM)	UVB
Octinoxate			Chemical
Octisalate (OCS)			Chemical
Para-aminobenzoic acid (PABA) *			Chemical
Octyl Dimethyl Paba (Padimate-O)			Chemical
Octocrylene			Chemical
Titanium Dioxide		Physical	Physical
Zinc Oxide	Physical	Physical	Physical
Avobenzone (Parsol 1789)	Chemical		
Oxybenzone (benzophe-none-3)		Chemical	

* Para-aminobenzoic acid causes an allergic reaction in many people and is no longer in wide use.

where from 10 to 20 years. UVA, which also causes aging, is also thought to be responsible for the oft-dreaded "age spots."

Like visible light, UV is reflected by many surfaces including water, sand, painted surfaces and snow. So it's very difficult to avoid altogether unless you are indoors. Still, UVA can pass through glass, so even if you are travelling (or work near a window) you should consider some protection.

UVA: Ultra-violet Ages & UVB: Ultra-violet Burns

Sunscreens work in two distinct ways but not all are created equal, and even the amount of protection isn't always as good as the manufacturer claims. Some creams (also called "organic" preparations) absorb UV rays before they hit your skin and re-radiate the energy off as harmless heat; the others actively reflect the UV away from our skin. However, the experts say, in either case, we need to apply the lotion a full 15 minutes before we step out into the sun and ideally, avoid the brightest times of day altogether unless we can get into shade. Note the terms organic and inorganic have a different meaning where sunscreen is concerned. Dermatoligsts now think we should use a daily moisturizer regardless of the weather with a SPF of around (or better than) 15. [6]

Despite this, tanning salons remain popular. There is a myth that the beds are less dangerous than sitting at the beach, probably due to the fact that the tubes create mostly lower energy UVA. Although UVA takes longer to cause a visible burn, it's doing damage deep inside our skin and every session increases the damage. Since the widespread use of powerful tanning beds is relatively recent, it's too early to predict just how many people are going to visibly age prematurely. But we can expect to see a rise in the next few decades.

But just when you thought it was safe to wrap up in a tin-foil suit and run screaming to the drug store, it pays to check just how effective the sunscreens are. Although the technology is improving (along with our understanding of it) it's important to know what those SPFs (sun protection factors) mean.

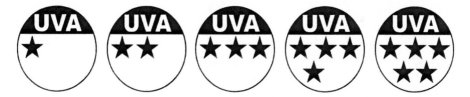

Created by Boots in 1992 and updated in 2004, the star rating is supposed to help consumers determine which suncreams offer the best protection against UVA. More stars is better. This simple system is now widely adopted.

Crucially, SPF determines a level of protection against UVB—the burning rays. So while you can help stop yourself from burning (and reduce the risk of cancer in later life) you may not be adequately protected against UVA. Perhaps surprisingly, SPF 30 isn't twice as effective against UVB as SPF 15. SPF 15 will protect you against 93% of UVB but SPF 30 will only protect against 97%. Even with the very best protection, a small amount of potentially damaging radiation is always going to get through. UVA is also split into two

---

6   http://www.consultingroom.com/treatments/sunscreen

British Association of Dermatologists

SKINDEX

HIGH RISK

TYPE 01 Pale skin, burns very easily and rarely tans.
Generally have light coloured or red hair and freckles.

TYPE 02 Fair skin that usually burns, but may gradually tan.
Some may have dark hair but still have fair skin.

TYPE 03 Skin that burns with long or intense exposure to the sun
but generally tans quite easily.

TYPE 04 Olive-coloured skin that tans easily, but could possibly
burn with lengthy exposures to intense sunshine.
Usually have brown eyes and dark hair.

TYPE 05 Naturally brown skin, with brown eyes and dark hair.
Skin darkens easily with sun exposure and only burns
with excessive exposure to the sun.

TYPE 06 Black skin with dark brown eyes and black hair.
Skin very easily darkens on exposure to sun and would
very rarely, if ever, burn.

LOW RISK

The images shown here are for illustration purposes and are not intended to be exact representations of the different skin types described.

Not everyone's skin offers the same level of protection in the sun. That's why you need to know your 'skin type'. It can help give you an idea of how much care you need to take in the sun. Your skin type cannot be changed and does not vary according to how tanned you are – it is determined by your genes.

NEVER LET YOUR SKIN BURN, WHATEVER YOUR SKIN TYPE!

SUN AWARENESS
British Association of Dermatologists

www.bad.org.uk | 020 7383 0266
Registered Charity No: 258474

© 2013

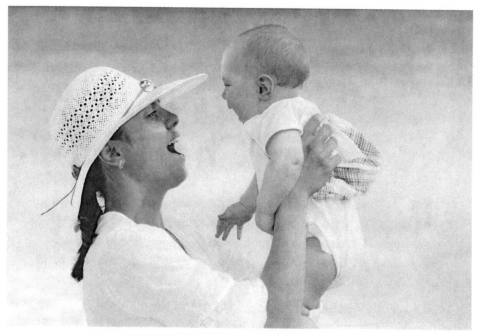

Fun in the sun. There's nothing quite like a relaxing day at the beach. Little ones are particularly sensitive and should wear a reputable factor 50 sunscreen. A well-ventilated, wide brimmed hat is a smart choice to keep that UVA at bay. Picture posed by models. (Petr Kratochvil/publicdomainpictures.net)

groups with the lower power rays 340-400 nM (ironically) doing the most damage.

Overcast days in the summer are almost as bad, if not worse. Although we can't directly see Mr. Golden Sun, almost all (about 80%) UVA radiation goes right through the cloud cover to damage our skin for decades to come. Medical science has yet to offer an ironclad solution. We can remove and treat many skin cancers (particularly the non-melanomas) and we can cover up the signs of aging; however, right now we are unable to fix the damage that's been done. Since this is so often considered just an unavoidable part of aging, pharmaceutical companies are not clambering over each other to find a solution. This may change in time, but right now the best we can all do is rely on credible information, stay out of the sun as much as possible, wear good quality sunscreen, and remember the mantra: ***no tan is a healthy tan!***

■

5

Trust Me...
I'm Charismatic

"History shows that charismatic rhetoric relies on the demonisation of an enemy to deflect blame and to continue to stoke the fires of emotion... Charisma is at once seductive, volatile and utterly compelling, yet often completely rejects rational logic. "—Dr. Elesa Zehndorfer, academic and writer [1]

Indulge us while we throw a few names out: Jim Jones, Adolf Hitler, Napoleon Bonaparte, Joel Osteen, Fidel Castro, Ronald Reagan, Bill Clinton, Tony Blair, Martin Luther-King, Gandhi, Malcolm X, Winston Churchill, Nelson Mandela, Eva Peron, Aung San Suu Kyi, Charles Manson, Marshall Applewhite, and David Koresh.

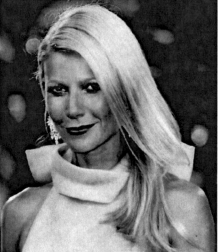

Now that might seem like a pretty mixed up bunch from civil rights heroes to cult leaders to political leaders, kooks, murderers and power-crazed despots. But they all share (or shared) one thing in common.

Charisma. Lots of it.

Actress and woo-promoter, Gwyneth Paltrow oozes charisma—but that collar and hairstyle is no accident. (Andrea Raffin/ Wikipedia)

Most of the bunch is also pretty easy on the eyes. Physical attractiveness is deeply connected to our need to breed—and the better looking someone is, the more attractive they are.

---

[1] http://www.bbc.co.uk/news/magazine-34021088

Outwardly we can connect facial features (he has a nice smile, she has nice eyes) but what we're really doing (thanks to millennia of evolution) is making a snap value judgement about how healthy that person is.

Our health (and even the state of our immune system) creates tell-tale signs in our physical features. Rather ironic when you consider that just as our bodies enter the stage when nature is preparing us to breed, acne kicks in! Every teenager dreads the appearance of zits at the time of their life when they're naturally their most conceited.

It should come as no surprise that our skin, the body's largest and most visible organ, is a primitive indication of internal health. We know instinctively if someone is sweating or flushed that they might be suffering from exertion or disease. Even skin tone, muscle tone, lip color, shape of the mouth and size of the lips, clarity of the eyes—these are just some examples of how our brain connects the dots when choosing a potential mate, and we do it in a fraction of a second without a conscious thought.

Evolution has a lot of explaining to do.

Attractive people are natural leaders. We are programmed to follow them and more importantly, we are programmed to listen to them. All humans have an internal "lie detector," but the instant we become enamored with someone, it gets turned down and we're often powerless to stop that from happening. Parents will see their teenagers hang on every word uttered by hunky movie stars, completely in the thrall of rock stars, and swooning over the cool kid in class. As Peter Day, the BBC's global business correspondent observes:

> *"The force-field of charisma and its impact on others is usually accompanied by huge self belief. Several of the American billionaires are convinced they will find a way of living forever, for example."* [2]

Social psychologist Dr Hanna Zagefka told the BBC in a separate article:

> *"Attractive people are treated better, are more popular and generally get better jobs. It is also assumed they are more intelligent."* [3]

---

2   http://www.bbc.co.uk/news/business-33977086
3   http://www.bbc.co.uk/news/health-32427178

The Fear Babe

But there is more to this than just sexual attraction; charismatic people of all genders affect us in just the same way. Men and women are equally taken in by charismatic people from Charles Manson to Bill and Hillary Clinton. Charisma is a drug. The more and the longer we're exposed to it, the easier we find it to pierce through the facade. By the time we regain sufficient cognitive resources for that to dawn on us, it's already far too late.

Sexual attraction is different. For example, a gay man can recognize a beautiful woman without being sexually attracted to her. This distinction in our ability to judge physical attraction (which translates to charisma) is deceptive. We naturally assume a heterosexual woman would not be swayed by an attractive woman, but quite the opposite is the case.

In her Food Babe persona, Vani Hari has been extremely canny in controlling her public appearance, particularly in professional photo shoots where she is frequently posed into the classic "open neck" posture appearing coy, demure and non-threatening. Yet in that chest beats the heart of a cold, calculating businessperson who knows what she wants and isn't afraid to use her disarming beauty and tenacity to get it. And she's used to getting her way—admitting, without apparent remorse or regret, to stealing candy as a child just because she wanted it. [4]

To demonstrate this, we created some artificial renderings of these poses so you can better understand how this works and compare them to Food Babe's pictures—in particular those used on magazine covers and blog posts.

This classic pose uses the head tilt—where the model's head is cocked to one side, typically to expose the neck, but the model's long hair disguises this somewhat here. Although barely perceptible, the body arches slightly forward, forcing the model to look up into the camera, exposing even more of the neckline, while forcing the observer to assume they are concentrating on her eyes.

You'll notice Hari usually wears V-necked or wide necked tops, which expose a large amount of this vulnerable area; occasionally with fine jewelry to force observers to notice this unconsciously. Photographers refer to this technique as "drawing the eye" or "drawing the gaze."

---

4   https://hbr.org/2012/11/the-dark-side-of-charisma

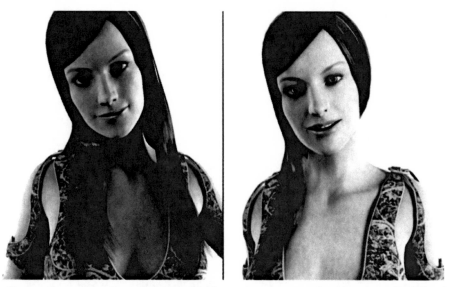

Two versions of the classic head-tilt. The hair swept over one shoulder to expose the neck. Food Babe often sports low necklines and pendants for fashion reasons, but they double up as making her appear more trustworthy at a very basic level. The variation on the right here is more egregious and has the same effect, and it works on all genders. Note how actress Gwyneth Paltrow uses a similar style at the opening to this chapter.

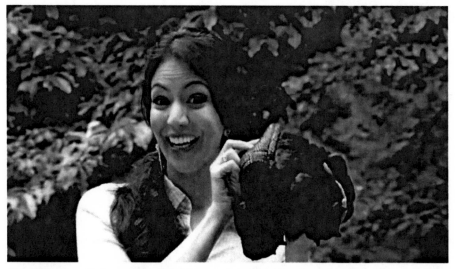

Consider this still, from Food Babe's beaver butt film. Note how the ponytail, swept over her right shoulder (together with the open shirt) expose and draw attention to the "unprotected" neck. This subtle use of body language makes us feel comfortable and less likely to question the speaker. (Food Babe LLC/YouTube)

The Fear Babe

This is crucial because the decisions or the judgments we make about a person's vulnerability (and, therefore, how trustworthy they are) happen in a fraction of a second.

The exposed neckline is another example, used by professional models for decades. Ladies with long hair such as Hari can employ several other techniques, but the most prevalent in still imagery is the side sweep, where the hair is swept over the left or right shoulder. This exposes even more of the neck, creating an even greater air of vulnerability.

Childlike innocence is disarming. Food babe occasionally employs this pose and close variations of it.

Even when it's faked, vulnerability engenders trust.

Another version is the "parent's perspective" or "parent's view" pose where the camera is angled down to the model – who looks up with a wide smile. Once again the emphasis is on the wide-eyed, childlike innocence, as shown here.

Dr. Tomas Chamorro-Premuzic, Professor of Business Psychology at University College London, offers this warning on the shared addiction of charisma:

> *"Leaders capable of charming their followers become addicted to their love. After the initial honeymoon effect is over, they continue to crave high approval ratings, which distracts them from their actual goals. Followers, on the other hand, become addicted to the leader's charisma, reinforcing displays of populism and perceiving unpopular decisions as deal-breakers. The result is a reciprocal dependence that encourages both parts to distort reality in order to prolong their 'high.'"* [5]

---

5   https://hbr.org/2012/11/the-dark-side-of-charisma

This will be an uncomfortable light-bulb moment for some, we're sure. Food Babe is a classic example of this psychological phenomenon, and to some degree she has even devolved some of the responsibility to her moderators.

In essence then, charisma is like a drug with larger doses becoming increasingly toxic. The world of those relying on their own charisma becomes one where everything is micro-managed in microscopic detail. They cannot afford to be seen to err because that might damage their perceived self-image in the eyes of their adoring fans. In this case, the distortion of reality is the cavernous gap between what Food Babe believes or claims and what a scientific consensus says is true.

> I give my moderators full authority to delete comments and ban insulting, harassing, or cyberbullying commenters. [6]

Misogynistic comments don't help anyone, and often have their roots in the (male) need to dominate by fair means or by foul. But it doesn't stop there—Food Babe or her moderators delete almost all dissenting remarks within minutes or hours, and on Facebook this will also earn the poster an immediate ban.

As with many others, the primary authors of this book have approached her with questions and either been ignored or banned from making further comments... earning her the nickname "Bani Hari" and giving birth to the popular Facebook group, Banned By Food Babe.

Contradictory science (read: consensus) is not allowed on her page, and her sycophantic league of followers, completely under the spell of this undeniably charismatic leader, will openly attack anyone who dares to discuss an opposing viewpoint. The love her followers espouse is undeniable with (as of this writing) over 1300 positive comments[7] on her post about criticism, urging her to carry on the fight.

Food Babe cannily refers to her legions of followers as the Food Babe Army, something not lost on a number of Internet jesters, but this is just another way to engender camaraderie usually only felt by troops in a real

---

6   http://foodbabe.com/2014/12/06/food-babe-critics/
7   http://foodbabe.com/2014/12/06/food-babe-critics/

battle. Everyone is pushing the same way; all following the leader without cause to question because the instant they do, the blinds come down and the truth will become apparent. Food Babe is in this for the money. The health of her followers is a secondary concern.

Charisma can be as addictive as it is toxic. Dr. Chamorro-Premuzic notes:

> *"... charisma facilitates ideological self-enhancement: our adoration for someone who expresses our own beliefs (usually better than we are capable of doing ourselves) is a socially acceptable way to love and flatter, not only ourselves, but also our 'tribe.' "* [8]

The Food Babe Army, like undead creatures under the control of a powerful necromancer, are willing to do her very bidding, all for the good of the cause. A simple wave of the mouse and they are jamming the switchboards, call centers and PR departments of companies, demanding to know or share whatever information Food Babe has encouraged them to.

Can You Even Trust a Doctor?

The word doctor implies a person of great learning. In common parlance, when we feel ill, we make an appointment to see the doctor; technically a doctor of medicine (MD) but there are many different doctorates awarded in both the sciences and the humanities. Some non-medical doctorates are honorific, meaning they are bestowed upon a person in recognition of something they have done. Some unscrupulous "universities" even award their doctorates for a price. This is, naturally, where it all gets rather confusing for the everyday mortals that make up the majority of the population because we rarely look beyond the title "Dr." –and we always should.

Above all else, what matters is the doctoral subject—the person's specialty. As soon as a specialist starts producing opinion (or worse, research) that both lies outside of their area of expertise and contradicts widespread expert consensus, you need to ask why. This is not to say that opinion is necessarily wrong. Science doctorates involve a lot of hard work and years of study—but the more someone opines on subjects outside of their field, the more cautious we need to be in evaluating the validity of the information.

---

8   https://hbr.org/2012/11/the-dark-side-of-charisma

Dr. Linus Pauling (1901-1994), the only person to date to have been singularly awarded two Nobels, was by any measure a clever man. Pauling became convinced (one might say obsessed) with the notion that ultra-high doses of vitamin C could treat the common cold, and also be used as a palliative treatment for cancer patients. Basing his beliefs entirely on anecdotal evidence and poor science, Pauling himself would take 3000mg of vitamin C every day. The continuing public perception that large amounts of vitamin C is good for us is almost entirely due to this error.

Pauling died from prostate cancer in 1994 at the age of 93 and is sadly more remembered for his poor quality later work than the genius of his younger years, which saw him win the Nobel Prize for chemistry in 1954.

That such a brilliant man can wander so far from the path of hard science is testimony to the frailty of the human mind and our capacity for self-delusion—so much so that this must surely serve as a warning that our most deeply held beliefs are always subject to revision. Even the best of us can fall prey to this most human of failings.

> *"All lies and jest.*
> *Still, a man hears what he wants to hear.*
> *And disregards the rest"—Paul Simon, "The Boxer"*

Scientists like Pauling fall prey to a set of cognitive biases where they seek out only that data which supports their theory. We're all subject to these effects, and there are a great number of them. The scientific method is designed to circumvent such problems and scientists are taught rigorous methods to avoid this trap. Even so, some fall into these mental black holes from which they are unable to escape. Intelligence, it seems, offers no protection against our innate humanity.

Our natural ego has a lot to do with this. No one enjoys being criticized for their beliefs, but we love having our ego stroked. This isn't just about telling your significant other how much you're attracted to them or how good their cooking is; it goes to the very heart of the human condition.

Tell a smoker that smoking is bad for them, and they will almost certainly recall some family member who smoked unfiltered full strength cigarettes well into their 90s. Or tell an alcoholic that their addiction to ethanol is slowly destroying their liver and they will similarly recount stories of "old so and so" who was drunk all his life and died at the ripe old age of 93 still clutching a bottle of Scotch. Or the drug addict who claims they can quit at any time, only they don't want to quit.

We've used extreme examples here, but this effect can be far more subtle.

Al Capone, for example, believed that he was an honest businessman; a Robin Hood of his time. During a time of prohibition, he delivered illegal booze to a grateful public through the underground of speakeasies. An outlaw and criminal to the authorities, Capone was worshiped as a hero, and that drove him deeper into the belief he was pursuing a righteous cause. Capone was a charismatic and complex character—as much a ruthless gangster as he was a talented businessman.

An unfortunate example of this black hole bias is Dr. Stephanie Seneff, who holds degrees in biophysics (MIT 1968) and electrical engineering (MIT 1980) plus a doctorate in electrical engineering and computer science (MIT 1985).

She's a smart cookie when it comes to her field of artificial intelligence and natural language processing, but more recently she's become the poster child for "researcher bias," a group of cognitive biases that afflicted Linus Pauling in his quest to prove megadoses of vitamin C were good for us.

Dr. Seneff firmly believes that glyphosate (the chemical in herbicides like Roundup) is responsible for all manner of ills, putting her ideas into peer-reviewed research papers that have made her popular with the likes of Dr. Mercola and Jeffrey Smith. Smith interviewed Seneff for one of his presentations and the accompanying YouTube note *falsely* link glyphosate with:

> *"autism ... gastrointestinal issues such as inflammatory bowel disease, chronic diarrhea, colitis and Crohn's disease, obesity, cardiovascular disease, depression, cancer, cachexia, Alzheimer's disease, Parkinson's disease, multiple sclerosis, and ALS, among others."* [9]

To the layman, this sounds like scary findings with lots of ifs and maybes, not to mention a ton of confirmation bias for the likes of Mercola and Smith. Indeed, uncertainty is scary.

---

9   https://www.youtube.com/watch?v=h_AHLDXF5aw

Dr. David Gorski (MD) has this to say of Seneff's "research" method, which amounts to statistical modeling to test the hypothesis:

> *"The sine qua non [essential condition] of a good study demonstrating an association between an environmental exposure and a condition requires the actual verification and quantification of the environmental exposure under study in the cases."* [10]

What Dr. Gorski means is you can't take a bunch of people who at one time lived near a nuclear power station, then assume they have been exposed to higher than normal levels of radiation.

It might sound logical, but in terms of science it's utter bunk—and you'd get better results by getting these people to strip naked in a dark room to see which ones glow. (The glowing ones are aliens because a human exposed to that much radiation wouldn't survive for long.)

Dr. Seneff has at some time fallen into the anti-Monsanto, anti-GMO mantra, i.e.,

```
var Monsanto = "Bad!"
function check(Monsanto) {
  if (Monsanto == true) {
  var KemKill = Mass_Panic("Monsanto causes autism!");
  check(KemKill);
  return("shillbux");
  }
}
```

(This is a programmer's joke since Dr. Seneff is a computer specialist—roughly it translates to "if you want to make money, use the *argumentum ad monstantium* and just blame a hated corporation.)

While the papers may be hard to follow, demographics are not, and Seneff has some nice ones to demonstrate this link. She is confidently predicting that this unstoppable trend is going to result in half of all children being diagnosed with some form of autism by 2025, making MMR look like a snowflake in a blizzard.

---

10   http://scienceblogs.com/insolence/2014/06/25/pesticide-exposure-during-pregnancy-increases-autism-risk-in-the-child-not-so-fast

The Fear Babe

That's some scary looking sh*t—but the reality is this: statistics is more of an art than a science and with the right data sets you can prove (as others have) that organic food causes autism or game consoles are responsible for ADHD. A correlation (matching pattern) in the data is just that. Something worth looking at but that's all. Drawing any conclusions from statistics alone (no matter how pretty your graph is) is a recipe to become a laughing stock. Using readily available data, experts have correlated the uptake of organic food with the increase in autism rates over a decade and found...

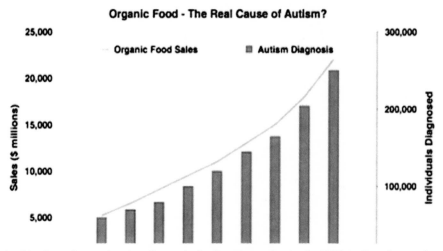

As this chart shows, the rise of organic food consumption in the USA is directly correlated to the rise of autism. Wait...what?

A fact that should show you just how utterly useless pretty graphics are when an expert has let their bias run out of control and (worse) when the peer-reviewers have failed to do their job properly. We could, for example, say that the number of prescription medications Kavin Senapathy takes rose after the birth of her first child, and rose again after she had another. Therefore, should we say that having kids causes an increase in prescription meds? Nah, it's just a correlation.

> *"[Glyphosate] ...is one of the most extensively studied chemicals in our environment. But the authors fail to cite the hundreds of papers and reports that address the safety and biological activity of glyphosate. This leaves me with the impression that the authors have*

little interest in an objective analysis of the available information."—
Dr. Peter Olins, Ph.D. [11]

Poor peer review was almost single-handedly responsible for the 1998 crisis over the Lancet's MMR paper, erroneously linking vaccination to metabolic problems and autism, which could (in retrospect, it's easy to say should) have spotted the sloppy research methods, although the full extent of Wakefield's financial incentives were not revealed until much later. [12]

■

---

11   http://ultimateglutenfree.com/2014/02/does-glyphosate-cause-celiac-disease-actually-no/
12   http://briandeer.com/mmr/st-mmr-reports.htm

6

Rich Man, Poor Man, PR Man

"A lie can travel half way around the world while the truth is putting on its shoes."—Mark Twain, American Journalist and Author

Mark Twain died in 1910, nearly a century before the age of modern telecommunications made it possible to lie to millions of people at the press of a button. His words then are as relevant now as they ever were.

Science used to be done in labs, behind closed doors, by smart people we trusted to find answers. It's a methodology, developed and refined over many centuries, a systematic set of techniques for assimilating new information and correcting previous assumptions. In medieval times, scientists were attacked by established religions for daring to question the word of God, but in this enlightened era, religion and science keep a respectful distance and rarely cross swords. In the 21st Century, science's biggest enemy is the very public it serves.

World War PR

PR is a modern war for our hearts and minds, and the battle is fought on every street corner, in every blog, every magazine, and newspaper; anywhere we have access to information. PR is an information virus, and the best PR spreads faster than a pyroclastic flow. Like a charging grizzly, you can't outrun it, you can't avoid it; it's just a matter of time before it catches you.

As crazy as it seems at first, humans (most animals, in fact) are hard wired to transmit bad information. It's a survival instinct that appeared long before truth and lies.

The most basic form can be seen when a wild animal detects a predator; flocks of birds are particularly good at this. The instant one flock member perceives a threat (real or imagined) it takes flight, and the rest follow suit without a second thought. Stopping to consider if the threat is real is a great way to become someone's next meal.

Crying in pain is another form of alarm. A stricken animal will cry out, which serves it no purpose, but acts as an alarm call to the surviving herd to run like hell.

Fire! Fire!

Humans are no different. In the right circumstances, we react without thinking. Our animal instincts kick in, and crowds of people will often panic, with the weakest, often children and elderly, being trampled in the rush. Such obvious displays of mass panic are, thankfully, rare these days, but there is a more subtle effect going on here. It affects our daily lives and is entirely down to our need to communicate fear. This instinctual behavior allows Food Babe, Alex Jones and their ilk to thrive.

It's important to note that animals don't think when they spread alarm. As we've said, doing so could cost them their lives. There isn't time to consider if the threat is real, just assume it is and act.

In the same way, when we hear about something "dangerous" we don't stop and think, "Is this true?" We act on instinct. Most of us simply spread the news to the next person (or people we meet) and thus panic spreads through a population. It's in our nature. Though it has evolved from the town crier to the gullible friend forwarding every alarming email meme, the underlying instinct is the same.

For this reason, we can't blame the Food Babe "Army" for disseminating these ideas. The buck stops with Food Babe (and any other commercial organization that feeds anti-science ideas to the general public for its gain).

Compared to advertising, PR is a relatively new idea. Its father is unquestionably Edward Bernays [1891–1995], a nephew of the famed Austrian psychoanalyst Sigmund Freud. Bernays' genius was in recognizing the power of a crowd to act on instinct and as a group using just the slightest nudge, however imperceptible. Once done, this nudge is sufficient to get things moving, and the rest is left up to our innate nature.

In one example, Bernays was charged with getting women to smoke. While this idea seems preposterous now, at the time only men smoked, leaving 50% of the US population in lost revenue for big tobacco. Working on advice from psychoanalyst *A.A. Brill*, Bernays persuaded a group of women to light up during a march on Easter Sunday in New York calling them "torches of freedom." The rest, as they say, is history.

Bernays' work in PR is more apparent in the work of Nazi propagandist Joesph Goebbels, who organized huge rallies to fire up people and their imagination based largely on Bernays' ideas.

When Freud developed these ideas, he meant them as a warning: something to be prevented. Bernays and Goebbels operated in the (mistaken) belief they could control it. Goebbels knew that in the right set of circumstances the love of the crowd is delivered to the leader and its hate is directed at all those who oppose him.

By accident or design, Food Babe has achieved a modern-day version of the same effect, even referring to her followers as an "army." In a cynical manipulation called the *appeal to emotion* or the "help!" card from Senapathy's *Deck of Deflection,* many Food Babe web pages end with a statement imploring the reader to help.

> Posts may contain affiliate links for products Food Babe has approved and researched herself. If you purchase a product through an affiliate link, your cost will be the same (or at a discount if a special code is offered) and Food Babe will automatically receive a small referral fee. Your support is crucial because it helps fund this blog and helps us continue to spread the word. Thank you.

Narcissists crave attention—they thrive on it and must be the center of attention at all times. It's a psychology that develops in childhood but can be nurtured quite unwittingly in adulthood too. The Internet and its associated plague of selfies have made narcissists of many—but Food Babe shows signs that it's beyond healthy levels—her face is everywhere. She needs to be seen and controls her image with almost hammer-like authority. On her "blog" (which is really a store-front by another name) almost every image is carefully posed—often "photoshopped" and she's shown everywhere from grocery stores to exotic locations, funded, presumably, by the spoils of being a successful blogger and speaker.

Posts and emails are often signed as if they are from a close friend like this:

"Much Love, Vani"

… and often with hugs and kisses (O and X). Consciously or otherwise, she loves the attention her followers give her and she reciprocates, though most of them have never even met her. She's like a pop star or famous actress but as a blogger she's several steps closer to the ordinary people and goes out of her way to appear to be like them. We like people who are like us and this retains a connection that is almost familial in its nature.

Vani desperately needs to be loved.

Backed into a corner under well-deserved criticism from SciBabe (Yvette d'Entremont), Food Babe responded. Her opening remark, emblazoned on a smiling portrait, read:

> I'm full of heart, love and hope for a better future and I know you are too. [1]

This is another appeal to emotion. In other words, it serves no purpose other than to make you feel sorry for her. Hard-nosed skeptics look at this and snort, but many find it difficult to disconnect the emotion (empathy) from the message and take Food Babe's side: particularly if you're sitting on the fence.

Food Babe was on the run following SciBabe/Gawker's evisceration and subsequent mainstream media bashing. Her page "likes" dipped noticeably for several days before climbing again, with many suspecting that the dip was fallout from the article, as the vultures gathered to heap disdain on this person who was so careless with her science and carefree with her accusa-

---

[1]   http://foodbabe.com/response-to-gawker-the-food-babe-blogger-is-full-of-shit/

tions. Hari doesn't enjoy being challenged. She wants to be front and center like a dictator bathing in the love and adoration of her followers.

It wasn't long before the "Army" fought back—posting unpleasant and demeaning messages to their own sites—even to the point of *ad hominem* (personal) attacks against d'Entremont—rather ironic given that Food Babe cries foul when this very tactic is used against her. But does she decry it? Not so much as a "hush" to date.

A Meme, A Meme, My Kingdom for a Meme!

Richard Dawkins coined the idea of memes in his 1976 book, The Selfish Gene, defining them as an idea that spreads between people through a variety of means from simple stories to rituals and mimicry. Memes on the Internet spread via Facebook, Twitter, and email—although the word itself has evolved to include satirical posters, short videos of cute pets and so on.

A real meme is far more taciturn. Moving like a thief in the night, many engage with our mind's internal filter: an effect called confirmation bias. Take any polarized argument from anthropogenic climate change [man-made global warming] to politics or creation vs. evolution, and people will invariably pick one side or the other, largely dependent on which side got to them first.

> *"Give me a child until he is seven and I will give you the man."*— Jesuit motto.

Science has evolved a system of checks and balances in recognition of this in an attempt to ameliorate this bias, but most of us are not trained in science and are entirely reliant upon our judgment; colored by our perception and pre-bias. Ego has a huge part to play here. We like to be told we're correct, so we tend to pay attention to, and even seek out, arguments that support what we already believe. Worse, we tend to reject (out of hand) arguments that disagree with what we already believe.

When we are born, our minds are like an empty castle at the top of a hill. As we learn, all sorts of notions populate the castle. As new ideas arrive, they enter the castle and take up residence—so long as an opposing idea isn't already living there.

The mind castle nurtures the ideas and they grow stronger, fortified by the many other supporting ideas that we are culturally exposed to. When an opposing idea assaults the castle, resident beliefs have the advantage of defensive walls and invariably prevent the contradictions from entering. Even if those ideas are a powerful and well-reasoned argument, the resident ideas have the upper hand.

Long term, deeply entrenched ideas work like this and easily defeat the attacker. In essence, this is how confirmation bias works.

It is possible for an attacking force to enter the castle either by laying siege (exposing us to opposing ideas for a long time) or by weight of sheer force. As this happens, we experience a mental battle as the two memes duke it out in our minds because ultimately, this castle isn't big enough for the pair of them.

Psychologists refer to this as cognitive dissonance—the deep discomfort felt when people try to simultaneously rationalize two diametrically opposing ideas. These battles are invariably won by the home team as it has the advantage of knowing the territory.

Food Babe @thefoodbabe · 4h

Why Are We Being Attacked? The Gory Details On A Dirty PR Campaign Finally Revealed. foodbabe.com/2015/02/12/dir…

Food Babe's February 2015 tweet promised to shine a spotlight on what some claim is a concerted effort to discredit her on the part of the biotech industry. (Food Babe/Twitter)

The reality is rather more nuanced, for those who can be bothered to read the articles Food Babe herself is referencing. For example, using one from Nature, Food Babe refers to courageous scientists being attacked by the "biotech industry's PR minions" as if there were some vast army of men in suits trawling for any dissenting voice. Writer Emily Waltz observes in the cited Nature article:

> *"Many of the critics have been studying biotech crops since they were developed commercially in the late 1980s, and some were involved*

with the first regulatory approvals. They have specific ideas about how the risks of these crops should be scientifically assessed. And they worry that papers that fall short of high standards will give anti-GMO activists ammunition to influence policy, just as the monarch butterfly study did." [2]

To look at the history, it's worth remembering that around 1998 a now infamous health scare erupted when Andrew Wakefield, the disgraced British MD, published a paper that appeared to link the MMR vaccine with inflammatory bowel disease and autism. Despite The Lancet's retraction, [3] [4] naive reporting in the wider press led to a global health scare that continues to resonate to this day.

In early 2015 measles erupted in parts of America, [5] where people like Jenny McCarthy continue to parrot Wakefield's fraudulent research. As a reader of this work fearful of the MMR vaccine or vaccination in general, we urge you to look at the other side of this story and decide for yourself. Vaccination is not without risk, but balanced against the alternative, there is no contest. It is by far the lesser of two evils and these infections can be very evil indeed. Consider that Dr. Andrew Wakefield's research was withdrawn at the earliest possible opportunity after rapidly being shown to be wrong, yet caused a crisis of fear that resonates today. Now read on to see how GMOs got dragged through the mud in the public's eye while the science community collected its marbles in the wake of equally bad science.

In 1999, just a year after the MMR fiasco broke in England, a team at Cornell University studying the effects of pollen from GM maize on larval monarch butterflies reported that 50% of the insects died within four days of consumption. [6] A hungry media erupted with alarm and Greenpeace staged protests over what would later transpire to be poor experimental design. [7]

The EPA (Environmental Protection Agency) demanded answers and, by 2001 six papers had been produced demonstrating that in nature, the most

2   http://www.nature.com/news/2009/090902/full/461027a.html

3   http://www.thelancet.com/journals/lancet/article/PIIS0140-6736(97)11096-0/abstract

4   http://www.bmj.com/content/340/bmj.c696

5   http://www.cdc.gov/measles/cases-outbreaks.html, accessed 17 April 2015

6   http://www.news.cornell.edu/stories/1999/04/toxic-pollen-bt-corn-can-kill-monarch-butterflies, accessed 17 April 2015

7   http://www.pnas.org/content/98/21/11937.full

common forms of GM maize were no more toxic to the monarch caterpillars than ordinary maize.

In most other areas of science, this is a good thing. Researchers find anomalies and use them to develop new and exciting theories. Where health is concerned, and maverick information leaks out, the results can be as far reaching as they are devastating. Losey and the Cornell team had used much higher concentrations to demonstrate toxicity, but the genie was already out of the bottle.

GM took another slap in 2007 with little more than some poorly chosen words in a paper led by Dr. Jennifer Tank and Dr. Emma Rosi-Marshall. In the paper, their first foray into GM research, they noted that debris from the Bt GM crops was finding its way into nearby streams. In laboratory tests, they observed that the fly larvae fed GM corn developed at half the rate of those fed conventional corn, and the larvae fed high concentrations of the debris died out at twice the rate. Co-author Todd Royer thought, "So what? We're going to lose a few trichopterans [caddis flies]."

This slightly devil-may-care attitude was to be the paper's (and almost GM science's) undoing. The concluding line of the (damning) abstract states:

> "Stream insects are important prey for aquatic and riparian predators, and widespread planting of Bt crops has unexpected ecosystem-scale consequences." [8]

Fellow scientists were enraged—since the conclusions and negative projections were drawn from poorly controlled experimental conditions—something experts in the GM field were quick to note. This led some to question if PNAS (Proceedings of the National Academy of Sciences) was even fit for purpose any longer.

One of the clearest objections to the experimental techniques was that Dr. Tank and Dr. Rosi-Marshall had failed to negate other variables in the control, such as using isogenic lines (identical strains of corn without the inserted genes) and controlling just how much the larvae consumed. Controls such as these are so basic in science they are taught almost as soon as experiments are performed in elementary education.

---

8   http://www.pnas.org/content/104/41/16204.abstract

The Fear Babe

A bigger question is posed by PNAS editor-in-chief Randy Schekman, who observed of the strongly worded abstract,

"Why this would have escaped the attention of the referees beats me." [9]

Referees are the experts that respected journals such as PNAS and The Lancet use to check the validity of scientific papers. This process of peer review seeks to ensure that the most obvious mistakes (and often less obvious ones) are spotted before the paper risks its reputation on it. Science comprises such a myriad fields, no editor could ever hope to staff their journal with the experts required to check everything they publish. This process of rigid review ensures that, by and large, poor phrasing or lousy science doesn't make it into print in the first place.

Abstracts are particularly problematic since they are often the only part of a paper available to the general public (and the only part busy journalists have time to read). A little overzealous hyperbole leaks faster than a bottomless bucket.

The Internet has created a new form of journal—those where authors pay to see their work in print, often known as "pay-for-play" journals. Even experts sometimes find it difficult to know if they are reading something in a respected journal or one of the vanity-publishing outfits that think peer review is something written about in Victorian seaside attractions. A joke that should be so obvious that it sticks out half a mile (and if you got that second, truly awful pun, you're probably a fan of British WWII sitcom, Dad's Army). It's impossible to be sure if Food Babe read the piece in Nature, but if she had, it's unlikely she would have referenced it or used the phrase "biotech industry's PR minions" since it's very clear from the article that quite the opposite is true, and the biggest dissenters are from the science community itself.

The loudest voices were primarily concerned that a vital area of research has been sabotaged by a few instances of sloppy peer review and some poor methodology, just like the MMR debacle beforehand.

So many self-important "investigators" either don't read or don't understand the paper or don't understand where a single paper fits into volumes

---

9   http://www.nature.com/news/2009/090902/full/461027a.html

of research that go to establish a body of evidence. (See "Scientific Consensus" on page 381.)

Pop Goes the Weasel

> Seemingly reputable news organizations even linked to the hate groups—quoting one of their spokespeople and repeated their ridiculous and biased messages as if they have any merit. [10]

The entire message here, from her response to a critical story entitled "*Is The Food Babe A Fearmonger? Scientists Are Speaking Out*", in NPR's *The Salt* blog is one of derision and rather than attacking the argument, does an effective job of undermining it without any substantiation.

Right off the bat here, Food Babe takes an undeserved swipe at NPR.

The source is either reputable or it's not—but using the weasel word "seemingly," she instantly creates doubt in the uncritical reader's mind over any story from any source that doesn't follow Food Babe's agenda to the letter.

When it comes to ridiculous and poorly sourced data, there is an oft-repeated claim that azodicarbonamide can land someone with a huge fine and a 15-year jail term in Singapore. But to date, no reliable sources have been able to verify this, despite the claim being repeated more virally than an amusing picture of a miserable cat.

For the uninitiated, weasel words and phrases are a PR (or an advertising) pro's dream. Weasel words are fallacies, used to obfuscate the fact the speaker is misleading you (although not necessarily deliberately). They are common in natural language, particularly in interpersonal discussions where you can ask for clarification. The same is not true when you're reading an article, book, or blog, making it more important to learn how to spot them. See the panel "A Weasel Word Primer" on page 178 for a more detailed explanation.

A Call To Action

Writer and science popularizer Kavin Senapathy[11] has certainly come under scrutiny. Like Food Babe, Senapathy is a first generation Indian-

---

10   http://foodbabe.com/2014/12/06/food-babe-critics/

11   This section was developed just before Kavin joined the team.

A Weasel Word Primer

A 2009 study of Wikipedia[1] found that weasel words fall into several broad categories.

- *Vague qualifiers*: Words such as "could," "may," "might," "probably," and "seemingly" undermine the argument being put forward. Note how in the quote on page 70, Food Babe uses the phrase "could be lurking".

- *Euphemisms*: In the castoreum example, "beaver butt" is used to implicate the anus or anal sphincter as a "gross-out" tactic to make people feel nauseous.

- *Vague expressions*: "could be lurking in your food" or "may cause cancer" or even "caused cancer in laboratory animals." (We're not lab rats so indicators in rodents don't necessarily indicate toxicity in humans.)

- *Non sequiturs*: A Latin phrase meaning, it does not follow, commonly used to imply something that isn't necessarily true. An example is when Food Babe says, "There are many other things that are called 'natural flavors' that could be lurking in your food." [2] Natural flavor could easily be the fresh orange juice and nothing as gross (or hideously expensive) as ground up beaver's anus.

- *Generalization*: "Many people believe…" when there is no way to know how large that number is. Although phrases like this imply a majority, in truth it might be just the author and their friends who hold this belief.

- *Anonymous authority:* "Scientists claim…" Great—but which scientists?

---

1   Viola Ganter and Michael Strube (2009), "Finding Hedges by Chasing Weasels: Hedge Detection Using Wikipedia Tags and Shallow Linguistic Features," Proceedings of the ACL-IJCNLP 2009 Conference Short Papers, p. 175 (online) http://www.aclweb.org/anthology/P09-2044

2   http://foodbabe.com/2013/09/09/food-babe-tv-do-you-eat-beaver-butt

American woman and is highly critical of the way Food Babe plays (fallaciously) to her heritage. She has been known to call these tactics the "Deck of Deflection," and in the tweet on page 180, Food Babe skillfully employs the "Liar, Liar" generalization.

Food Babe has frequently courted controversy and has her fair share of detractors, some of whom have written unfounded and plain nasty things about her on Twitter, Facebook, and around the web in general. They are, thankfully, in the minority but that doesn't stop Food Babe from using hyperbole to make a point.

In contrast, there are a large number of people now committed to exposing the lies and fear-mongering that Food Babe delivers at almost every turn. This book was born from a need to discuss the methods she employs in more detail than Internet media allows for.

> My friend is being attacked, threatened, cyber-bullied and harassed because of her recent critical work in exposing Monsanto's glyphosate in popular food products that children eat. Unfortunately, I know all too well what's happening to her because it's happening to me too. This is why I think it's absolutely critical for us to stick together and not be afraid to tell the truth. These bullies want to intimidate us into submission. They want us to be too scared to write, investigate and share our findings. So scared, that we quit. [12]

Glyphosate is produced by a large number of companies. The last relevant patent expired in 2000, but tag a hated mega corporation in there and you're engaging the *Reductio ad Monsantoum* fallacy, which is enormously effective.

---

12   http://foodbabe.com/2015/02/12/dirty-pr-campaign/

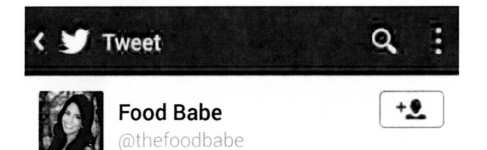

Another baseless allegation now removed from the twitter feed. (Food Babe/Twitter)

She knows that unless the companies bend to her will she can keep up the pressure until they do, and then stand triumphant on the smoldering remains of the scientific evidence as the company caves in because it's simply too expensive to fight. The sheer mob mentality is perverse in its irony, stating,

> These bullies want to intimidate us into submission. [13]

Every contributor to this book has, at some time, been silenced or attacked by Food Babe, her "moderators" or members of the army for challenging the "truth." This is also an appeal to emotion; playing the victim under pressure from bullies. No one on the side of good science wants to stop people questioning accepted wisdom: science progresses by doing just that. Publishing unfounded, fallacious claims is neither science nor investigation. It's the sort of thing that's going to annoy both science advocates and scientists alike.

To quote that oft-used line from *The Princess Bride*.

---

13   http://foodbabe.com/2015/02/12/dirty-pr-campaign/

"You keep using that word. I don't think it means what you think it means."

Food Babe: we don't want you to quit, we just want you to stop misleading and fear mongering for your own gain, leaving a trail of critical thinking failures for others to clear up!

The PR Men Who Stare at Goats

Food Babe is often vaunted as a one-woman crusade, forcing changes to the food system. The reality is that while some companies have buckled under the pressure of having their switchboards jammed and communications systems overloaded by a tirade of angry (but misinformed) consumers, food technology is a moving target. That doesn't stop Food Babe taking credit wherever and whenever a change is announced.

> The industry is listening to what we want and are making changes—whether they admit it's because of us or not. [14]

This claim is typical of Food Babe's manipulative tactics. Claims like this are very difficult to prove since so many people are involved. Food processes and technologies change all the time and a correlation does not a causation make. In other words, just because someone started a campaign to have a class of coloring removed from food and such a change is subsequently announced, we cannot logically infer that one caused the other. That may have been the reason, it may be product development, or it may be a cheaper alternative was found… there are any number of reasons to consider.

These claims were creating such a stink among scientists, bloggers and others, it was only a matter of time before someone pulled the rug from under Food Babe's feet. As of this writing, the largest salvo so far has come from Yvette d'Entremont, also known as SciBabe. [15] Yvette is a member of the Facebook group Banned By Food Babe [16] and consulted the members there for their favorite Food Babe pseudo-scientific and anti-scientific "gotchas." This resulted in a tough-talking piece that didn't pull punches.

---

14 http://foodbabe.com/category/most-controversial/
15 http://www.scibabe.com
16 https://www.facebook.com/groups/BannedByFoodBabeOpen

You can read it at Gawker.com. [17] Within just days of publication the page had nearly four million views and the fallout reverberated across the wild internet world, being picked up by the online presence of Elle [18] and Cosmopolitan. [19]

This was big. Really big.

For the first time ever, Food Babe's home crowd was starting to take issue with the "sky is falling message." They were finally able to come out and say as much. Hordes of science advocates (and a few trolls) started to overwhelm the Food Babe's Facebook page with sarcastic remarks.

The Food Babe PR machine sprang into action almost immediately and produced a rebuttal that you can read from the links in the quotes.

> I want a safer and healthier food system, and some people want to keep the food system just like it is today—broken, corrupt and full of unregulated food additives and chemicals that only improve the bottom line of food and biotech companies and not our health. This is a desperate attempt to stop the food movement. [20]

Food is a chemical. More specifically, food is full of chemicals. Chemicals can be delicious. As we've already implied, any chemical can be harmful or helpful. It's all a matter of dosage. To suggest than an entire industry comprising millions of people across the world is corrupt is both alarmist and unethical.

All businesses exist to make money for their shareholders or owners – even Food Babe LLC. Food additives are very highly regulated, and this is another case of Food Babe bending the truth for her own ends. Businesses evolve and change according to pressure from their customers—if they don't, they don't last very long.

As for this allusion to the biotech companies, this is another unwarranted swipe with no real substance. It's ironic that improving the health of millions has been a positive force for many biotech discoveries. Golden rice [21]

---

17   ttp://gawker.com/the-food-babe-blogger-is-full-of-shit-1694902226

18   http://www.elle.com/culture/a27692/food-babe-problem/

19   http://www.cosmopolitan.com/health-fitness/news/a38750/food-babe-blog-vani-hari-criticism/

20   http://foodbabe.com/response-to-gawker-the-food-babe-blogger-is-full-of-shit/

21   http://www.goldenrice.org

in particular is designed to reduce the awful consequences of vitamin A deficiency in parts of Asia and Africa where it causes blindness and maternal mortality. Pest resistant crops are similarly useful because they can reduce the requirement for harsh pesticides, and also help reduce dangerous mycotoxin infections that enter plants via pest damage, and subsequently infect consumers: including us.

The claim that "this is a desperate attempt to stop the food movement" [22] is just Food Babe complaining about taking flak herself. Ms. d'Entremont did not take pot shots at any "food movement"; she simply eviscerated Food Babe's most egregious claims: personally. The real danger with Food Babe and her ilk is that this pretense creates a smokescreen through which very real dangers can slip. Just recall that the woman who wants *a safer and healthier food system* [23] also espouses drinking raw milk (in India nonetheless, where raw milk consumption is particularly risky).

Returning to the Food Babe PR Engine—she continues like this:

> There's (sic) plenty of scientists and consumer organizations [24] that back this message and this writer completely ignores the mountains of evidence that synthetic, carcinogenic and neurotoxic insecticides are bad for human health and the environment.

Carcinogens are bad for us—the name means something that can cause cancer—but there are many other factors to consider. Factors such as neurotoxic insecticides. You know that caffeine is a neurotoxic insecticide, right? But sure, this is another straw man argument that's entirely meaningless and should be obvious to anyone.

Gasoline is toxic too, but you don't go around drinking the stuff. Glyphosate, probably the most hated and derided (not to mention, commonplace and broadly safest) herbicide around, is mildly toxic and perhaps even carcinogenic in *large* quantities, but you're not supposed to drink it! IF there is any left on the produce you get in your market, it's easily washed away when you clean your fruits and vegetables as advised. Indeed, according to the Environmental Protection Agency's toxicity values, caffeine is about twenty-five times more toxic than Glyphosate. Again, the dose makes

22 http://foodbabe.com/response-to-gawker-the-food-babe-blogger-is-full-of-shit/
23 http://foodbabe.com/response-to-gawker-the-food-babe-blogger-is-full-of-shit/
24 http://livingmaxwell.com/what-the-media-food-industry-wont-tell-you

the poison and these authors are not giving up their cups of Joe, tea, Diet Mountain Dew, and Diet Coke.

This next quote is unusually large to keep it in context. Quote mining (using selective passages out of context to change their meaning) is another tactic employed by some writers and is one that this writing team has taken steps to avoid:

> My statement that "There is no acceptable level of any chemical to ingest ever" was taken from my book on page 40 from the section regarding ractopamine and growth hormones. My critics took it out of context (after The Atlantic [25] decided to highlight the quote as a side bar). My point was in the context of hormone mimicking chemicals and growth stimulants. Extremely low levels of compounds that mimic hormones work in the body like hormones. That is why I don't believe there is any acceptable level of these chemicals to ingest, ever. Certainly reducing all synthetic, artificial chemicals is best, but it is difficult to avoid each and every one of them in all amounts. [26]

We checked, and this is what she says in The Food Babe Way:

> The Russian consumer protection agency, Rospotrebnadzor, backed a study on ractopamine. In 2014, the agency issued findings showing that eating products with traces of ractopamine leads to an unacceptable level of risk of diseases of the cardiovascular system. This tells me–again–that there is just no acceptable level of any chemical to ingest, ever. [27]

Now let's make sure we have this right. She's clear this was about ractopamine but at the end of this quote, she states, quite clearly and in context:

> *"This tells me–again–that there is just no acceptable level of any chemical to ingest, ever."*

Sorry Food Babe– but your rebuttal holds no water. If we followed this advice to the letter, we'd be dead in a matter of days because everything is a chemical. Clearly, Food Babe doesn't mean any chemical literally. No one could be that daft and still be able to write a coherent sentence. That doesn't

---

25   http://www.theatlantic.com/health/archive/2015/02/the-food-babe-enemy-of-chemicals/385301/

26   http://foodbabe.com/response-to-gawker-the-food-babe-blogger-is-full-of-shit/

27   The Food Babe Way. p. 40

excuse her claiming one thing and saying another. Accepting a mistake is fine, claiming you didn't and then hoping no one checks is eventually going to come back and haunt you. Just like this:

> Obviously I don't use the word "toxic" to say something will kill you instantly, rather I'm using this term in its common sense and my readers understand that. Sugar is addictive and too much is toxic in the common use of the term. [28]

What precisely is the common sense? Toxic, like carcinogenic, is a very loaded word with a very specific meaning. If either of these words has a less invidious meaning in common parlance, we'd love to know what they are. The *Oxford Dictionary of English* defines it (in this context):

> Poisonous: *the dumping of toxic waste | alcohol is **toxic to** the ovaries.*
>
> - relating to or caused by poison: toxic hazards | toxic liver injury.
> - very bad, unpleasant, or harmful: a toxic relationship.

and to be thorough, here's the definition of *carcinogen* also from the Oxford:

> a substance capable of causing cancer in living tissue.

So whichever way you cut this, there is no way Food Babe can rightfully deny her gaffe. Toxic things are poisonous and we all know that poisons are bad for us. So either Food Babe has:

(a) been using some internalized definition of toxic all the time and assumed we're all on the same page or

(b) knows exactly what she was doing and has been caught red-handed with her fingers in the cookie jar. Again.

---

28   http://foodbabe.com/response-to-gawker-the-food-babe-blogger-is-full-of-shit/

The Fear Babe

To reiterate, any chemical is toxic in the right dose and administered in the right way; but the chemicals we're exposed to in our food and drink are regulated in such a way that they are not toxic. Caffeine will wake you up in the morning, but get too much of it and it will kill you just as quickly as a dose of arsenic.

Food scientists know this, and we suspect Food Babe knows it too. But telling someone that it's ok to drink a Starbucks Grande Latte isn't going to make you any money. Scaring the hell out of them over the same drink? Show me the money!

Now for the news: read by Straw Man

> Organic crops cannot be grown with synthetic pesticides, and contain much lower pesticide residues overall. [29]

The second half of this statement, from her blog post claiming to explain the difference between organic and conventional farming, is demonstrably silly, and it's fairly clear Food Babe has not spent much (if any) time with farmers, despite the Kansas Farm Bureau and other farms' gracious invitations to take Ms. Hari on farm visits. Farmers who don't use pesticides, herbicides, fungicides, etc. will go out of business. Rapidly. The idea of a farmer with his weathered skin and rolled up sleeves tilling the earth in some rural idyll is the stuff of fantasy and perhaps distant history.

Organic farming is a big business, accounting for $35.1 billion [30] in 2014, a rise of 11% on the previous year, and slated to grow to over $60 billion in the US alone by 2017. In business, the aim is to make money, not throw it away. A failed crop is a crop you can't sell. Unfortunately, farmers can't stand in the field waving their arms, hoping the pests won't descend and ruin everything. Pesticides are a must, and "organic" pesticides are, in many cases, worse for the environment than their synthetic equivalents.

What people don't seem to get is how dangerous mycotoxins (poisons produced by molds) are. If organic farmers truly didn't use some amount of insecticide and fungicide on their affected crops, the chances of mycotoxin residue ending up in the food supply are very real indeed. Aflatoxins,

---

29   http://foodbabe.com/2015/02/26/difference-between-organic-non-gmo-labels/
30   https://www.ota.com/what-ota-does/market-analysis

for example, are common in grain and can pass through the cattle and end up in the milk produced for human consumption. Aflatoxin B is one of the most potent hepatocarcinogens (causing cancer of the liver) known to man.

Big organic agricultural concerns rely on this cute idea of local produce with "no man-made pesticides" as a USP (unique selling point) but the reality is that it's little different from its more evolved cousin, conventional agriculture. If anything, some organic potions are more dangerous to the environment and other life than ones created in labs.

The difference is, people like Food Babe profit from promoting the organic ones.

■

7

Fear and
Loathing of GMOs

"So much of the public is clueless, paranoid, and knows nothing about basic biology. This is why folks like US-RTK must silence and intimidate scientists. If anyone learns, they lose their power to influence them." [1] *Kevin Folta, PhD.*

The great GMO debate rages on. In this chapter we're going to look at what GMO is and what it's not. As of publication, none of the writing team work for any corporation developing GMOs for market. This book was inspired entirely in response to Food Babe's quest to make money by terrifying an already misinformed and fearful public.

A GMO, short for Genetically Modified Organism, is a living thing that has been modified slightly to give it an improved feature or function that already occurs in nature. Often the trait comes from a related organism. Food Babe describes the process thus:

> Genetic modification occurs when genes, viruses, or bacteria from one organism are artificially injected into a fruit or vegetable in a process that occurs in a laboratory and not in nature. [2]

While an awful number of people believe this to be the case, the idea that something is injected into a plant on animal with some kind of hypodermic syringe is utterly preposterous. Opinions differ as to whether a virus is a living thing or not because it consists primarily of DNA or RNA, but is itself made up of genes. Viruses are special because they live inside other organisms, including bacteria. Regardless of the technical description, this isn't how genetic modification, which is achieved by a number of methods,

---

1   http://kfolta.blogspot.com/2015/02/this-is-what-we-are-up-against.html
2   The Food Babe Way, p. 27

is performed. It's just plain wrong. Injecting a live virus or similar pathogen willy-nilly into another living organism is likely to make it sick and die: assuming it has any effect at all.

> Genetic modification is done to make a fruit or vegetable more hardy or impervious to the application specific pesticide. These pesticides are linked to myriad diseases. [3]

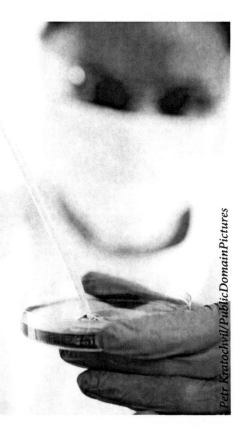

Petr Kratochvil/PublicDomainPictures

That's partly true at least, except the part about pesticides and disease. It's true that pesticides may cause ill health at very high doses because they are, by nature, toxic, but this has nothing to do with GM technology. Crucially, the amount of pesticide residue consumers are exposed to is far too low to cause harm.

> We have a right to know what's in our food just like people in countries like China and Russia do–especially when studies have linked GMOs to a wide variety of diseases like infertility and cancer. [4]

Gee. That sounds bad and such studies do exist. But just because someone writes a paper doesn't necessarily make it true. Scientists work outside of their field, experiments are badly designed, and rarely, people flat out lie.

Take, for example, her claim that GMOs are linked to infertility. We believe that she's referring to a study linking glyphosate to male infertility, though the link is weak if not non-existent. *"Roundup: The sneaky and cheap contraceptive hiding in your food."* a 2013 headline from *Natural News* declared

---

3   The Food Babe Way, p. 27

4   http://anokhimedia.com/magazine/q-a-with-vani-hari-the-food-babe

about the study. Then again, *Natural News* is infamous for fudging science at best, and at worst, actually making stuff up.

The study in question was an *in vitro* rat study, and its conclusions in no way demonstrate that glyphosate in our food causes infertility. The results showed that "*acute Roundup exposure at low doses (36 ppm, 0.036 g/L) for 30 min induces oxidative stress and activates multiple stress-response pathways leading to Sertoli cell death in prepubertal rat testis.*" [5]

Crucially, the study wasn't done on live rats, it was done on rat testiclular cells in culture. And the most important part? 36 ppm (parts per million) is way higher than the typical residues found on crops, around one ppm. Suffice it to say, don't pour Roundup on your genitalia guys, though even that would be unlikely to render you infertile. If you want sterility, stick with a vasectomy. And ladies, keep your IUDs, pills, implants, and other birth control.

No matter how you look at this, we know that every living thing on the planet contains a unique blueprint called genes. Genes are essentially instructions that tell the organism how to build itself into a complete, working offspring of its parent(s). Be it plant, animal or fungus, we all have genes.

Vertical GMOs

At the simplest level, genes travel vertically from generation to generation. You got your genes from your parents, they got theirs from their parents, and so on. This is sexual reproduction and occurs in all but the simplest of creatures. (Yes, even plants reproduce sexually.)

We don't usually think of plants mating but in biological terms they usually have male and female organs just like animals. The difference between a plant and an animal is how the material is transferred. Animals need no explanation, but plants rely almost entirely on everything from insects to the wind for fertilization.

Very simple organisms such as bacteria have been shown to transfer genes from another species (horizontal gene transfer or HGT), allowing them to develop new traits more rapidly than by random mutations. Although first

---

5   http://www.ncbi.nlm.nih.gov/pubmed/23820267

described in 1951, it's still an active area of research outside the scope of this book and is something you might wish to explore for yourself.

Genetic engineering mimics this natural process by horizontally transferring genetic material in higher organisms.

Humans have been modifying plants and even animals for millennia using a painfully slow process of selection, and selective breeding, and more recently hybridization, wide-cross hybridization (in which genes from "unrelated" species are forced into a plant) and mutagenesis. None of these methods result in what regulatory agencies or industry call GMOs, though we would argue that they're all very much genetically modified. The best example of this is our canine cousin, the pet dog.

Selective breeding has given us a broad range of breeds—over 330 generally recognized by the *Fédération Cynologique Internationale* (the World Canine Organization) with more being added periodically.

All modern dogs in their mixed up range of shapes, sizes and skills are the result of selective breeding. This includes the terriers that catch rats, collies that round up sheep and labradors working as gun dogs, retrieving fallen game birds for their master, etc.

Plants too, have been modified by selectively breeding and cross breeding the strains we desire. Wild carrots were a deep purple before the Dutch started selecting the paler shades and eventually creating the common orange color we see today.

This genetic "modification" by vertical gene transfer (sexual reproduction) is a clumsy process prone to failure, which makes it slow and difficult. Plants like root vegetables may take a year or two to bear fruit. Trees, on the other hand, typically require far more time. Even when you have created a strain you're happy with you still have to make sure it's stable and capable of reproduction.

Over time, the breeding process can create inbred varieties, with very predictable traits. Certain corn strains have very regular characteristics, the same way a dalmatian has black spots on white fur. Though inbred strains are predictable, they can be prone to health problems. Plant and animal breeders alike will mate two different inbred strains to mitigate these problems and create a more robust offspring. Like a "puggle" is a cross between a pug and a beagle, plant breeders will cross inbred strains of corn to make a more robust crop. Though the crop might be stronger, it is also less predictable. Our Kavin jokingly calls it "slamming two inbred genomes together willy nilly." This process, typically called hybridization, is a very simple form of genetic modification. We don't call it that because the mechanism could (in theory) happen in nature all by itself. We just help it along a little: lead it by the nose if you like.

Modern molecular GMO technologies use microsurgical-precision to move just single instructions, rather than less focused methodology, and herein lies the fear and confusion. It sounds like scientists are playing God. Before you know it, we're presented an image of the fictional Baron Victor Von Frankenstein creating his vile monster from the body parts of deceased victims.

It's a powerful concept and it couldn't be more wrong.

Would the Real Dr. Frankenstein, Please Stand Up?

Genetic modification doesn't take parts of a plant and graft it on to other plants although, ironically, humans have been doing this for over 2,500 years, and no one bats an eyelid! [6]

If you have a rose bush in your garden, particularly if it's store bought, there's a very good chance that its root system doesn't belong to it and was grafted on to support the flowering bush we enjoy.

Just like Victor Frankenstein, folks!

Professional growers do this because rootstocks are easy to produce, and the pretty flowers we want are easier to grow on a rootstock. One parent plant can produce many clones—branches that can be easily grafted to the easily grown rootstocks. This is particularly useful for shrubs and trees that don't breed true, are hard to breed, or have poor roots that won't tolerate poorer quality ground.

There's a practical reason for this when it comes to plants such as fruit trees. Trees grown from a seed (such as an apple pip) take many years—often decades—to mature sufficiently to bear fruit. However, take some

6   Mudge, K., Janick, J., Scofield, S., Goldschmidt, E.E., A History of Grafting, Horticultural Reviews, Volume 35, 2009

easily grown rootstocks and graft mature, fruit bearing branches (called scions) and you have a productive plant within a year or two. Another technique (there are many) derived from grafting is to create self-pollinating trees–and even decorative trees– from many variant species.

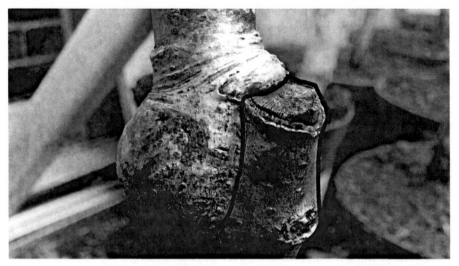

Grafting in action. We've outlined the root stock to make it easier to see. This graft is already well vascularized where the mature cutting connects to the rooted donor.

Some disease resistance can be created with the correctly selected rootstock. For example *Meloidogyne* (the root knot nematode) affects around 2,000 different species including peaches; closterovirus causes CTV in citrus and *Erwinia Amylovora* is the bacteria responsible for fire blight in apples and pears. Indeed, fire blight spreads so rapidly, it can destroy entire orchards before the appropriate treatments can be administered.

These chimera-like organisms share a vascular system, but they are not capable of interbreeding because their DNA (their genotypes) are so different. While this is much closer to Shelley's fictional doctor, the organism is never artificially resurrected by electricity or any other strange voodoo. If this is what scares you about GMOs, you can rest easy, because grafting isn't considered a GM technique. But Dr. Frankenstein? He was and is the stuff of fiction.

Read The F-F-Friendly Manual

Genes are what makes you you; a complete set of instructions on how to create and sustain a living thing from scratch. Using these instructions, your body can repair itself as parts wear out.

Your skin, for example, is a layer of dead tissue that constantly sheds itself as new skin is created just under the surface. The pink, sensitive stuff that appears when you scrape your knee or elbow is living skin—the largest organ in your body.

Your unique genetic makeup was created when the egg that was destined to become half of you fused with the sperm that was destined to become the other half.

Those instructions are still there in almost every cell in your body. In the future, we may be able to take a single cell and grow another you: a clone. However, the world's most famous clone, Dolly the Sheep, proved that cloning is rather more difficult than we had anticipated. [7]

Cloning long-dead creatures is the stuff of science fiction, with Spielberg's Jurassic Park representing the fictional pinnacle of what might be possible in the future. Right now, no one has managed to find enough DNA from an extinct creature to even attempt to grow one from scratch.

DNA in a genome is an instruction book like the directions in a kit of parts; not so much a thing as instructions on *how to make* the thing.

To put this into perspective, let's imagine you're making a cake—a nice easy Victoria sponge; light, quick and simple.

We have the following ingredients available:

Eggs, self-rising flour, plain flour, caster sugar, butter, cocoa powder and vanilla essence.

To make a simple sponge cake:

1. Blend together the 4oz/100g butter and 4oz/100g sugar

2. Beat in two eggs

3. Fold in the 4oz/100g flour

7   http://www.roslin.ed.ac.uk/public-interest/dolly-the-sheep/a-life-of-dolly/

4. Place in a 8" cake tray

5. Bake in an oven at 220°C/Gas 7/425°F for 20-30 mins.

It's that simple. DNA creates a set of instructions that tell the ingredients how to assemble themselves. The result of this experiment is a rather burnt sponge cake. It's edible but not very good.

To explain how evolution (or selective breeding and vertical gene transfer) works, imagine that the recipe has to be passed on to someone else, perhaps over a bad telephone connection and something goes slightly amiss at step 5.

Bake in an oven at 180°C/Gas 4/350°F for 20-30 minutes.

This is pretty neat—by complete accident we've discovered how to make a better cake—and we pass that information around to all our friends and they make better cakes. This version survives and becomes the accepted norm because it's better. This form of selection created our wide variety of dogs (from their native wolf—*Canis lupus*—ancestors) and even orange-colored carrots (to name two examples).

Another page in the recipe book contains instructions to make delicious fudge brownies using plain flour, sugar, vanilla and cocoa powder. Some of the ingredients are the same, others are not.

Now imagine that we like the taste of chocolate (from the cocoa powder) but we want it in a cake. It's not a great leap of imagination to deduce that you add the cocoa powder to the Victoria sponge and, hey presto, chocolate cake.

So the instructions now read:

1. Blend together the 4oz/100g fat and 4oz/100g sugar

2. Beat in two eggs

3. Fold in the 4oz/100g flour

4. Fold in 30g/1oz of cocoa powder.

5. Place in an 8" cake tray

6. Bake in an oven at 180°C/Gas 4/350°F for 20-30 minutes.

Voilà, we've got ourselves chocolate cake (and we're hungry).

That remarkable change occurs because we've added a single instruction from a different recipe.

At the most basic level, this is what genetic modification does. Lift away the curtain of ignorance and fear-mongering and what you're left with is an uncomplicated, rather bland reality behind this breakthrough technology. Truly, it's not that big of a deal. If it were, the authors, scientists, farmers and other experts wouldn't feed GM ingredients to their children.

Achieving this in reality is a lot harder—and that's the soup where the crazy unscientific ideas are allowed to thrive. Luddites (people who are so afraid of change they want to go backwards) and people with vested interests are keen to sabotage these developments.

If we look back through history, much of what we accept today without so much as a second thought was at one time regarded with fear and derision. People are resistant to change and the Internet has bestowed the ability to spread terror to millions without ever leaving their office.

Fahrenheit 451

In Ray Bradbury's 1953 science fiction vision of a dystopian future, firemen destroy prohibited books. The title supposedly alludes to the temperature at which paper burns. Animals fear what they cannot understand. That's why most animals flee from fire. We widely agree that harnessing fire is one of the things that gave us an advantage. Like other animals, we fear the technologies we don't understand—particularly if they are couched in obtuse language. Bradbury writes, almost prophetically:

> *"If you hide your ignorance, no one will hit you and you'll never learn."—Fahrenheit 451*

Organizations like US Right To Know and Moms Across America promote the idea that GM is bad, but none of them can clearly explain why. They want to terrify you with bogus stories of deadly toxins produced by innocent plants when GM has gone horribly wrong. They want to "burn the books" and prevent you from acquiring the knowledge to make an informed decision.

They don't want you to know just how beautifully simple GM techniques are, or how much good they're doing and have the potential to do.

Since their introduction into the food chain, GM technologies have been directly implicated in precisely zero deaths or poisonings. The same cannot be said for organic farming. As recently as 2011, an outbreak of listeria claimed the lives of 33 people and sickened many more– the largest case of food poisoning in the USA since 1924. The farmers responsible, brothers Ryan and Eric Jensen, had contaminated cantaloupe melons by poor hygiene in their processing facilities. USA Today quotes [8] the FDA as saying this is:

> "..the latest illustration of the continuing need for a strong food-safety program."

Traditional agriculture has a stake in agricultural biotechnology because it allows for greater profits and better management of difficult problems such as pests, disease, and waste. The organic movement is vested in preserving the *status quo,* and in charging a premium for lower efficiency. Like the original saboteurs, they're looking to throw a metaphoric clog into biotechnology's works.

Pesticide resistant plant strains that produce their own insecticides against common pests aren't created at random. They are carefully designed and reduce, not increase, the use of man-made pesticides, by letting the plants do the heavy lifting. Paradoxically, this creates plants that are even more organic than organic farmers could dream of. Many plants are naturally toxic to some pests: potatoes and the coffee plant, for example. Remember our discussion of caffeine toxicity? Yep, it's an insecticide.

This anti-GM campaign has done so much harm it's given the proverbial dog a bad name. In the short term at least, people live in fear that plants are going to do them harm and that natural is somehow better.

But here's the thing: no matter how you believe we (life) got here, there are a lot of plants out there that can either make you seriously ill or even kill you, and the vast majority of what we eat is far from "natural." We've even harnessed some of the toxins to produce useful medicines. The dose makes the poison—or the remedy. Ask yourself: what benefit is there to any large

---

8   http://www.usatoday.com/story/news/nation/2014/01/28/sentencing-of-colorado-cantaloupe-farmers/4958671/

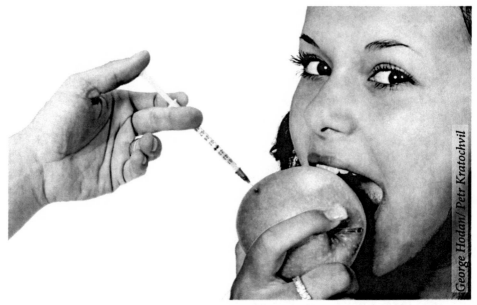

The idea that GM is performed by injection is a powerful (entirely false) concept, often promoted using deeply emotional images relying on the fear of vaccination. In reality, a GM organism is indistinguishable because it simply bypasses millions of years of evolution.

biotech corporation in killing us all off? What possible good is that going to do?

The counter-argument here points to the tobacco industry. "Look," the naysayers protest, "big tobacco has been killing people for years, and yet no one stops them!"

This is an example of a straw man fallacy. It sounds plausible, but the comparison isn't accurate. Tobacco, specifically nicotine, is highly addictive. The nicotine delivery system (smoking) is what kills people through the inhalation of multiple other toxins. [9, 10]

Is it possible to make toxic plants? Sure—we only have to isolate the toxin-producing genes from, say rhubarb (oxalic acid), belladonna (atropine) or wolf's bane (aconite and aconitine).

---

9   http://www.cancerresearchuk.org/about-cancer/causes-of-cancer/smoking-and-cancer/how-smoking-causes-cancer
10   http://www.quitsmokingsupport.com/whatsinit.htm

Assuming some crazed scientist thought this would be a good way to murder people, how many people is this going to kill? This is a very convoluted example because it can't happen. But let's assume that it did.

Accidental poisoning from plants is quite rare. We evolved a taste sensation (bitter) that detects many forms of poison, so we tend to spit these things out at first bite. Plant-produced toxins taste nasty, so accidental poisoning of this kind is rare. It's this very taste sensation that causes children to turn their noses up at vegetables like broccoli and sprouts.

Real poisoners have to get close enough to their victims to adulterate their food. Or, at least, to get the poison into their system. Products like ricin (derived from the castor plant) are entirely natural. The most potent toxin known to man is produced by nothing more than a simple bacteria, *Clostridium botulinum*. The nasty little bug creates the botulinum protein that could (conceivably) be inserted into a food organism. This sounds terrifying, and could perhaps be the plot of a blockbuster movie.

Assume a scientist was able to insert the correct genes, managed to bypass the checks and balances that GM food has to go through and got this stuff into our fields... so we find our farmers growing botulinum-laced strawberries!

It sounds like a nightmare scenario, but the reality is rather dull.

The first few innocent people to try the fruit would get sick quite rapidly and the source discovered within hours. Mass poisoning through food is the stuff of bad science fiction and (unfortunately) websites that promote organic products, lifestyles, etc.

Just like the snake-oil salesmen of yesteryear, we want to buy solutions to the problems we didn't even know we had. Telling people GM food is safe to consume isn't going to make Food Babe rich. But repeating poor-quality research and ignoring the hard facts? Now that's a different story!

Give my apologies to Shakespeare

> *Alas, poor Ratty! I knew him, Horatio; a fellow of infinite jest, of most excellent fancy... He suffered the most terrible fate and did die of the neoplasms.*

Aside from massacring Hamlet, what's not generally known outside of animal research is inbred lab rats, like the Sprague–Dawley and Lewis rat, are known to suffer terribly with cancer. Lewis rats are albino (white fur, pink eyes) and therefore quite easy to spot. There are at least 20 other similarly inbred rats in general use, and many are extremely prone to developing tumors.

Since rats are prone to cancer this makes them extremely useful for studying the disease –and particularly useful for a researcher with an axe to grind! Here's a sample of the more common tumors these creatures commonly develop. [11]

- *Keratoacanthomas*: *skin tumors found on the back, chest, and tail.*
- *Mammary Adenocarcinomas*: *a breast cancer that, because of the rat's unusual physiology, can occur anywhere on the animal's underside,*
- *Mammary Fibroadenomas:* *a form of breast cancer found in both genders.*
- *Pituitary tumors*: *found mainly in females and causes rapid death.*
- *Testicular tumors*: *in the testes of male rats.*
- *Zymbal's tumors*: *a rare form usually found in older rats.*

As with cancers in humans, cancer has the potential to spread if not treated (metastasis) but does not always kill the animal.

This is not to say that we can't use rats to study cancer (we can, and we do), but some researchers have claimed that rats given GM food have developed cancer, as if the GM food had something to do with that. (Much the same can be applied to carcinogenic effects from any compound; rats are a poor experimental model if not selected with care.)

GM isn't an inherent threat to organic agriculture, but it's been perceived as such by some vocal groups within its ranks and they have attempted to sabotage the science at every step. Ironically, since GM improves crops and reduces pesticide use, it benefits all of us. One of the most aggressive anti-GMO papers "*Long term toxicity of a Roundup herbicide and a Roundup-tolerant genetically modified maize*" [12] by Gilles-Eric Séralini and colleagues

---

11   http://www.cldavis.org/cgi-bin/download.cgi?pid=788
12   http://www.sciencedirect.com/science/article/pii/S0278691512005637

became known as the Séralini Affair, and was broadly panned for being wrong.

Not just a *little* wrong; but *a complete whitewash,* not unlike the MMR scandal led by Andrew Wakefield several decades earlier. [13]

As Jon Entine notes in a 2014 Forbes article:

> *"If Séralini's data were real and 80% of food was poison, animals and people would be dropping like flies."* [14]

Séralini's problem was in experimental design, as is often the case, and not a deliberate fraud as Wakefield perpetrated, at least initially. In this case, it was found that a major concern was with the breed of rats used, which are known to be prone to tumors. As the investigating editor notes in the retraction:

> *"Given the known high incidence of tumors in the Sprague–Dawley rat, normal variability cannot be excluded as the cause of the higher mortality and incidence observed in the treated groups."* [15]

So every time you see a website claiming that "weird sounding chemical" gave this rat cancer, ask yourself this: did it really?

Here's Food Babe in spectacularly hypocritical and self-serving form:

> GMOs don't benefit customers, just the biotech industry's pockets. [16]

Really? Just whose pockets is Food Babe benefiting with the constant battery of misinformation? Things look awfully different when you step outside of the goldfish bowl. Food Babe is making huge amounts of money exploiting the natural fear people have of the things they don't understand. Ignorance is a big money-spinner if you can keep one step ahead of your public—and keep them in the dark. Once you have them scared, you can emerge as a leader in the fight against this fictional threat. Senator Joe

---

13   http://geneticliteracyproject.org/glp-facts/gilles-eric-sralini/

14   http://www.forbes.com/sites/jonentine/2014/09/17/the-debate-about-gmo-safety-is-over-thanks-to-a-new-trillion-meal-study/

15   http://www.sciencedirect.com/science/article/pii/S0278691512005637

16   http://foodbabe.com/2015/02/12/dirty-pr-campaign/

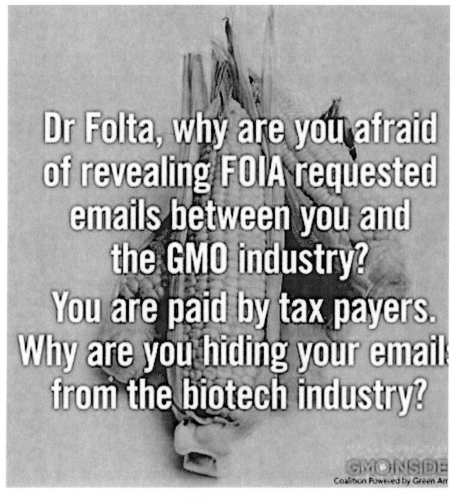

This misjudged piece nearly landed GMO Inside in hot water by pointing fingers and was rapidly deleted, but not before a fair amount of damage had been done. (GMOInside/ Facebook)

*Dr. Folta had **nothing** to hide, but this posturing made it look like he did.*

McCarthy employed a similar leverage to further his political career in the 1940s and 50s.

Food Babe claims to have demonstrated twice at the 2012 Democratic convention in North Carolina, first:

> To bring attention to this issue, during Michelle Obama's speech, I whipped out my lipstick, a shade called True Blood, and marked the back of my program in big, bold letters: LABEL GMOs! [17]

Infamously (and, frankly, rather rudely), repeating the same stunt interrupting Tom Vilsack, Secretary of Agriculture, as he took the stage:

> Within 20 seconds cameras besieged me," she says. "I mean, completely took the focus off of his speech and completely besieged me. I was on C-SPAN, and people were writing on my Facebook page. 'Oh, my God! Food Babe's protesting at the Democratic National Convention.' It was crazy. [18]

Curiously, it was this second piece of self-promotion that is so widely preserved: an attractive woman holding these hastily made signs was sure to hit the headlines.

> For the rest of the convention, a dedicated security guard watched over me, and they banished me to the back row, a punishment that was well worth it in my eyes. If a convention isn't the time to speak up and stand up for your rights, I don't know what is! [19]

Ah, the old, "*Stand up for your rights*," cliché. Food Babe isn't standing up for a right; she's shamelessly promoting her personal agenda, and it is working brilliantly. From her gleeful re-telling of the story, it's apparent to us she enjoyed her moment in the media glare.

She's not the only one to use aggressive PR stunts.

The biotech industry is big business. It can only make money by creating products that people want to buy. It's not rocket science to understand that if people don't benefit from GMOs, they won't buy it and they go out of business. However, some parts of the *organic* industry (also big business) are happy to create a climate of fear when conventional advertising isn't working.

---

17 The Food Babe Way, p. 27
18 http://articles.mercola.com/sites/articles/archive/2013/07/07/van-hari-food-babe.aspx
19 The Food Babe Way, p. 27

The Fear Babe

On February 20th 2015, GMO Inside, a well-organized and active anti-GMO lobby group, shared a since-deleted hysterical post on Facebook. GMO Inside describes itself as such:

> GMO Inside is a new coalition of businesses and organizations that are launching the biggest safe food campaign ever. It's designed to capture people's energy from the fight for Prop 37 in California and to catapult it to the next level, bringing greater awareness to the public about GMOs and the right to know.

Its mission statement is patently wrong in science terms:

> "GMOs, or "genetically modified organisms," are plants or animals created through the gene splicing techniques of biotechnology (also called genetic engineering, or GE). This experimental technology merges DNA from different species, creating unstable combinations of plant, animal, bacterial and viral genes that cannot occur in nature or in traditional crossbreeding. We want to see GMOs labeled and ultimately removed from the food system."

Molecular genetic engineering technologies aren't experimental, they are highly specialized, and are no less safe or 'natural' than varieties created by other means. Indeed, the term 'unstable' here is misleading. 'Stability' isn't a good way to describe plants. They have shown themselves to be enormously useful both in reducing pesticide use and improving health and wellbeing across the globe. All GMOs available on the market are completely safe. Additionally, crossbreeding is not at all the only breeding technique used to create so called non-GMO crops. Radiation and chemical mutagenics, wide-cross hybrids, and chemically-induced polyploids can be sold as non-GMO or organic. And if those techniques' names sound unnatural, it's because they are. People who have money invested in competitive businesses don't want you to know that.

Ironically, the businesses behind these advocacy groups seem to miss the fact the knife cuts both ways. You can't go around slagging off commercial (non-organic) agriculture and pretend you're different. A pressure group is a pressure group, regardless of where its funding is coming from. If you're an anti-GMO pressure group funded by the organic and natural food industries, then you are, in very real terms, a shill.

Alongside the February 2015 image above, GMO Inside made argumentative, defamatory and potentially libellous claims against a professor known for his tireless dedication to public education and the public's understanding of science.

> "*US Right To Know is attempting via FOIA requests to understand the work professors such as Kevin Folta AKA "Monsanto activist" did for Ketchum, as well as agrochemical companies Monsanto, Syngenta, Bayer, BASF, DuPont and Dow; trade groups like the Grocery Manufacturers Association, the Biotechnology Industry Organization, and other PR firms like Fleishman Hillard and Ogilvy & Mather to shape the public dialog. Professors are public employees. They are paid by the taxpayers to work for the public good; their university affiliations give them the status of "independent" experts, and they are often quoted in the media as independent experts. #stopmonsanto #food #GMOs #nonGMO*"

Dr. Folta's (prohetic) response follows after the rather paranoid and grandiose letter from USRTK reproduced in full on page 215.

USRTK expanded its search using further FOI requests but, after trawling through thousands of pages of emails, it found one that appeared be a smoking gun: a $25,000 grant from the Monsanto company to be used in any way he saw fit.

That was all it needed to know: a transfer of funds from a hated corporation right into Dr. Folta's hand and so the USRTK's PR machine went to work without apparently questioning where the funds went or what they were for. All that served USRTK's agenda was an exchange of money between Monstanto and their nemesis, Dr. Kevin Folta.

> "*Real knowledge is to know the extent of one's ignorance.*" - *Confucius*

So let's shine a light into these murky dealings.

Thanks to the open nature of publicly funded institutions like the University of Florida, it's entirely possible that USRTK already knew about the donation but chose to hold back so it could claim to find something hidden in the closet making it sound like a bribe, surreptitiously passed under a

Part IV	List of Officers, Directors, Trustees, and Key Employees (list each one even if not compensated—see the instructions for Part IV)				
	Check if the organization used Schedule O to respond to any question in this Part IV . . . . ☐				
(a) Name and title	(b) Average hours per week devoted to position	(c) Reportable compensation (Forms W-2/1099-MISC) (if not paid, enter -0-)	(d) Health benefits, contributions to employee benefit plans, and deferred compensation	(e) Estimated amount of other compensation
Juliet Schor				
Chair, board of directors	1	0	0	0
Lisa Graves				
Member, board of directors	1	0	0	0
Charlie Cray				
Member, board of directors	2	0	0	0
Gary Ruskin				
Executive Director	40	22479.09	0	0

Of the staff at USRTK in the 2014 return, only Gary Ruskin is listed as receiving any compensation and has done the lion's share of the work.

table, which is far more damaging than finding it out in the open for all to see. As Dr. Folta writes:

> *"It never was a secret. At universities, our records are public, and people know where our funding is from. You can probably find it online if you look hard enough, but just ask and I'm glad to tell you about who sponsors my research or who sponsors my outreach."* [20]

In a statement made as recently as August 10, 2015, Dr. Folta stated that not only had the payment gone to the university but it was to fund a 12-event educational outreach program. By that date only $9,000 had been used.

Even if the guest speakers at the three-to-four hour events had not been paid, there were still numerous, quite legitimate, expenses to cover such as taxis and hotel bills: not to mention refreshments.

What appears to be happening here is a underhanded PR trick called *exclusionary detailing (see page 335)*. This means you tell the truth but omit anything that aids clarification. Once it's clear that the money (in this case) wasn't hidden or for some devilish research, the story loses all traction.

USRTK is keen to flourish its stated aim which is: [21]

> *U.S. Right to Know is a new nonprofit organization, working to expose what the food industry doesn't want us to know.*

---

20 http://kfolta.blogspot.co.uk/2015/08/contributions-funding-and-outreach.html
21 http://usrtk.org/about/

We do research and communications on the failures of the corporate food system. We stand up for the right to know what is in our food, and how it affects our health.

We unearth the political economy of our food system, and how big food companies buy political influence in a quest for profit that has led to an epidemic of food-related diseases.

We believe that transparency – in the marketplace and in politics – is crucial to building a better, healthier food system.

We believe that, together, we can create a food system that makes us healthy and strong, one that works better for all of us, our children, families, other loved ones, communities and our nation.

Laudable indeed, and one might expect this organization to be helmed and staffed by nutritionists, biologists and other experts in food science. Unfortunately, quite the opposite is true - the following biographies are edited slightly (for space) but comprise the salient details of the minds running USRTK. The complete details are available at the USRTK website. [22] Some details here are from the IRS filings available here. [23]

US Right To Know Staff

Gary Ruskin:

In 2012, Gary was campaign manager for California Right to Know (Proposition 37), a statewide ballot initiative for labeling of genetically engineered food in California. For fourteen years, he directed the Congressional Accountability Project, which opposed corruption in the U.S. Congress. For nine years, he was executive director and co-founder (with Ralph Nader) of Commercial Alert, which opposed the commercialization of every nook and cranny of our lives and culture. He received his undergraduate degree in religion from Carleton College, and a master's degree in public policy from Harvard University's John F. Kennedy School of Government".

Stacy Malkan:

In 2012, Stacy was media director for the historic California Right

---

22   http://usrtk.org/about/
23   http://usrtk.org/wp-content/uploads/2015/06/2014-IRS-990.pdf

to Know ballot initiative to label genetically engineered foods, and she is the former communications director for Health Care Without Harm, which got mercury out of hospitals and closed down medical waste incinerators around the world. Prior to her work as an environmental health activist, Stacy worked as a journalist and published an investigative newspaper.

USRTK's Board of Directors

Juliet Schor, Chair

Juliet Schor is Professor of Sociology at Boston College. Before joining Boston College, she taught at Harvard University for 17 years, in the Department of Economics and the Committee on Degrees in Women's Studies. A graduate of Wesleyan University, Schor received her Ph.D. in economics at the University of Massachusetts.

Charlie Cray

Charlie has been a member of Greenpeace USA's research department since 2010. Between 1989 and 1999, he also worked with Greenpeace as a member of the Greenpeace Toxics Campaign, organizing campaigns to shut down toxic waste incinerators and phase out PVC plastics.

Lisa Graves

Lisa is executive director of the Center for Media and Democracy. She has served as a senior advisor in all three branches of the federal government and other posts.

She has also worked as a leading strategist on civil liberties advocacy in the area of national security and as an adjunct law professor at one of the top law schools in the country.

Not food scientists, nor RDs, not even biologists… These are clearly driven and intelligent people but are they really interested in food safety as defined by actual experts or food safety as defined by vested interests?

According to its own website (which does not disclose donations below $5000) the single largest benefactor for USRTK is the Organic Consumers Association: which has (so far) donated $114,500.

So USRTK is funded, at least in part, by an association which is directly opposed to genetic engineering which, to put it mildly, comes over as something of a conflict of interests. Particularly as its stated aims include:

- A global moratorium on genetically engineered foods and crops.
- The conversion of American agriculture to at least 30% organic by the year 2015, including major reforms in agricultural subsidies and appropriations to help family farmers make the transition to organic, develop local and regional markets, and adopt renewable energy practices.

In practice this means that an organization intending to shut down agricultural genetic engineering food is supporting USRTK. Further, while the Monsanto grant was demonstrably used to further education, USRTK specifically targets experts for its own agenda.

Food Babe notes of this story (also alluding to Dr. Folta) in this quote from 12 February 2012 (coincidentally the same day as Gary Ruskin's letter to Dr. Folta):

> If you are not following U.S. Right To Know (USRTK) on Twitter, please do here – they are doing some great things and really need our support! They just filed a Freedom of Information Request for correspondence from science professors employed in public universities who write for the GMO Answers which is a website funded by the biotech companies. U.S. Right To Know wants to better understand how these professors (including one that has attacked me personally) are working with biotech companies and PR firms, such as Monsanto, Syngenta, DuPont, Dow, Ketchum, Fleishman Hillard, Ogilvy & Mather. [24]

Further, like Food Babe, the non-experts at USRTK continue to parrot misinformation about aspartame and sucralose using weasel words and vague claims that are not supported by evidence:

> *"Meanwhile, artificial sweeteners such as aspartame (NutraSweet) and sucralose (Splenda) have health risks as well. Aspartame (used in Diet Coke, Diet Pepsi, Diet Dr Pepper and many other popular*

---

24   http://foodbabe.com/2015/02/12/dirty-pr-campaign/

products) appears to cause cancer in laboratory animals, and to make people gain more weight even than eating sugar." [25]

Similarly, its stance on GM consists of hysterical ramblings from ill informed people and does not source any credible scientific information:

"During the last two decades, agrichemical companies have been genetically engineering many of our most important food crops. This fact has been largely kept out of public discourse until recently, when efforts to label genetically engineered food (or GMOs) reached ballot boxes and legislatures across the country. Since 2012, when the first initiative was placed on the ballot in California, the agrichemical and food industries have spent more than $100 million on a vast PR and political campaign to undermine our right to know if our food contains genetically engineered ingredients."

This would be the campaign (California Proposition 37) managed by Gary Ruskin no less.

People are rightly frightened by things they do not understand but knowing something is not the same as understanding it. Knowing that (for example) glyphosate is deadly to plants is not the same as understanding the mechanism by which it operates.

Glyphosate blocks the action of the enzyme (5-enolpyruvoyl-shikimate-3-phosphate synthetase or EPSP) plants need to produce their amino acids *tyrosine, tryptophan*, and *phenylalanine* through the shikimate pathway.

Crucially - we don't produce this enzyme - so glyphosate has no effect on us. Acute toxicity is only achieved through massive, self-administered doses of the pure product.

USRTK doesn't want you to know this. It only wants you to know what suits its agenda. Science is different and while it's often very difficult, the information is readily available and there for the taking. You just have to be careful who you get it from. As of August 2015 USRTK "Sweeteners" list of "key documents" [26] still includes Mark Bitman's long-debunked claims about sugar [27] and many other non-scientific or poor sources.

---

25   http://usrtk.org/sweeteners/

26   http://usrtk.org/sweeteners/

27   http://opinionator.blogs.nytimes.com/2013/02/27/its-the-sugar-folks/

Stacy Malkan similarly tweeted [28] what amounted to lies by omission (exclusionary detailing) over the WHO status of glyphosate.

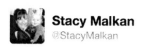

Stacy Malkan
@StacyMalkan

ok, actually astounded by false reporting on @GeneticLiteracy by @ksenapathy - WHO says glyphosate probable carcinogen; she reports opposite

RETWEET FAVORITE
1   1

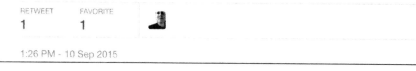

1:26 PM - 10 Sep 2015

Claiming astonishment, Malkan uses typical PR fallacies to paint a cloud of confusion around the safety of glyphosate and to undermine Kavin Senapathy's reputation.

The quote to which Malkan was presumably referring, within Kavin Senapathy's article titled "Anti-GMO activists use FOIA to bully mother-scientist nutrition and lactation expert" [29] reads (emphasis ours):

"The US Environmental Protection Agency, the European Commission and a joint panel of World Health Organization and the Food and Agriculture Organization of the United Nations, … among dozens of global science oversight groups, have determined that glyphosate is mildly toxic to humans, not carcinogenic and perfectly safe *as used by home gardeners and farmers alike.*"

Malkan fails miserably at understanding the difference between hazard analysis and risk assessment, and doesn't seems to grasp the central tenet of toxicology, "the dose makes the poison". The WHO's statement on the difference between "hazard" and "risk" reads as follows:

---

28 https://twitter.com/StacyMalkan/status/642071698481774592 (live Sept. 13 2015)
29 http://www.geneticliteracyproject.org/2015/09/10/anti-gmo-activists-use-foia-to-bully-mother-scientist-nutrition-and-lactation-expert/

"Scientific studies of the potential health effects of hazardous chemicals, such as pesticides, allow them to be classified as carcinogenic (can cause cancer), neurotoxic (can cause damage to the brain), or teratogenic (can cause damage to a fetus). This process of classification, called "hazard identification," is the first step of "risk assessment". An example of hazard identification is the classification of substances according to their carcinogenicity to humans carried out by the International Agency for Research on Cancer (IARC), the specialized cancer agency of WHO.

The same chemical can have different effects at different doses, that depends on how much of the chemical a person is exposed to. It can also depend on the route by which the exposure occurs, e.g. ingestion, inhalation or injection." [30]

The WHO (based on information from the IARC) recently placed glyphosate into class 2A a probable carcinogen; but the IARC's definition of "probable" is barely a distant relative to Malkan's simplistic and unscientific viewpoint. This (briefly) is what it actually says:

"For the herbicide glyphosate, there was limited evidence of carcinogenicity in humans for non-Hodgkin lymphoma. The evidence in humans is from studies of exposures, mostly agricultural, in the USA, Canada, and Sweden published since 2001." [31]

Readers are encouraged to study the entire paper at the IARC website for more detailed information but as you can see the risk is tenuous for most of us, and even then, only one cancer type is even suspected.

Jack Payne, University of Florida's Senior VP for Agriculture and Natural Resources and leader of the Institute of Food and Agricultural Sciences wrote in the *Tampa Bay Times*:

"What we've previously learned from episodes such as Climategate is that scientists' emails can be cherry-picked and used out of context to confuse the public about issues around which there is solid scientific consensus. In Folta's case, the emails are being used to unfairly paint a public servant in science as a corporate stooge. U.S. Right to Know,

---

30   http://www.who.int/features/qa/87/en
31   http://www.iarc.fr/en/media-centre/iarcnews/pdf/MonographVolume112.pdf

the anti-GMO activist group that obtained the records, has also driven the narrative of their interpretation." [32]

So what's so bad about organic produce anyway?

On the face of it, organic produce seems a great solution. The hugely fallacious notion is that we haven't tinkered with it, that it's natural and untouched just like our ancestors enjoyed for millennia.

But organic or not, factory farming is still factory farming and it uses the same basic methods with a few notable exceptions. The problem is not with the method it's with the pests. Humans are not the only ones who find strawberries and tomatoes just delicious or potatoes scrumptious... All life on Earth is competing for a slice of the pie and we've become rather good at keeping most of it at bay using toxic chemicals. Some of those chemicals can be refined from nature (and are therefore organic) others are created in laboratories. GM scientists took a natural insecticide (*Bacillus thuringiensis*) used since the 1920s[33] and have used it to increase pest resistance in cotton reducing the need for spraying since the plants produce their own insecticide. Like many (but not all) modern pesticides, Bt has no effect on humans since it is destroyed in the acids present in our gut. Insects have an alkaline digestive system which leaves them vulnerable.

Take away these measures and the insects have a field day destroying crops.

It seems a reasonable argument to suggest that more insects means more insectivorous birds. While this is true, it ignores the problem that birds require a lot more land than is readily available and our industrialized agricultural developments are entirely to blame.

We've destroyed much of habitats the birds need to survive and therefore, we can't rely on natural predation. Ironically, the growth of farming is part of what drove insect populations up in the first place. Nature is a very delicately balanced scale and the *law of unintended consequence* is never far behind. We can't go back to the old ways because there are simply too many people on the planet and many are already suffering crippling starvation and famine-related disease. The Great Famine of Ireland was caused

---

32   http://www.tampabay.com/news/perspective/perspective-records-requests-hijack-scientists-time/2245131
33   http://www.bt.ucsd.edu/bt_history.html

by potato blight and killed approximately 1,000,000 people over a seven year period from 1845.

When people become enamored with an idea - organic produce or GM foods - they tend to become blind to the problems. But more people are attracted to the organic proposition simply because it's easy to understand. Dig hole, insert seed, wait for plant and harvest. They don't see all the failures that have led up to this point.

Truly organic farms as many people fallaciously perceive the industry, those which did not use toxic chemicals from any source would be obliterated today as they were in the 19th century.

As an example, organic (or conventional) farmers can freely use a fungicidal/bactericidal called Bordeaux mixture which is created from lime, copper sulfate and water. As you might expect from something containing lime (calcium oxide), metal compounds and water, this is very nasty stuff.

Bordeaux mixture is corrosive, causes eye and skin damage and irritates the respiratory tract. The regulatory information [34] lists it as both an immediate and a delayed health hazard. Farm workers using the product would normally be expected to wear chemically protective overalls, eye protection and even respirators.

It's also highly toxic to bees and worms and unlike the alternative, Dithane 945 for instance, Bordeaux mixture persists in soil for a considerable length of time.

This isn't to say that organic farming is necessarily bad - but just to point out that many of those who are promoting it are either unware of the real risks or are so deeply invested they need to kill off, rather than embrace, any and all viable alternatives.

■

---

34   http://www.pbigordon.com/pdfs/BordeauxMixture-MSDS.pdf

Posted on February 12, 2015 by Gary Ruskin

Dear Professor Folta

Yesterday there was some news coverage and commentary about our use of the state Freedom of Information Acts to obtain the correspondence of professors who wrote for the agrichemical industry's PR website, GMO Answers. We're glad to have a public conversation about this topic with the professors involved. We believe that transparency and open dialog are fundamental values by which we must operate in a democratic society and a truly free market. To that end, I thought it would be useful to explain why we FOIA.

Since 2012, the food and agrichemical industries have spent at least $103 million dollars on a massive PR and political campaign to deceive the public about genetically engineered foods. As the public relations firm Ketchum bragged in a recent video, "positive media coverage had doubled" on GMOs following this PR campaign, and it has put agrichemical industry spin front and center in the debate over GMOs. The purpose of this PR campaign is to repel grassroots efforts to win GMO labels that are already required in 64 countries, and to extend the profit stream from GMOs, and the pesticides that go with them, for as long as possible—not to foster an authentic public dialog about GMOs.

This anti-consumer campaign has been dirty in more ways than one. It has been packed with numerous deceptions and well-documented efforts to trick voters. In connection with such efforts, the Washington State Attorney General is suing the Grocery Manufacturers Association for the largest instance of campaign money laundering in the history of the state.

At US. Right to Know, we believe the food and agrichemical industries must have a lot to hide, because they spend so much money trying to hide it. We try to expose what they're hiding.

As part of our effort, we made the state FOIA requests to obtain the correspondence of professors who wrote for the agrichemical industry's PR website, GMO Answers.

These professors are public employees. They are paid by the taxpayers to work for the public good; their university affiliations give them the status of "independent" experts, and they are often quoted in the media as independent experts. But when these professors are closely coordinating with agrichemical corporations and their slick PR firms to shape the public dialog in ways that foster private gain for corporations, or when they act as the public face for industry PR, we have the right to know what they did and how they did it.

Through the FOIA requests, we are attempting to understand the work these professors did for Ketchum, (as well as agrichemical companies such as Monsanto, Syngenta, Bayer, BASF, DuPont and Dow; trade groups like the Grocery Manufacturers Association, the Biotechnology Industry Organization and the Council for Biotechnology Information; other PR firms like Fleishman Hillard and Ogilvy & Mather, and the political firm Winner & Mandabach) on the GMO Answers website which was created as a PR tool for the agrichemical companies.

There are reasons to be concerned about GMO Answers. The website was created by and is run by the public relations firm Ketchum, which also represents Russia and its president, Vladimir Putin. Ketchum is linked to an espionage effort conducted years ago against non-profit organizations concerned with GMOs, including the Center for Food Safety and Friends of the Earth. Ketchum also targeted Greenpeace with espionage.

The professors whose documents we requested are using the prestige of our public universities to burnish the image of an industry that has repeatedly hidden from consumers and workers the truth about the dangers of their products and operations. Entire books have been written documenting their reprehensible conduct. Public relations on behalf of private corporations is not academic work. It is not work for the public good. It is the use of public funds for private gain.

Federal and state Freedom of Information Acts exist, in part, to uncover such potential misuse of public funds for private ends.

We are also interested in failures of scientific integrity. To use one obvious example, one of the professors whose records we requested closely mirrored industry talking points in an op-ed he wrote against GMO labeling for the Woodland Daily-Democrat. Did that professor write the op-ed himself? Or was it written by a PR firm hired by the agrichemical industry?

Repeating industry talking points is not integrity in science; in fact, it is the opposite.

We believe that transparency and openness are good remedies for the lack of integrity in science.

We are glad to live in America, where the tools of the FOIA are open to all citizens. And so our work is guided by the ideals of James Madison: "A popular Government, without popular information, or the means of acquiring it, is but a Prologue to a Farce or a Tragedy; or, perhaps both. Knowledge will forever govern ignorance: And a people who mean to be their own Governors, must arm themselves with the power which knowledge gives."

Sincerely,

Gary Ruskin, Executive Director, US. Right to Know

Dr. Folta responds:

Not afraid at all. No big deal. I'm glad to talk to anyone, as I have few dealings with these companies. Aside from a few old friends and former students, there's not much to talk about. Our university is happily providing all materials requested.

The big question is one of what the FOIA system is for. Should someone that has done nothing wrong, who simply taught science consistent with the literature, be subject to having private emails probed? Worse, it discourages scientists from interacting with the public.

It also discourages the public from asking scientists for help or assistance. Would you ask a scientist to help with a project, if you knew that your name, or your child's name, would become public and smeared on the Internet?

It also opens up a public scientist, that did nothing wrong, to having phrases lifted, items taken out of context. I don't have time to read everything for alternative interpretations.

As a public employee my records are all public, folks scan for any way they can to try to harm my reputation all the time.

Keep in mind that these laws are wonderfully important for finding cases of illegal action, etc. They should not be used to harass or intimidate scientists that do nothing wrong, other than teach science.

Thanks for the space to comment, Next time contact me directly, and I'd be glad to answer any questions. It does not take an expensive FOIA action to motivate me to tell you about what I do in science.

Kevin Folta ∎

8

What Makes Us Fat

"If we don't somehow stem the tide of childhood obesity, we're going to have a huge problem."—Lance Armstrong, professional cyclist

The advertising blurb for The Food Babe Way asserts that chemicals sprayed on a juicy peach could be "triggering our body to store fat." It's a neat little weasel sound bite, but the reality is far more complex. Silly assertions like this are just paying lip service to the organic industry and the frenzied readers who flock to pages such as Food Babe's.

> *"Did you know that your fast food fries contain a chemical used in Silly Putty? Or that a juicy peach sprayed heavily with pesticides could be triggering your body to store fat? When we go to the supermarket, we trust that all our groceries are safe to eat. But much of what we're putting into our bodies is either tainted with chemicals or processed in a way that makes us gain weight, feel sick, and age before our time."* [1]

In this chapter, we're going to look at the real reason some of us seem to pile pounds on just by visiting the donut shop.

Food is The Drug That I'm Thinking Of

Addictions develop because something we experience triggers a pleasurable sensation in our brains. Some people, such as adrenaline junkies and high-stakes gamblers, derive pleasure from risks. Others get a kick from nicotine, the potent drug in tobacco argued to be more addictive than cocaine (it's not)[2] . There are those who take pleasure from illicit drugs, and so on.

Anything that makes us feel better has the potential to become addictive. Food is such a basic need. It is by nature the mechanism that exists to keep

---

1   http://www.hachettebookgroup.com/titles/vani-hari/the-food-babe-way/9780316376464/
2   http://www.ncbi.nlm.nih.gov/pubmed/1859920

us alive and has the potential to lead us to an early grave. Our diet today consists of far more highly-processed, packaged food (GMO or not) with excessive amounts of sugars, unhealthy fats, and sodium than ever before, and this appears to be a large part of why an increasing and disproportionate number of people are overweight or obese.

The problem with highly processed food is that by design it delivers easily bioavailable calories, which means we get that natural rush that nature designed to reward us for finding food. Finding food at the local McDonald's is not quite the same as walking tens of miles to find a few ripe berries. While the reward is the same (or greater), the effort (loss of calories) is far less.

A 2014/2015 study in PLoS One [3] looked at the effect of these foods vs. perceived addiction, tabulating the results from most to least addictive. The results aren't particularly shocking. Here are the top 10.

1. Pizza
2. Chocolate
3. Crisps (UK)/Chips
4. Cookie
5. Ice cream
6. Chips (UK)/French fries
7. Cheeseburger
8. Non-diet sodas
9. Cake
10. Cheese

With the exception of cheese, all of these foods are highly processed and deliver a large amount of carbohydrates and sodium salts. This is unsurprisingly commonplace in fast food restaurants. Most of us will recognize one or more foods on that list we find difficult to resist. Many of us would find it difficult to take just one or two mouthfuls and not come back for a little more. The fast food mantras of:

"Would you like fries with that?"

or

"A large one?"

… tug at both the heart and purse strings of even the most resolute dieter when offered a "value meal" upgrade while enveloped by the enticing odors

---

3   http://journals.plos.org/plosone/article?id=10.1371/journal.pone.0117959

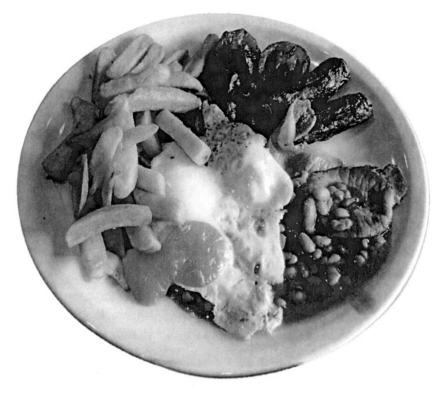

Would you like a heart attack with that? A large one? Some fatty food is not as bad for us as we once thought, but it's very high in calories. (Paul Lloyd/PublicDomainPictures.net)

of a fast food restaurant. "Oh, what the heck? Supersize me!".

Even when customers deliver a specific phrasing to their order, for example: "Just a small cheeseburger, please," staff are told to prompt them for something extra, and the shopper naturally feels the urge to oblige. This is remarkable, but it's a natural part of human behavior and one that McDonald's and other fast food companies are quick to seize upon.

This practice is the reality behind the false smiles delivered at the counter by workers entrenched in almost robotic servitude by these huge corporations. These companies are more interested in the bottom line than they are with our waistlines. They respond cynically to public pressures in ways that help them, such as McDonald's sourcing organic milk in the UK. Paradoxically, the larger people get, the more difficult we find it to refuse those extra-large helpings. Not only are the fast food restaurants feeding our addiction, their staff are instructed to encourage it.

Simplistic arguments that flavor enhancers (primarily MSG) are the root of all food addiction evils allow the real culprits to escape unnoticed, and the corporations laugh heartily, all the way to the bank.

We expend fewer calories today than we ever have, and yet many of us just keep putting on weight, not because of the additives that Food Babe loves to demonize, but because of continued intake of more calories than we expend. In 2003, the WHO calculated that over 1 billion adults are overweight and at least 30% of those are clinically obese. Not only is it the biggest epidemic of modern times, it's the largest epidemic in history. 17.6M children under five are overweight, and the United States Surgeon General estimated that childhood obesity has doubled in the last two decades of the 20th century. [4]

This is particularly problematic for health providers since obesity is directly linked to so many other maladies, such as heart disease and type II diabetes. It may also be implicated in a whole raft of hormonally triggered cancers.

In order to understand the problem, it helps to know what fat is, what it does, and why men and women (and ethnicities) are so different. Animals use fat as a long-term energy store and insulation from the cold. Ethnicities who have evolved to live in Northern climates, such as the Innuits, will normally be expected to carry more body fat than people whose lineage derives from the equatorial regions.

Fat is stored in a special cell called adipose tissue. We all start with a fixed number of cells, and each cell can only store a small amount of fat. In theory, once they are at maximum capacity, we stop getting fatter. You can think of fat tissue like one of those little sponges that expands when it's wet. At some point the material reaches saturation and won't accept any more water. Adipose tissue works in much the same way. But the more adipose tissue we have, the more fat we can store.

Women can store twice as much fat as men in preparation for childbearing and rearing. Our bodies are 15% and 30% fat respectively. Someone with

---

4   http://www.cdc.gov/healthyyouth/obesity/facts.htm

20Kg (44lbs) of fat is carrying about 33 billion fat cells. That said, not all fat sites are the same. Visceral fat (the stuff around our bellies) is more dangerous to our health than the stuff around the thighs and buttocks, because this fat is responsible for the free fatty acids (FFAs) in our blood. It's responsible for the metabolic diseases associated with obesity, in particular insulin resistance and, therefore, type II diabetes.

It's believed adults also create extra fat cells and continue to do so as long as the excess fat is being laid down. This might explain why, despite each fat cell being limited to what it can store, some people can reach enormous weights (morbid and super morbid obesity), putting their heath in serious jeopardy.

Dr. Michael Jenson and his team at the Division of Endocrinology, Diabetes, Metabolism, and Nutrition at Rochester's Mayo Clinic, found that just a gain of just 1.2Kg (2.6lbs) resulted in an increase of 2.6 billion new cells. [5]

When our fat cells become saturated like that sponge, and we add more fats through our diet, they leak the extra FFAs right back into our bloodstream, where they deposit around our visceral organs: the liver, heart and even around our muscles. These sites tend to store chemicals that interfere with normal hormonal signaling, creating obesity-related hypertension, insulin resistance, excess cholesterol, and hyperlipidemia.

> [Genistein] mimics the action of estrogen, fat forming hormone. [6]

Like many on the fringes of pseudo-science, Food Babe blames a raft of chemicals referred to as obesogens[7] a term coined by Felix Grün and Bruce Blumberg in 2006 to classify chemicals that they felt cause obesity. Among those mentioned by Food Babe is genistein, a phytoestrogen found in many legumes, but appears in greatest concentrations in Indian Bread Root (Psoralea Corylifolia) and soybeans, hence why it shows up in soy-based foods.

Estrogen is a group of hormones. Of those, genistein mimics the action of oestradiol, the primary estrogen found in all healthy women of childbearing age. Oestradiol performs a number of functions, including controlling fat stores required for pregnancy. It is essential in maintaining bone health.

---

5   ttp://www.mayoclinic.org/medical-professionals/clinical-updates/endocrinology/what-new-adipose-tissue
6   The Food Babe Way, p. 60
7   http://www.ncbi.nlm.nih.gov/pmc/articles/PMC2713042/

Notably, it's also found in "combination" contraceptive pills, which are not usually considered responsible for an epidemic of obesity among young women. Further, since oestradiol (and, therefore, genistein) is responsible for the development of feminine features such as breasts, it would be reasonable to expect epidemic outbreaks of gynecomastia (enlarged breasts in men) in Asia, where soy products are regularly consumed.

Genistein is also thought to reduce the risk of some cancers, but Food Babe's not done with "obesogenic" hormones yet…

> [Estradiol] synthetic estrogen given to dairy cows to increase milk production; may be in nonorganic milk. [8]

Although estradiol is a naturally occurring estrogen, it's likely a synthetic version that's given to cows. It's not given to milk herds, but rather to the animals destined for the table in order to improve meat production. Whatever estrogen gets into our milk supplies is more a result of over-milking to get the best yield than the pharmaceuticals the farmers are accused of slipping their herds.

Cows produce the largest quantities of milk when they are well fed and treated. Sure, we could pump them full of chemicals, but you can't get blood out of a stone, and dairy farmers know they won't get good milk/feed returns from unhappy cattle. Even the quality of the milk is determined by the feed: better pastures make for better milk.

> [MSG] flavors food to make it more appealing and addictive; customers wind up eating more calories than they need. [9]

Oh dear, poor old MSG gets another whipping. While it's true that MSG does make lifeless savory dishes taste better, so does salt. No one is seriously suggesting table salt causes us to eat more.

One of the reasons childhood obesity is so worrying is that children and young adults can make more fat cells than they were born with. This means an obese child has more storage space (free fat cells) to get even larger in

---

8   The Food Babe Way, p. 60
9   The Food Babe Way, p. 60

adulthood. This applies even if they lose weight because although the fat cells empty, they are not removed.

Evolution simply hasn't had time to catch up with the remarkable pace of change that we've seen over the last few thousand years; never mind the last few decades. We are hunter-gatherers that don't need to hunt or gather anymore and, for the most part, we spend our days sitting around the metaphorical campfire.

Fat is a high-energy, slow-release store. Animals evolved this trait to store up food when it was available for those times when it was less plentiful. Our ancestors couldn't just drive to the grocery store and grab bread, milk and a few vegetables. But with increasing urbanization since the industrial age, access to and availability of food has increased, and it keeps getting easier. Access to high-energy, great tasting food has never been more easy and there lies the first problem.

Nature designed our bodies to feast and fast. When food was plentiful, the excess calories we consumed were stored as fat for later conversion to energy during leaner times. Instant access to high-energy food destroys that system.

Food is so important to us that we've evolved mechanisms to make sure that we eat the right things and that we're rewarded for doing so. These functions—operating at the conscious level—can override the systems that tell us when we've eaten enough. So it's possible to overeat in order to store energy for a later, leaner time.

Taster For 10

Humans taste five distinct flavors. If that doesn't sound like much, consider that your television or computer monitor creates images from just three colors. Each of these flavors tells our brains what we're eating—from an evolutionary perspective you need to think like a caveman or woman.

Sweet: mother's milk is sweet. This is our first taste sensation; we retain it in order to detect simple sugars such as fructose, which will give us easily accessed energy to get us to our next meal.

Bitter: It's thought we developed an ability to taste bitter to detect poisons in nature, as most poisons are very bitter indeed.

Umami: human milk contains free glutamates (about 10x the amount found in cow's milk)[10], and this taste sensation tells our brains that we're getting something high in protein. We need protein to grow and repair every cell in our bodies so it's important we can taste it.

Sour: in varying combinations with sweet allows us to check fruits for ripeness.

Salt: We need a tiny amount of sodium and potassium in our blood. These elements create the electrolytes that allow our cells to function correctly, allow our hearts to beat, and maintain blood pressure.

The first direct evidence for the evolution of bitterness was only shown in 2006 when it was conclusively shown that glucosinolates, which are natural substances, can alter our thyroid's ability to absorb iodine, in turn affecting its ability to manufacture hormones. Remember broccoli? The authors noted that although our brains tell us to avoid such vegetables, they also supply many essential nutrients that may be missing from our diet and, therefore, should not be dropped from a healthy lifestyle, as the advantages far outweigh the disadvantages in a balanced diet.

Salts (sodium is the most common in our diet) are highly toxic in large doses, which probably explains why we are so sensitive to it. Too much salt causes a condition called *hypernatremia*, where the amount of salt in the blood reaches a level where the fluid is sucked from our cells, damaging our bodies. The shrinking organs (including our brains) are torn away from their support structures, rupturing membranes, and leading to internal bleeding, kidney damage, coma and, if untreated, death. (This is the reason you can dehydrate at sea if you can't get access to fresh water.)

Eating just a little too much salt on a daily basis also puts our cardiovascular system under pressure, increasing our risk of heart disease and stroke. Although it's possible to have too little salt (hyponatremia), our diets of highly processed food already deliver more than we need, so caution is advised.

Although many, many bloggers demonstrate a fallacious dislike of MSG, as a result of a single unproven incident, it's a much safer flavoring by volume

---

10   Sandell, M. A. and Breslin, P.A.S. Variability in a taste-receptor gene determines whether we taste toxins in food. Current Biology, 2006, 16, R792-R794.

than everyday salt, since it contains about 1/3 of the amount of sodium by weight.

Digestible Comestibles

Generally speaking, obesity has a lot to do with how much we eat. If we consume more calories in food than what we use in our day-to-day lives, some of those calories are going to be stored as fat. This is a very simple, crude measure and, although largely true, it's only part of the story. Most of us think of the earth as ball shaped, and that's good enough—it's roughly spherical—but it's technically an oblate spheroid. Sometimes those little details count.

Calories in our food are the same. What counts is the quality of those calories. A thousand excess calories of apple and a thousand excess calories of cake are still a thousand excess calories. But the apple calories are more nutritious bite for bite (although the cake bites are arguably far more delicious).

If you can set fire to something, you're converting some of it into heat energy. In this way, we can figure out how many calories are in a substance by burning a known amount and measuring how much energy is given off. These calculations used to be done using a device called the bomb calorimeter. [11] With the bomb method, the food item is sealed off and surrounded by water and burned. The rise in water temperature shows the total energy calories in the item, though that total includes components that aren't digested by the human body and therefore not absorbed. Now more precise techniques are used, so the calorie content listed on a specific food item is much closer to the actual calories your body will absorb.

If you'd like to experiment, you can see energy being released from sugar by setting fire to a sugar cube. This isn't something we'd recommend without adult supervision.

From this observation, we can establish that if you can burn something, it contains a store of energy. However, you can burn paper, gasoline, or even a branch from an apple tree—but you wouldn't eat it. The reason we don't eat these things is that our bodies can't break them down into useful energy that we can use. The energy they contain is not bioavailable.

11   http://www.scimed.co.uk/wp-content/uploads/2013/03/Introduction-to-bomb-calorimetry.pdf

Hopefully that should be a light-bulb moment, but don't worry if you're still puzzled. We had to light our editor's copy of the *National Enquirer* on fire before he got it. (He refused to eat it.)

A typical apple contains about 100 calories, most of which comes from its sugar content (around 10%). Apples contain a lot of water too—typically around 80%.

Weight is a better way to describe this. 4oz/100g of apple delivers about 50 calories. By comparison, 4oz/100g of white table sugar (sucrose) contains a staggering 387 calories: nearly eight times as much. 50 apple calories will fill you up far more than a spoonful of 50 table sugar calories.

This is one of the numerous reasons that excess sugar is bad, the forms it comes in often don't satiate our hunger as much as more nutritious options, and prompt us to eat more to be satisfied. Another reason is that by forcing our bodies to produce large amounts of insulin (the carbohydrate and fat regulating hormone) over a long period, we wear out the system and our bodies can develop a resistance to it. This is analogous to the way a deep wound develops into tough, scar tissue, and a repeatedly damaged scar gets tougher each time it re-heals.

Most of the processed foods we eat today are very calorie-dense, meaning they have more calories per volume and mass than other foods. For this reason alone, we have to be careful how much highly processed food we eat. As the example of sugar vs. apple shows, you can't tell how fattening something is just by looking at it.

Be it calories or nutrition: bioavailability and calorie density matter. Highly processed food—fast food, white breads, non-diet soft drinks, and packaged snacks in particular—are very dense in empty calories; nutrients take a distant second, and your body will notice. But it's not the oft-demonized food additives that make us gain weight—it's the calories.

Keeping Up With The Endocrines

Most of us are familiar with our nervous system even if we're not consciously aware of it all the time. The peripheral nervous system looks after our limbs and connected organs, sending impulses over nerve fiber to the central nervous system, then onward to our brain. So when you stub your toe on a door (or someone sets fire to your magazine), signals rapidly pass from the affected organ into your brain and register pain or discomfort. Although our main sensations (pain, pressure and temperature) travel at slightly different speeds, the impulses reach our brains in a fraction of a second.

That's only part of the story though. The rest of our body communicates using chemical messengers that travel through our blood at much lower speeds. The advantage is they can affect any other part of our body; or even several parts at the same time, with different functions, without ever having to involve our brain. If nerve impulses work like telephones (delivering to a single destination), hormones are more like a scent—the further we are from the source of a smell (be that a perfume or cologne, or coal fire) the longer it takes us to detect it. Anyone in range will be able to.

We talk about hormones with little deference. However, consider they were only discovered at the beginning of the 20th century and we're still discovering new ones, and new functions of the ones we know about. As of 2014 there are around 80 known hormones; up from the 50 or so discovered up to the 1990s.

For example, the male sex hormone, testosterone, once considered to be a hormonal bad guy, is now thought to be more useful than first thought. Like all chemicals, the dose makes the cure or the poison. Men who are producing too little testosterone tend to have a lowered libido and tend to gain fat easily whereas men who have too much (often added through artificial means) can be overly aggressive and are prone to testosterone-sensitive cancers.

Food Babe, like many of the modern-day promulgators of miracle cures, makes a big deal of kale (also called borecole). It's brassica (a type of cabbage) and related to the cauliflower, bok choy, broccoli, and Brussels sprout.

> It [kale] is a superfood ingredient that has completely transformed my health and my life and the one food I added to my diet that got me in tip top shape and beautiful for my wedding day (and ever since). [12]

---

12 http://anokhimedia.com/magazine/q-a-with-vani-hari-the-food-babe

Like most foods, kale is harmless in moderation. However, along with other cruciferous vegetables, it contains a chemical called goitrin, a gluco-sinolate [13] which can affect the function of our thyroid by lowering production of thyroxine.

Aside from affecting our metabolism, a diet too high in kale (and similar cruciferous vegetables) leaves the consumer prone to cabbage-goiter. [14] Women and in particular women over forty years of age are susceptible. [15]

Leptin and ghrelin are the hunger and satiety hormones. One of the best known hormones of all, insulin, regulates the amount of sugar (glucose) in our blood. Our bodies function best in a fairly narrow window of blood sugar levels. They constantly monitor and adjust it through a process called homeostasis. (This is a general term that covers all of our self-monitoring functions, not just blood sugar.)

The level of glucose in our blood rises quite naturally after a meal, particularly one with lots of complex carbohydrates such as starches and pasta or simpler ones like table sugar. This change is detected by the pancreas, triggering a small patch of dedicated cells to release insulin. Insulin reaches all parts of our body and instructs "target" cells (primarily muscle and fat cells) to absorb glucose from our blood. Insulin also causes our liver to convert glucose into glycogen, in effect removing the glucose and restoring the levels to normal. This change is sensed in the pancreas, thus lowering the production of insulin.

People with diabetes either don't produce sufficient insulin or have developed a resistance to its effects. This causes the concentration of glucose in their blood to rise, thickening it and forcing the body to drain water from the tissues to maintain the correct viscosity. This is what gives untreated diabetics a raging thirst as the body cries out for increased water intake, and causes detectable glucose in our urine as our bodies try to evacuate the sugar via our kidneys. Clever things, bodies!

---

13   De Vries, J. Food Safety and Toxicity, Taylor & Francis 1996, pp. 44-45
14   Greer, MA., Goitrogenic Substances in Food, American Journal of Clinical Nutrition. (http://ajcn.nutrition.org/content/5/4/440.full.pdf)
15   http://www.mayoclinic.org/diseases-conditions/goiter/basics/definition/con-20021266

Enter Disruptors

Endocrine Disruptors, one of Food Babe's demons, sound scary. Such things do exist but what exactly are they? Let's take a quick look at two very familiar ones.

Normal urination is controlled by another hormone called vasopressin. There is a very real endocrine disruptor that affects our vasopressin levels, and yet many of us imbibe it on quite regular occasions; often to excess.

Alcohol!

Vasopressin, also known as antidiuretic hormone, is secreted by a tiny structure (about the size of a pea) near the base of our brain called the pituitary gland. This busy little gland, separated into three lobes, produces a huge amount of the basic hormones we need to survive, including growth hormones, hormones for blood pressure and salt regulation, and even for some aspects of reproduction, pregnancy, and nursing. One of the world's tallest men, Christopher Greener (who sadly died while this text was being prepared) was a veritable giant standing at 7ft 6¼. Mr. Greener reached that height as a direct result of a benign tumor putting pressure on his pituitary gland. Christopher's growth was only stopped when the tumor was detected, aged 27.

For such a tiny structure, this little pea packs a lot of punch. Alcohol slows it down, causing our natural vasopressin levels to drop, forcing us to run to the bathroom; again and again. (Nerves in the bladder are irritated as the breakdown products of what we've been drinking reach them—so once you "break the seal," you can't stop.) Vasopressin regulates the amount of water in our blood by instructing the kidneys to reabsorb water rather than pass it directly to our bladder.

As the level of water in our system falls, our blood starts to thicken and water is stolen from our organs, including our brain (except Marc, whose brain is in a jar at a secret research facility pickling in glyphosate and MSG—Ed.). As our bodies steal water from our brains, it pulls on the membranes of the walls of our skull contributing to the familiar hangover pain and general malaise.

Alcohol is not the only endocrine disruptor in common use. Another one is caffeine, found in coffee, tea, and many soft drinks. Like alcohol, caffeine (which is very mild neurotoxin designed by plants to kill insects) affects the pituitary gland, suppresses the release of vasopressin, and in effect forces us to need the bathroom more.

Chemically, caffeine is sufficiently similar to a chemical in our brains called adenosine, which is the stuff that makes us feel sleepy as the day wears on. When caffeine enters our brain, it competes with adenosine, causing us to feel less drowsy and disturbs our sleep. It's worth noting that caffeine's effects are still detectable six hours after ingestion. It has other effects too: including dilating blood capillaries in our brain (which may ease a headache and is probably why it's a commonly used hangover remedy); causing our liver to convert glycogen into glucose—part of our "fight or flight" reflex. It increases dopamine levels, making us "feel" better and releasing the hormone epinephrine (also called adrenaline) causing our heart rate to increase in readiness to run from danger.

The reason we mention these two everyday drugs is to demonstrate that while we can't afford to walk around with our eyes closed and hope for the best, we equally don't need to run for the hills when Food Babe uses buzz phrases like "endocrine disruptors" as if the sky is falling.

It's not.

Our bodies are under constant attack from all manner of foreign chemicals throughout our lives. By and large, we never even notice. For every breath you take, your lungs are assaulted by airborne pathogens so small they are only visible under an electron microscope, and dust particles that are still invisible to the naked eye. But they're there, and our lungs brush them away as they always have, using the mechanisms nature has provided. Even with dangerous endocrine disruptors, unless we are exposed for a long period to larger doses, our bodies cope like they've been doing for thousands of years.

The real danger in fearing the things that can't hurt us is we risk running headlong into those things that can.

Leptin & Ghrelin—Twins of Eating

The next part of this puzzle is perhaps the most difficult to understand:

hormones. Most of us have heard of the common ones such as testosterone, estrogens, and progesterone.

Hormones, those chemical messengers, tune our bodies in very subtle ways. While we're not directly aware of them, we can feel their effects very quickly, because they are transported by our blood. A hormone can get from the cells that produce it to the cells it acts upon in around a minute. Two main hormones, leptin, and ghrelin, are responsible for how we eat.

> *Ghrelin*: the hunger hormone, is released from cells in our GI tract (stomach, intestines) when there is no food left to process. As we eat, our ghrelin levels drop, so we feel less hungry. Some people are unable to respond correctly to ghrelin, making them constantly hungry.

> *Leptin*: (one of a recently discovered group of hormones, the adipokines) the fullness hormone is primarily excreted by our fatty tissues and should (note *should*) tell us when we've had enough. Some people produce mutated leptin variants, which do not trigger the correct reaction in the brain. Affected people are obese as children and may have insatiable appetites, occasionally with strange eating habits.

The discovery of leptin and ghrelin is leading to new understandings of both childhood and adult obesity, as part of complex reasons why some people are naturally unable to control their appetites.

One thing that is making us fatter is sugar in all of its forms; and one of the best sweeteners out there is aspartame. Strange to think, that the very people who claim to have our health at heart, are spreading fear and loathing about a product that could help us all maintain a healthy weight.

Ultimately, the vast majority of us are entirely responsible for our weight. Fast and convenience foods are a creation of market forces, feeding on our natural addictions.

It's easy to wag an accusing finger at the fast food chains, but they are only responding to a demand that existed in us since our ancestors dragged themselves out of the primordial ooze. Metaphorically, these chains farm us like cattle. But unlike cattle, we have a choice. We can learn to make better choices. We can learn to cut down on the junk foods that we crave which deliver little practical nutrition (and in some cases are slowly deteriorating our health.) ∎

9

Love Yourself Fit

"Your body is the church where Nature asks to be reverenced."—
Marquis de Sade, 19th C. French author and aristocrat.

You are unique. If you never remember another thing—you need to grasp this idea with both hands. In order for you to be here, your parents had to be born and, their parents before them, and so on. In each generation, both of your parents had to survive accidents and disease long enough to even have you—and like you, each generation won against all seemingly insurmountable odds, even to be born! [1] Infant mortality just 150 years ago was around 10% and up to 30% were dead before they reached age 16 [2]. Working class people (servants, laborers, etc.) would be lucky to see their 25th birthday.

Your existence is remarkable.

The chances against any given person being conceived are so stupendously astronomical, that experts in probability can use them to demonstrate how easy it would be to win the lottery.

Every week.

For the rest of your life.

Try to wrap your head around it. This is why you are what you are and who you are. Your body was created from a set of unique blueprints fused at the very moment sperm and egg merged.

Like a snowflake, there has never been anyone quite like you and there never will be another you, even if we start cloning people. Indeed, we now know that even identical twins aren't 100% identical. Your body is a finely tuned, autonomous biological machine capable of repairing much of its

---

1   http://isites.harvard.edu/fs/docs/icb.topic1377262.files/Health%20and%20Mortality/ferrie%20troesken.pdf

2   Lynda Payne, "Health in England (16th–18th c.)," in Children and Youth in History, Item #166, http://chnm.gmu.edu/cyh/primary-sources/166

systems without so much as a conscious thought. If you look after it, with luck, you should get around 80 trouble-free years out of it.

Even if you feel pretty ordinary, even if you're in bed with a cold, take it from us, you are amazing, and it's exceptional to be what you are. Fundamental change is only possible when you let go of the mental chains others have created. Family, society, and worst of all celebrities, all contribute to our sense of self and insecurities.

Food Babe is a wonderful example of this very modern, and very ugly phenomenon. She spends so many "column inches" bragging about her mission to be healthy and change the food system that she makes you feel ashamed. In every post, you see her happy, slim and smiling for the camera, often cuddled up to celebrities, politicians and fellow health bloggers, basking in the glow of celebrity. As Kevin Folta noted, "Vani likes Vani." [3]

Take a moment to give yourself permission and say this out loud to yourself, "*It's OK to be me!*"

This feels a bit silly at first. But there's a powerful psychological function that comes into play when we adopt mantras like this. Although we're speaking the words to ourselves, the fact that we hear them back creates a "feedback loop" that bolsters our confidence.

Self-improvement gurus like Food Babe charge lots of money to create and then exploit fabricated insecurities. For the price of this book (or for free if you're reading this in the bookstore or library), we're trying to undo what she and her ilk have done to our collective psyches. It's called positive reinforcement, and we all respond to it. Rather bizarrely, it works– even if we're both the instigator and the recipient!

The same works in reverse too. If you've ever ridden in a car with an angry driver cursing at every other jerk on the road, you have experienced a form of feedback that raises tension and makes you increasingly upset. The more you do it, the angrier you get.

The World According to Google

This is the Information Age. Never before have we had access to so much information right at our fingertips. Search engines like Google and Wol-

---

3   http://kfolta.blogspot.co.uk/2014/10/food-babe-visits-my-university.html

fram Alpha allow anyone in the world with an Internet connection to access seemingly limitless knowledge. Some of it is good, some bad, and some is downright dangerous.

Worse still, people in the developed world are becoming increasingly obsessed with celebrity. Just walk into a supermarket and glance at the magazine rack: beautiful celebrities blessed with perfect lives stare back at you

From Kim Kardashian's butt to Ryan Reynolds' abs and Gwyneth Paltrow's gluten-free diet; we want to emulate them, as if to believe that some of their glamor will spill into our humdrum lives. We're obsessed with them in much the same way the Victorians became obsessed with death. [4]

Like it or not, charisma is a powerful force and the pressure to emulate successful people is enormous. In the past, the worst pressure a growing child would likely encounter would be from parents, elder siblings or other people in their community. Today, like it not, every one of us is pressured by society and the media to emulate our icons and achieve things that are realistically outside of our grasp. The young boy wanting to be the next David Beckham or the young girl dreaming of being Katy Perry... the names change over time, but the drive remains the same. With our celebrity culture we are no longer allowed to grow out of youthful dreams and be ourselves: we have to be something out of the ordinary.

By the time we reach adulthood, we're resigned to the idea we're not going to reach those dizzying heights of fame, fortune, and stardom. But the unhealthy, unrealistic messages don't stop—they just change.

Women are bombarded by the idea that they have to be perfect mothers and beauty queens—perfectly attired and beautifully proportioned (remember those supermarket tabloid cover girls?). Men feel the need to have a rock-hard six pack, masculine features, and perfect biceps. In 2014 some male "hipsters" took to growing extravagant, bushy beards. But not every man can grow one, giving those who could a distinct advantage just through luck of biology.

Look in the mirror for a moment. Your worst enemy is staring right back at you. Stop and think for a moment—do you love yourself?

---

4   http://www.gresham.ac.uk/lectures-and-events/the-victorians-life-and-death

The Fear Babe

If your answer was an emphatic no, go back to the beginning of this chapter, do not pass Go and do not collect 200 Monsanto Shillbucks. Joking aside, remember, you're unique, and it's OK to be you.

The only people who genuinely love themselves are narcissists and if you're one of those, you won't be reading this. We all have a degree of narcissism. It's necessary for healthy psychological function but when it gets too low, we start to feel bad about ourselves and develop a cycle where our self-esteem falls into a black hole.

Fat shaming, a relatively recent form of psychological bullying, plays to this.

The rise of simplistic measurements like Body Mass Index (BMI) have only served to make a bad problem worse. A BMI of 18.5 or lower means you're underweight; 25 or higher and you're overweight; over 30 is obese.

BMI is great if you happen to have an average muscle/fat ratio, but many of us don't. Women naturally have more fat, typically around 6-10% more than men, but every one of us is slightly different!

It's fair to say that since we're all human, we're all based on the same basic outline. It's the little details that make all the difference. It sounds obvious, but consider that we can instantly recognize the basic form that makes us human (as opposed to a dog, cat, fish, monkey, and so on). We can recognize friends and family from nothing more than a photograph, and often recognize famous and familiar people from just their eyes or mouth.

Despite being similar, we're all different enough that we can identify a familiar individual from the billions on the planet just from something subtle in their gaze in just an instant.

Your brain is truly amazing.

Modern Day Dorian Gray

Oscar Wilde's 1890 novel is as frighteningly prophetic today as it was spine chilling in its day. In Wilde's story, Dorian Gray is forever youthful while his portrait, hidden in away in an attic room, begins to age.

As if in juxtaposition, we look at pictures of our famous heroes and imagine that's what they look like right now, in real life. We look in the mirror and want to be them.

We trust the veracity of these images without stopping for a moment to consider the photographer and celebrity took advantage of the best lighting, clothes, hair, and makeup, all topped off with professional image editing. And this is exactly how industry wants us to perceive them. If we believe that these unrealistic standards can be achieved, we're convinced to buy the latest beauty lotions and potions, diet supplements, and makeup. We're persuaded to try the latest glitterati fad diets.

To borrow from the French, *vive la différence* (long live the difference). The cult of celebrity has created the very antithesis of variety. Celebrities didn't get to be celebrities without some, *je ne sais quoi* (I don't know what), that little spark of something that sets them apart from the rest of us. More often than not, the magic factor is largely charisma. The Food Babe has blogged *ad nauseam* about food chemistry and yet labored under the misapprehension that air is primarily oxygen (it's nitrogen!) She claims rainbow chard (a member of the beet family) will give you night vision and sells products with the very same ingredients she says are dangerous. She's been shown to be wrong on almost every claim she has ever made –and yet –because of her undeniable charisma, her followers don't question her.

An actor's career is a good barometer of their acting skill vs. their charisma. The true greats get regular work well into their twilight years, but those who relied on their looks fade into obscurity as the years drag on. Unfortunately it's women who fall harder and faster into this trap.

Much the same rule can be applied to health & fitness gurus. Very few retain their status as the 20s give way to the 30s, 40s and beyond, as there are always others, hungrier and younger and ready to fill their place. There are exceptions of course. To some extent these are the most dangerous examples of all, since they often attribute their amazing figure to hard work, clean living, exercise, and a privileged lifestyle the rest of us could only dream of.

Genetics are never mentioned despite being a huge part of the equation.

> *"Want to know what a person's going to be like in 20 years? Look at their parents"*

The Fear Babe

That's a well-known phrase that accounts for more than just genetics, but it's a good guide. We're more a product of our genetics and our environment than we allow ourselves to believe. In much the same way as your skin color will be similar to your parents', so will your overall build and even your eating habits. Children learn how (and what) to eat from their parents and, therefore, learn the same basic rules of nutrition, good or bad. This is something we can overcome, but it's only part of the equation.

Despite all of Gwyneth Paltrow's bizarre dietary claims and their supposed benefits, take a quick look at her mother, actress Blythe Danner. She looks lithe and gorgeous despite being 30 years older. Consider, if you will, Tippi Hedren (famous from Hitchcock's The Birds) and her celebrity daughter Melanie Griffith– mother of 50 Shades of Gray star Dakota Johnson. Look them up. Those examples alone should convince you that genes are a major player.

Not all fat is that obvious and we all need a small amount to stay healthy. Where you store your fat is as visually important as how much you have. That's the fat you see when you measure your muscle definition (although this is something that applies primarily to men). Women's natural fat stores are most obvious in their thighs and hips.

Even the most developed six-pack in the world will be quickly disguised with a comparatively thin layer of soft, pliable and perfectly normal belly fat. The guys you envy for their well-defined six-packs are as much a product of different fat reserves as they are diet and exercise (and often, strategically applied abdominal contouring makeup in photoshoots).

We assume that because a model looks the picture of health as she struts her stuff down the catwalk little more than a human clothes horse, that she must be in bad health. For all we know, she's subsisting on a diet of lettuce leaves, chocolate, and illicit drugs and will collapse and die from a heart attack before she's forty. Then again, it's hard to say. Her lifestyle may be healthy. We cannot pass judgement based on appearances alone.

At the other end of the scale, there are super plus models. Perhaps most famous as of this writing is Tess Munster, better known as Tess Holliday. At size 22, and at just 5'5," she is the largest model currently signed to a professional agency. At 260lbs and a BMI of 42, Holliday is morbidly obese, but that has not prevented her from garnering thousands of faithful followers.

Holliday's claim to be a "body positive activist" and her "#effyourbeautystandards" hashtag are another example of this "Look, I'm OK so you can be too!" faux positivity that regrettably, has no basis in reality and is just as unrealistic as the example set by the stick-thin models. The instant glamor pose takes an instant in time, but long-term the human anatomy isn't designed for it. Still, we can see the need for these kind of images to throw a wrench in the overly homogenous beauty standards that bombard us.

It's entirely possible for some people to carry huge amounts of sub-cutaneous fat and yet not suffer from any of the traditional obesity woes of sleep apnea, dyslipidemia, hypertension and type II diabetes. Not to mention a dramatically increased risk of congestive heart failure, cancer, hemiplegia (a type of paralysis), liver and kidney disease, as well as severe skeletal stress. The risk increases as the years march on, and some of these conditions are difficult to control, life-threatening and often irreversible. The long-term prognosis is often bleak.

People who reach a BMI in excess of 40 by middle age can expect to lose, on average, eight to ten years of their lives—roughly the same as a lifelong smoker. The effects of childhood and young adult obesity have not yet been correlated, as the problem is too new for reliable data to have become available.

You are *not* Tess Holliday, Gwyneth Paltrow, David Beckham, Ryan Reynolds, Kate Moss or Dakota Johnson.

Unless you are Vani Hari, you're not Food Babe either.

You are you and you're unique!

When you look in the mirror, you're not looking through a camera's lens, soft light or judicious post production. Don't judge yourself by their measure. They have not lived your life; they have not walked in your shoes.

Give yourself permission to be yourself.

Do it now, and do it often.

The Fear Babe

Beauty Through Nature's Eye

There is something to be said for Tess Holliday's approach to eschew beauty female standards set by eccentric (and often male) fashion designers. Using clothing to accentuate our looks is a relatively recent development in human history. For the majority of our time on earth, clothing offered us warmth and protection.

At its most basic level, physical attraction is about the need to reproduce the next generation of humanity. People in the prime of their reproductive lives dress in skin-tight and often revealing outfits to accentuate their health and readiness to accept a mate. Girls preen while the guys stretch their muscles and strut, unconsciously drawing attention to their chests, arms, groin and buttocks. (Obviously, there are exceptions to these rules as we learn more about the fluidity of gender and sexuality, but these are topics for another day. For the purposes of discussion, we'll stick to the generalization.)

This anthropological view is hard to accept through the complex fog of modern society, but it's something very primordial and essential to our survival because for much of our time on the planet we didn't wear clothes at all.

We selected our breeding partners primarily on visual cues and secondarily on chemical cues (scent, taste), just as we do today.

A healthy weight is naturally attractive because those around those proportions are statistically most fertile. Women are particularly affected. Ovulation becomes more unreliable as they slide to either side of the ideal weight– nature's way of protecting us against the physical stress of pregnancy at times when our bodies are unable to cope. (Clever old thing, Mother Nature.)

To our ancestors, our ability to produce and nurture healthy offspring (women) or care for the family (men) would dwindle with age. We can recognize these signs in our potential partners as muscle loses tone, skin and hair lose luster, and so on.

The need to reproduce was a powerful instinct. Competition for partners was fierce, and humans are unique in their ability to cheat nature's cues.

We call it cosmetics but a rose by any other name…

From something as simple as lip gloss to the complexity and dangers associated with cosmetic (plastic) surgery, most of us suffer from such sexually derived vanity that we will do anything to look "good." Celebrities and ordinary public alike have suffered at the hands of botched and sometimes illegal procedures. Botched– but probably entirely legal– procedures are responsible for the new visages on Pete Burns, Donatella Versace, Janice Dickinson, Joan Rivers, Jocelyn Wildenstein, and many others.

Women in particular feel pressure from the cosmetics industry to keep their youthful looks for a long as possible. As we're living longer, that pressure increases to the point where it becomes almost humorous – unless you're the butt of the joke.

Going Loco for Coco

Right up to the end of the 19th century, what we now think of as healthy tan (an irony in its own right) was considered rather vulgar and working class because the lower classes in society frequently worked outdoors. Middle and upper-class women in particular, would apply lotions including lead-based pigments and arsenic compounds– unwittingly risking poisoning for their perceived refinement.

The effect of sunlight on our skin was not fully realized until the early part of the 20th century when Neils Finsen, a doctor and sufferer of Niemann–Pick disease, [5] was awarded a Nobel for medicine for his Finsen Light Therapy. Finsen's therapy recognized the role of UV light in the production of vitamin D (a curative therapy for rickets and lupus vulgaris, [6] a rare condition caused by skin infected by the tuberculosis pathogen).

This discovery and its subsequent popularity led to an uptake of what was called heliotherapy in the day. Although immensely popular with those who could afford it, it's thought the current standard of tanning began with the French fashion designer Coco Chanel when she was accidentally sunburned on vacation in the 1920s.

Although we've known for decades just how dangerous tanning is, many

---

5   http://www.niemann-pick.org.uk/niemann-pick-disease
6   http://www.ncbi.nlm.nih.gov/pmc/articles/PMC3109836/

people still believe it's a sign of healthy skin. Dermatologists say any amount of tanning represents skin damage, leading to premature aging and skin cancers that may prove fatal.

As far back as 2011, in a post ostensibly about sugar, Food Babe advised her readers to go outside without sunscreen. [7] The effects can be devastating for people with sensitive skin conditions and over time, may result in potentially fatal skin cancer. We've covered this in more detail in Chapter 4, but this point is worth reiterating.

Too much unprotected exposure could kill you and it *will* age your skin.

Tiger Got Her Stripes

Mothers are often made to feel uncomfortable after pregnancy leaves their skin covered in stretch marks and are unable to return to their pre-baby tone. Different genetics are at work here—primarily the amount of collagen you have.

Collagen refers to a group of proteins that make up part of our connective tissues (tendon, ligaments, skin). You might think of it as the rubber-band protein, elasticity is its function. To check your skin's turgor, pinch a loose "tent" of skin. The back of your hand is a good place to try this. As long as you're well hydrated, you should be able to pinch a little and watch it snap back almost immediately when release. If you're sick or otherwise dehydrated, your skin becomes less flexible, and the "tent" doesn't return right away.

Most people can pinch about 1/2 inch of skin without too much discomfort. The greater the height, the more flexible your skin is, but note that our skin becomes less flexible and thinner as we age. People with connective tissue disorders such Ehlers–Danlos syndrome can pinch a lot more because their skin is much more elastic.

Although Ehlers–Danlos is an extreme dysfunction, there is a wide range of natural skin flexibility—just as we're all around the same height but with some people very tall and some very small. Women on the far end of the skin flexibility scale (but fall short of a condition severe enough to cause other complications) simply don't show stretch marks and can return to

---

7   http://foodbabe.com/2011/09/22/seize-your-sugar-cravings/

pre-pregnancy shape with little less effort.

If you are not the girl with the so-called perfect figure after having children, it doesn't matter. Her perfect life is only as perfect as the image she projects to the world. Behind closed doors she could have her own insecurities. You're you and that's perfectly fine. As we all know, the grass is often greener on the other side.

The Calorie Connection

When fitness gurus cry mantras like "feel the burn" they may not know it, but they're being literal. The burn they're likely referring to is the unpleasant feeling that you've overdone it as excess. This is lactic acid building up in our muscles faster than our bodies can shift it.

If you're sitting here thinking, they've got that wrong, it's lactate that causes the burn: there's a difference between the chemical burn that makes us warm up (thermogenesis) and sweat and the lactic acid that causes the discomfort. Lactic acid builds up when our muscles burn glucose, making pyruvate (pyruvic acid), which is metabolized to lactate (lactic acid).

If you were to burn a sugar cube (outdoors and away from children and animals) you could see this effect for yourself: as the sugar burns it releases energy as heat, and a similar chemical process is happening inside your muscles.

We don't smoke like the sugar cube because our muscles are much more efficient at converting the chemical energy locked away in the glucose than can be performed by a simple garden variety, outdoor experiment.

That said, we do use oxygen (just like the sugar cube does), and we do exhale carbon dioxide gas (CO_2) and water vapor (H_2O)—just like the sugar cube does. You can't see either of these—but you'll see the smoke (mostly ash), carbon, and particles of sugar. The gooey remains comprise almost all carbon, with a few trace elements.

But the heat it gave off… that's energy. You don't need to stick your pinkie into the burning cube or smoldering remains to see how much heat that tiny white cube gave off.

If you were to burn the sugar cube in pure oxygen, as a scientist might do in a lab, you could measure its calorific content. The energy it contains is about 12 Kcals (12 Cals).

This confusion ("cals" vs "Cals" vs "Kcals") is an awkward thing. What a scientist calls a calorie and what we call calories live on a different scale– by a factor of 1000x in fact. Fortunately, when it comes to dieting and food, calories in terms of what we need to live are always the same.

Technically, a calorie is the amount of energy required to raise the temperature of one gram of water by 1°C at one atmosphere (sea level). Which is a lot when you think that 1g of water is only a drop. (Just to add even more confusion into the mix, you occasionally see kilojoules (kJ). 4.2kJ is roughly equivalent to 1Kc. Scientists can be awkward devils.

When the rest of us think of calories (our imaginary sugar cube has 12 calories in it), we're working in kilocalories, the energy required to raise the temperature of 1Kg of water by 12°C.

We know instinctively that a little sugar cube is never going to produce anywhere near enough heat to do that, so something must be going on here. The sugar cube experiment is very inefficient and while it produces a fair amount of heat, a huge amount of carbon goes up as smoke and ash, and a great deal more ends up in a smoldering black mess on the surface you burnt it on. Scientists measuring calories use pure oxygen to make sure all the chemicals in the sugar cube get burned up, and special equipment to capture as much heat as is practical.

Like that equipment, your body is hugely efficient at capturing that energy. Life has spent millions of years evolving a huge array of systems to make the best use of the limited food supplies and what it can't use can always be stored away for another day.

As fat.

Fat is your long-term energy store. We all need a small amount of it.

The ability to store fat is so basic to our humanity it's thought there are only around eight people in the world living with a condition called muscular fibrositis disproportion[8] or MDP—the more common condition of lipo-dystrophy. Now these conditions, where our bodies are unable to store fat,

---

8   http://www.dailymail.co.uk/health/article-2029930/Mother-eats-like-horse-muscle-condition-stops-piling-pounds.html

might sound like a dream come true but as sufferers will tell you, they're nightmarish.

In the Victorian Golden Era (1850-1880) people consumed twice the calories we typically do today and rarely became overweight. Men were lithe and muscular with a typical manual laborer capable of shifting a ton of earth in a day. Women naturally carried more fat, but they were rarely overweight. Adulteration aside, the Victorians had an excellent diet: high in fresh fruit, fish and vegetables, low in salt and alcohol. Easy access to processed food was still a century or more away.

In the 21st Century, we're facing different challenges.

We're bombarded by advertisements telling us what to eat and how easy and quick a given food is, while at the same time receiving contradictory standards of what's OK from celebrities, models, magazines, film and television, and popular bloggers like Food Babe who have the PR down to a fine art.

It's difficult to know what to believe but it's easy to fall into the trap of finding a celebrity we want to emulate and to follow whatever fad diet they happen to be promoting, without any idea what sort of long-term effect that diet is having on their health (let alone our own). We don't even know if they're cheating. Professional cyclist and cancer survivor Lance Armstrong demonstrated this in his denial of using performance-enhancing drugs for years, finally coming clean in 2013. [9] Precisely what effect, if indeed any, that will have on Armstrong's future health is unknown.

We do know from analyzing the effects of chronic smoking that it takes around ten years for the long-term effects of an acute condition to fade. When cells wear out, are damaged, or otherwise need to take one for the team and die, they self-destruct through a process known as apoptosis. This allows new ones to form. Parts of our bodies are replaced at different rates, with the slowest tissues being those of the heart (1% per year at 25) and fat cells (which exist for about eight years). Our skeleton is renewed entirely over about ten years. For this reason, cancer survivors invariably have to wait a decade after completion of treatment before doctors can give them the "all clear." (It's now thought that some cancer cells can "hibernate"

---

9   http://www.theguardian.com/sport/2013/jan/15/lance-armstrong-admits-doping-winfrey

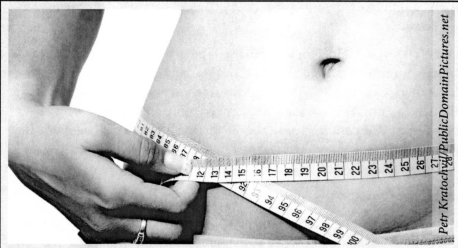

Petr Kratochvil/PublicDomainPictures.net

Beat the BMI

We've used BMI as the canonical example of weight and fitness in this chapter because it's so widely used. The truth is, unless you happen to conform to a very average body type—and few of us do—BMI is essentially misleading [1] as a measure of physical health or fitness.

A much simpler and accurate way to figure out if your weight is affecting your health is to check your visceral fat. This fat around our organs has been shown to be the most deleterious to health. Large buttocks (typically on women) are completely normal and thought to be fat stores for use in pregnancy and lactation: which is why men don't have them.

To check your visceral fat simply measure your waist size around your middle (at the belly button) and double that number. Now check your height. If 2x your waist measurement is more than your height, then you need to dump a few extra pounds. Amazingly, this works just as well for men and women and you can even do it with a piece of string!

A better, electronic solution, is offered by body composition monitors which can determine our fat to muscle ratio very accurately and help us decide if that overweight BMI reading is actually just all the muscle we've grown from our exercise regime or fat from too many doughnuts.

---

1   http://www.medicalnewstoday.com/articles/265215.php

for decades, so some sufferers may never be truly clear.)

Our health is a moving target and ten years is a long time to see the effects of any change we make. Celebrities, however, can sometimes act as a useful barometer, as the Internet features sites exposing how our favorite stars have aged. Just like the rest of us, some have aged well, others, not so well. Case in point, the buff figures of Val Kilmer (now 55) and Tom Cruise (now 52), whose aspirational physiques in 1986's Top Gun were the envy of men the world over. Three decades on, Kilmer has been subject to notable weight gain and a supposed cancer scare while Cruise remains an apparent picture of health. Cruise's fictional love interest, Kelly McGillis, now 57, looks very different from the waspish beauty of her 1980s heyday.

None of these stars were promoting fad diets. That's a more recent phenomenon. Besides that, they are no different from the stars of today. Until we figure out how to reverse the aging process, life is going to catch up to all of us sooner or later, and that includes Food Babe.

We only have Food Babe's word for it that her diet works, and we don't have the luxury of hindsight to know for sure that it will. By the time the results are in she will have doubtless been replaced by some other vacuous celebrity.

If we can learn anything from the Victorian Golden Era, it's that physical effort is key to maintaining a healthy weight.

The amount of energy we expend is determined by a number of factors, but as baseline daily measure, women expend around 2,000 calories and men 2,500. These rates vary quite dramatically depending on your frame size and level of activity. Compare that to Food Babe's claim:

> I got back to an attractive normal weight, and I've stayed there—
> even by eating up to 2,000 calories a day, normally a lot for a
> woman with my frame. [10]

So you can see that what she considers a lot is quite normal for a healthy woman of her age and activity levels. Remember she alludes to working out and doing yoga. She's not a couch potato who has discovered the secret to staying thin while binge-watching Netflix.

10   The Food Babe Way, p. 58

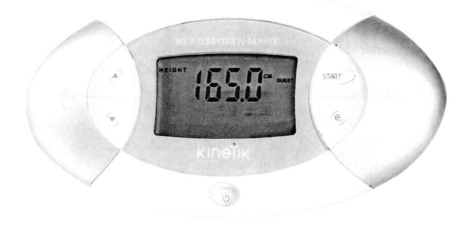

Figure 9.1: Simple, low-cost devices like this can give an accurate insight into how effective an exercise or diet program really is, by calculating our body fat and muscle ratios. (Kinetik Medical Devices Ltd.)

Men use more calories because their bodies comprise relatively larger amounts of muscle and it's muscle that burns the most calories. Even while we're sitting down, some of our muscles are working and using energy. Fat cells, on the other hand mostly just sit there acting as insulation and helping us to maintain a normal body temperature.

Ironically, the greater the percentage of body fat we have, the less energy we expend to keep warm in cooler environments and (pound for pound) the less muscle we have to use those extra calories.

When we're not exercising, two metabolic factors come into play. The first is the basal metabolic rate (BMR), which is the amount of energy our body uses just to stay alive. The second is the resting metabolic rate (RMR), the energy we expend doing everyday tasks while we're awake and not actively pushing ourselves.

Although an accurate measurement of our BMR is impossible without specialist equipment, for the purpose of weight loss, we can use the Harris-Benedict principle to provide a very rough estimate. From that, we can decide how many calories we need to expend in order to achieve a healthy weight.

To determine your total daily calorie needs (RMR), multiply your BMR by the appropriate activity factor, as follows:

Example 1: Bob is about 6 feet tall, 45 years of age and weighs 15 stones (210lbs). This gives him a BMI of 30.1, making him slightly obese.

$= 88.362 \quad + (6.08 \times 210)$

$\qquad\qquad + (12.19 \times 72)$

$\qquad\qquad - (5.677 \times 45 \text{ years old})$

$= 88.362 \quad + (1276.8 + 877.68 - 255.465)$

$= 1987.377$

So, Bob's BMR is approximately 2000 and since he sits on his butt all day, that means he needs to consume fewer than 2400 calories per day. Ideally, somewhat less than that.

Example 2:

Jo, a 30-year-old woman. 5'5" (65 inches) tall, weighs 139lbs and does moderate exercise about three times a week.

$= 447.593 + (4.19 \times 139) + (7.87 \times 65) - (4.330 \times 30)$

$= 447.593 + (582.41) + (511.55) - (129.9)$

$= 1411.653$

Note that Jo's BMR is considerably lower than the editor's but she does a little light exercise, giving her a total recommended calorific intake of 1900 calories per day. We should stress these calculations are an estimate and your true BMR/RMR is unlikely to match any of these exactly.

If your goal is to lose weight and keep it off (or just maintain a healthy weight) these figures in the "RMR for Weight Loss Calculator" on page 252 will help calculate safe, comfortable and achievable daily limits to help you through.

Despite the myriad claims, there are no magic bullets and no quick fixes to weight loss. Understanding your own body and its individual requirements is essential. We can't stress this enough and that's why we're providing these examples. Calculating your actual resting metabolic rate (RMR) is the first

Basal Metabolic Rate Calculator: US/Imp. version

Male			Female		
88.362	+	6.08 x Lbs)	447.593	+	4.19 x Lbs
	+	12.19 x Inches		+	7.87 x Inches
	-	5.68 x Years		-	4.330 x Years

Basal Metabolic Rate Calculator: Metric version

Male			Female		
88.362	+	13.397 x Kgs	447.593	+	9.247 x Kgs
	+	4.799 x cms		+	3.098 x cms
	-	5.677 x Years		-	4.330 x Years

Daily Calorie Calculator (RMR)

Daily Activity	BMR multiplier
Sedentary (no exercise)/desk job	1.2
Light exercise/sports 1-3 days	1.375
Moderate exercise/sports 3-5 days/week	1.55
Hard exercise/sports 6-7 days a week	1.725
Athletic/endurance training or very physical work	1.9

RMR for Weight Loss Calculator

Weight Loss Zone	RMR Multiplier
Max Weight Zone (BMI >30)—12 weeks max.	0.85
Slow Weight Loss (BMI >28)	1.0
Gentle Weight loss (BMI >25)	1.3
Maintenance Zone 1	1.4-1.6
Maintenance Zone 2	1.6-1.9
Maintenance Zone 3	1.9-2.5

step, as shown above before we modify it using the adjustments to match our own lifestyles. At the highest rate—designed for people with a BMI in excess of 30 (or a belly/height ration >0.5) you should be dropping no more than 1.5lbs per week over a period of no more than 12 weeks. Any more than this risks putting your body into a yo-yo cycle where any weight lost is immediately regained.

As your BMI drops, you can begin to increase your calorific intake slightly and slowly until you reach a comfortable weight and then work out your maintenance intake. However, it's important to realise that as we age, our metabolism slows so you need to re-calculate your RMR as you age.

This is the reason diets don't work in the long term—because once you return to your previous daily routine, the weight just jumps back on. The key is to adjust your everyday calorific intake to something you can stick with. Don't call it a diet—think of it as a change for life.

Following a plan like this an obese person such as Bob from the first example might drop 30lbs over 52 weeks which doesn't sound much but it's both achievable and manageable. Losing weight this way prevents us from setting impossible goals, which invariably results in a cycle of weight loss and rapid weight gain.

Food Babe has never really detailed her weight loss other than to boast about how fit and healthy she is—a shadow of her sugar-fuelled days of yesterday. We see the before and after pictures (blink and you'll miss them) and hear of her courageous struggle but we have no hard evidence other than anecdotes.

Trying to emulate this without guidance is a recipe for disaster.

Food Babe claims to have dropped 30lbs in her twenties simply by changing her diet. As we've just shown that loss can be achieved in around a year without too much effort other than a change in lifestyle: actively taking note of the calories we consume.

It's science, not magic.

Being sufficiently privileged to spend lots of time at the gym and preparing well-balanced meals—not to mention dumping sugary soda and sweets from her childhood—is what led to her "babe" physique. All of the other

Heart Rate Zones for Safe Exercise

- **50-60%**: the "walking the dog zone" zone. At this level your heart is just starting to push the blood a little faster than normal because your muscles are demanding slightly more oxygen to create the energy needed to move. Note that you can't usually get into this zone unless you start to walk slightly faster than normal. This is because your muscles use energy even at "rest", even though we're not actually aware of it. People who are just starting to exercise after a long period of sedentary existence, particularly those who are obese, should not usually exceed this level for at least the first few weeks of daily training. At this heart rate, experts suggest that we can lower our LDL cholesterol count, reduce the effect of emotional stress, and lower our blood pressure. So even this very light exercise is beneficial to our health.

- **60%–70%**: the recovery or "glow" zone. At this level your skin should be starting to redden slightly and you may start to sweat slightly as your temperature rises and your body compensates by exuding water to cool your skin. At this level you should be slightly breathless, but still able to hold a conversation without too much difficulty.

- **70%-80%**: the aerobic zone. The area most of us need to aim for to keep fit and live longer. At this rate we're starting to increase our endurance—the amount of time we can maintain exercise at the lower levels. This level is required to start to burn off serious calories from too much chocolate, chips and junk food. You will be sweating now as your muscles start to give off a lot of extra heat, and you will be quite breathless.

- **80%-90%**: the threshold zone: Once thought to be the upper limit for athletes, now recognized as achievable for everyone wishing to extend their endurance by increasing their tolerance for lactic acid production. Lung capacity is notably increased at this level, which may help with conditions such as asthma.

- **90%-100%**: Red zone. Few people need to exercise at this level— only the elite of the elite and even those athletes rarely push themselves to this limit, beyond which complete heart failure (and death) is likely.

Age		20	30	40	50	60	70
Z1		100 ⇕ 120	95 ⇕ 114	89 ⇕ 108	85 ⇕ 102	80 ⇕ 96	75 ⇕ 90
Z2	Aerobic zone	120 ⇕ 140	114 ⇕ 133	108 ⇕ 126	102 ⇕ 119	96 ⇕ 112	90 ⇕ 105
Z3		140 ⇕ 160	133 ⇕ 152	126 ⇕ 144	119 ⇕ 136	112 ⇕ 128	105 ⇕ 120
Z4	Anaerobic zone	160 ⇕ 180	152 ⇕ 171	144 ⇕ 162	136 ⇕ 153	128 ⇕ 144	120 ⇕ 135
Z5		180 ⇕ 200	171 ⇕ 190	162 ⇕ 180	153 ⇕ 170	144 ⇕ 170	135 ⇕ 160

tactics she touts are just window dressing.

To reiterate what we said at the head of the chapter, you cannot emulate her because you are not her. As Food Babe gets older, her metabolism will slow the same as ours. She will have to increase her energy output (exercise) and/or reduce her food intake, or she will get heavier. Age plays a cruel hand here too because as we age, our ability to exercise diminishes, so the only way to manage our weight is to watch what we eat more carefully.

This is the reason children and young people can eat almost non-stop and stay thin: they have much higher basal metabolic rate. When we reach our mid 20s, the slow, slippery slide begins, and we have to take more care of ourselves. Our health depends on it.

Walking the RMR

Ironically one of the most important things if you aim to lose weight is the amont of energy you actually burn. Your RMR is the amount of energy your body expends just sitting in a chair—but it's almost the same as the energy you expend walking the dog, driving to work or doing some light housework. Even though we know that sitting down for extended periods is bad for us, in terms of weight loss, it has little or no impact.

This is because the amount of calories we're burning is directly related to our heart rate and respiration. Our heart rate at rest (60-100 BPM for most of us [11]) directly reflects our RMR. Lower numbers indicate a better level of fitness. Adults with a regular resting heart rate over 100BPM should consult their doctor as this may indicate a condition called tachycardia which may be life-threatening.

You can see this for yourself with a simple experiment. Take your heart rate (or have a friend do it for you) when you've been sitting down relaxing for about 10 minutes. Now, get up and walk around for another 10, being careful not to push yourself. Walk the dog, make a cup of joe; that sort of thing.

Now, check your heart rate once more and see if it's elevated.

A difference of a few BPM isn't really relevant (you may even find that yours has dropped) since our heart rate changes all the time by small amounts as our bodies naturally adjust to a myriad small changes in demand. Simply eating a meal affects your heart rate as does what you eat and even the time of day.

The point to all of this is to demonstrate that although you may feel that you're active, you might find that your body is just "ticking over"—like a car sitting with the engine running. You can put your car into Drive and it will creep forward—albeit slowly—and your body is doing the same thing.

A simple guide to checking your energy usage is to check your breathing. If you're able to hold a conversation without feeling a little breathless, your body is still ticking over. In order to burn that extra weight, you need to make your muscles work harder—so they demand more oxygen and that drives your breathing harder. Just doing sufficient exercise to be slightly breathless four or five times per week (cycling, swimming, running etc.) is enough to improve your fitness level dramatically and increase your life expectancy.

For more accurate measurements without specialist equiment, heart rate remains the best indicator. Experts divide our exercise heart rates into five

---

11   http://www.mayoclinic.org/healthy-lifestyle/fitness/expert-answers/heart-rate/faq-20057979

broad ranges—each with specific benefits and purpose. Our maximum heart rate is usually estimated to be 220 minus our age in years. It's not perfect but it's quite close enough unless you're an elite athlete in training. Given that, the following zones apply: with details in the table on "Heart Rate Zones for Safe Exercise" on page 254. ■

10

Celiac, Gluten & You

"After I was diagnosed with celiac disease, I said yes to food, with great enthusiasm. Told I should never eat gluten again if I wanted to save my life, I vowed to taste everything I could eat, rather than focusing on what I could not." —Shauna James Ahern, Gluten-Free Girl and the Chef

Most people who claim to be gluten intolerant are self-diagnosed, driven by a strong desire to belong to the herd. The world is full of gorgeous celebrities who attribute their stick-thin figures to fad diets (that they frequently endorse), while at the same time, ignoring their excellent genes and designer clothes (not to mention the best makeup and hair money and studio lighting can buy). All of which conspire to make an average person look spectacular.

What we're seeing is a snapshot of how Jill Celeb looks right now, at this instant. Subject them to a few months of everyday life and the cracks will soon appear. (More of this in the next section.)

One pointed claim remains (touted by people like Dr. Joe Mercola and created by computer specialist, Stephanie Seneff [1]) : just how much influence does glyphosate residudes on our food have on, say, Celiac disease (gluten intolerance)? None whatsoever, as *Dr. Alessio Fasano, MD, Chief of Pediatric Gastroenterology and Nutrition, Massachusetts General Hospital for Children, Center for Celiac Research* & Treatment writes:

> *"Genetic predisposition plays a key role in CD and considerable progress has been made recently in identifying genes that are responsible for CD predisposition. It is well known that CD is strongly associated with specific HLA class II genes known as HLA-DQ2 and HLA-DQ8 located on chromosome 6p21."* [2]

---

1   http://articles.mercola.com/sites/articles/archive/2014/09/14/glyphosate-celiac-disease-connection.aspx

2   http://emedicine.medscape.com/article/1790189-overview

That means you inherit it from your parents. Though we don't recommend chugging Roundup on a Saturday night. If you haven't already tested positive for Celiac disease (only about 0.7% of the population has) you're probably not gluten intolerant—at least, not yet. You could, however, be sensitive to FODMAPs (more on this in the next section), which don't sound nearly as sexy as "gluten intolerant."

Although we don't know why people suddenly develop Celiac disease, we do know that sufferers all produce a faulty version of the human leukocyte antigen, and yet around a third of us are walking around with it, blissfully unaware anything is "wrong." What we don't know (yet) is why some people develop Celiac at a later age and others don't.

Adding to the problem is the delay between onset of symptoms and a final clinical diagnosis—up to 11 years just a decade ago, and still at least five years in 2014. Celiac disease remains very difficult to spot. Not everyone presents with the same symptoms discussed here.

Some of the blame is centered around popular books by physicians writing outside of their field of clinical expertise, such as *Grain Brain* (by neurologist David Perlmutter, MD), *Wheat Belly* (by cardiologist Dr. William Davies, MD), and further promoted by celebrities like Gwyneth Paltrow.

There's no question that both Perlmutter and Davies are qualified MDs in their own right, but there is a serious question if these books do anything other than exacerbate an already tense climate of fear over our food.

Persons with Celiac disease (gluten enteropathy) may experience some or all of the spectrum of complaints we've listed here. It is not a diagnostic chart and diagnosis must always be made by qualified health professionals. We can't stress strongly enough just how important it is, particularly as sufferers will normally need a blood test. Additionally, a biopsy is frequently called for in adult patients. They may also require experimental, professionally monitored changes in diet to confirm the condition.

Celiac disease is a highly complex, multi-systemic condition that even medical professionals find difficult to spot. Self-diagnosis is as ineffective as it is unhelpful, since eliminating gluten from our diet may mask symptoms of an entirely different disease. As a result of the placebo effect and our own cognitive biases, symptoms may be the result of other factors, or a reaction to FODMAPs.

Chest pain, for example, is often something simple like a bout of indigestion. But it could be something more complex like a gallstone, or even a potentially life-threatening condition such as a pulmonary embolism (a condition where a blood clot becomes lodged in the lungs) or a myocardial infarction (heart attack).

Medical professionals spend many years and very long hours to qualify and are constantly studying new diagnostic techniques as science provides new answers to age-old problems. Even the best "expert systems" are no replacement for qualified and experienced medical personnel, and relying on Google to check your symptoms is tantamount to self-flagellation.

Ironically, one of the worst things you can do if you suspect you might suffer from Celiac disease is to give up gluten. Pre-removing gluten from the diet actually makes a confirmed diagnosis and effective treatment more difficult.

Any person who thinks they can self-diagnose celiac disorder has a quack for a physician.

Hectic lifestyles, smoking, drinking too much alcohol, and general overindulgence take their toll on our bodies. It's tempting to pick up a book or listen to a celebrity like Food Babe and assume that you've found the problem. When combined with lack of adequate and regular exercise, these choices can cause a number of the ailments listed below, including all manner of digestive upsets: pain, loose stools, constipation, bloating; plus tiredness, headache, mouth ulcers, and poor immune response. This list is by no means exhaustive:

- Severe or occasional diarrhea, excessive gas and/or constipation
- Persistent or unexplained gastrointestinal symptoms, such as nausea and vomiting
- Hyposplenism (under-active spleen) in about 30% of cases, which *may* manifest as a poor immune response.
- Poor quality (pale/greasy) stools
- Recurrent stomach pain, cramping or bloating
- Any combination of iron, vitamin B12 or folic acid deficiency

caused by the poor absorption of some minerals
- Type 2 diabetes
- Anemia
- Tiredness and/or headaches
- Mouth ulcers
- Unexplained hair loss (alopecia)
- Skin rash (dermatitis herpetiformis) in about 1% of patients.
- Tooth enamel problems
- Liver abnormalities
- Joint and/or bone pain
- Neurological problems such as ataxia (poor muscle coordination) and peripheral neuropathy (numbness and tingling in the hands and feet)

Infants and children may additionally suffer from these symptoms

- Failure to thrive
- Diarrhea
- Muscle wasting
- Poor appetite
- Abdominal distension
- Lethargy
- Change of mood and emotional distress

If the above looks like a laundry list, that's because it is. While any permutation of these symptoms might be caused by food sensitivities, they are just as likely if not more likely to be due to other culprits. This is why it's important to address any troublesome symptoms with your doctor, and not self-diagnose and make sweeping dietary changes without consulting a professional. Don't simply listen to the Gwyneth Paltrows of the world. Indeed, we provided the lists above not as medical advice because we're not qualified to give it. The list serves to make a point: that it's easy enough to attribute health problems to food scapegoats. But easy answers are rarely right answers.

FODMAPS

FODMAPs is an acronym for "Fermentable, Oligo-, Di-, Mono-saccharides And Polyols" (enough to give our editor IBS). FODMAPs have become a huge part of our western diet and are considered to be far more likely culprits in the poor digestion than natural gluten or additives. FODMAPs include things as simple as fructose (a fruit sugar) and lactose (a sugar found in milk). Also found in this group are indigestible sugar alcohols such as xylitol, erythritol, isomalt, and maltitol.

Susceptible individuals are unable to process FODMAPs correctly, leading to bacterial fermentation, bloating, pain, gas (flatulence) and other symptoms associated with FGIDs (functional gastrointestinal disorders), such as irritable bowel syndrome.

The bad news for anyone thinking they may want to claim FODMAPs as a sexy new ailment to brag to their friends about is it really requires a medical referral to a dietician, because the dietary changes are dramatic and tailored to the individual patient.

FODMAPs are a relatively recent discovery and the best person to advise is a qualified physician. It's worth repeating that any one attempting self-diagnosis has a quack for a physician.

■

Foods suitable on a low-fodmap diet

fruit	vegetables	grain foods	milk products	other
fruit	**vegetables**	**cereals**	**milk**	**tofu**
banana, blueberry, boysenberry, canteloupe, cranberry, durian, grape, grapefruit, honeydew melon, kiwifruit, lemon, lime, mandarin, orange, passionfruit, pawpaw, raspberry, rhubarb, rockmelon, star anise, strawberry, tangelo	alfalfa, bamboo shoots, bean shoots, bok choy, carrot, celery, choko, choy sum, eggplant, endive, ginger, green beans, lettuce, olives, parsnip, potato, pumpkin, red capsicum (bell pepper), silver beet, spinach, squash, swede, sweet potato, taro, tomato, turnip, yam, zucchini	gluten-free bread or cereal products **bread** 100% spelt bread **rice** **oats** **polenta** **other** arrowroot, millet, psyllium, quinoa, sorgum, tapioca	lactose-free milk*, oat milk*, rice milk*, soy milk* *check for additives **cheeses** hard cheeses, and brie and camembert **yoghurt** lactose-free varieties **ice-cream substitutes** gelati, sorbet **butter substitutes** olive oil	**sweeteners** sugar* (sucrose), glucose, artificial sweeteners not ending in '-ol' **honey substitutes** golden syrup*, maple syrup*, molasses, treacle *small quantities
Note: if fruit is dried, eat in small quantities	**herbs** basil, chili, coriander, ginger, lemongrass, marjoram, mint, oregano, parsley, rosemary, thyme			

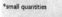

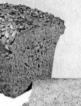

Eliminate foods containing fodmaps

excess fructose	lactose	fructans	galactans	polyols
fruit apple, mango, nashi, pear, tinned fruit in natural juice, watermelon	**milk** milk from cows, goats or sheep, custard, ice cream, yoghurt	**vegetables** artichoke, asparagus, beetroot, broccoli, brussels sprouts, cabbage, fennel, garlic, leek, okra, onion (all), shallots, spring onion	**legumes** baked beans, chickpeas, kidney beans, lentils, soy beans	**fruit** apple, apricot, avocado, blackberry, cherry, longon, lychee, nashi, nectarine, peach, pear, plum, prune, watermelon
sweeteners fructose, high fructose corn syrup	**cheeses** soft unripened cheeses eg. cottage, cream, mascarpone, ricotta	**cereals** wheat and rye, in large amounts eg. bread, crackers, cookies, couscous, pasta		**vegetables** cauliflower, green capsicum (bell pepper), mushroom, sweet corn
large total fructose dose concentrated fruit sources, large serves of fruit, dried fruit, fruit juice		**fruit** custard apple, persimmon, watermelon		**sweeteners** sorbitol (420) mannitol (421) isomalt (953) maltitol (965) xylitol (967)
honey corn syrup, fruisana		**miscellaneous** chicory, dandelion, inulin, pistachio		

IBS Self Help and Support Group - www.ibsgroup.org

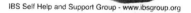

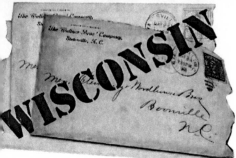

11
Letters from the Trenches

*I like the scientific spirit—the holding off, the being sure but not too
sure, the willingness to surrender ideas when the evidence is against
them..."* [1] *–Walt Whitman, American poet, essayist and journalist*

In many ways, Food Babe is a symptom of the growing dearth of critical
thinking in the information age; a lethargy of the brain, if you will. We've
all experienced the wildfire spread of scare stories and too-good-to-be-true
miracle cures. From the well-meaning aunt forwarding the latest article on
a frightening yet benign chemical in our household products, to that friend
always touting the latest superfood, it's hard to separate the truth wheat
from the myth chaff.

The following are pieces adapted from blogs and articles that originally
appeared online. Kavin published them as she encountered certain Food
Babe gaffes, with the intent to highlight the lack of, well, factual information in Vani Hari's claims.

In her first letter, Kavin takes a look back at the beginning of the Big Organic camp's crusade against Starbucks, arbitrarily demanding the company switch to organic milk in its drinks. To date, Starbucks hasn't complied
with this request.

Speaking of compliance, we sincerely hope nobody heeded Food Babe's
advice on trying to "prevent cancer naturally". In the next piece, we'll delve
into the world of Food Babe's cancer snafus. Cancer is the worst C-word,
yet the public discourse on the very complex disease is rife with misinformation. This letter explores just one instance of Hari's spreading dangerous
myths about cancer, and BRCA mutations in particular.

---

1   http://www.whitmanarchive.org/criticism/disciples/traubel/WWWiC/1/med.00001.37.html

Another myth that Food Babe loves to spread is that she's a victim: of sexism, racism, and even "hate groups". As an outspoken woman of color, Kavin knows what it's like to be on the receiving end of those "isms", but pulling those cards to defend against valid, even-handed criticism seems like a cheap shot. The next piece dissects Food Babe's retort to a 2014 NPR exposé. Needless to say, her accusations aren't pretty.

Also not pretty are Food Babe's gross misrepresentations of India, her parents' (and Kavin's parents') country of origin. In addition to the sweeping, inaccurate brush Hari has used to paint India, she even went as far as to state that her name, Vani, means "voice" in "Indian,"[2] though there is no such language, with the majority of Indians speaking Hindi, Bengali, Telugu, and Tamil, among several other languages. The piece explores some of the most egregious instances of "exotification" in the Food Babe Way.

The final letter explores Food Babe's victim card, with the addition of the "hater", "sexist", "racist" and "shill" cards among others, which Kavin collectively terms the "Deck of Deflection". Keep in mind, other charlatans also play these cards to deflect from valid criticism, and you'll soon see why it's such an effective albeit cheap tactic.

After all, if you don't have facts to back up your arguments, the second best thing is painting your opponents as haters, am I right?

Kavin Senapathy, Madison, Wisconsin

---

2   The Food Babe Way, p. 7

The Fear Babe

Dear Reader,

I've been reading in my free time again when I'm not writing. I regret to report that while I have never been a Starbucks connoisseur, I must side with the company in this newest battle. Wielding figurative torches and pitchforks and shouting "Organic Milk Next!," Vani Hari and her cronies are burning Starbucks at the stake. Fortunately despite social media fuel, Starbucks refuses to catch fire.

Here are the details:

Food Babe (Vani Hari) went after Starbucks for its Pumpkin Spice Latte. According to her in-depth investigation, [1] these lattes not only contain "no real pumpkin," and a "toxic dose of sugar," but also use dairy from "Monsanto milk cows fed GMO" fodder.

This is so absurd it's laughable. Twitter users had a blast jokingly lambasting products with similarly misleading names a la, "no kids in sour patch kids," "no fruit in Fruity Pebbles," and "no beans in jelly beans." Furthermore, any customer buying a decadent Starbucks latte without the faintest notion that it's high in sugar has more serious problems than the sugar itself.

Although Food Babe implored Starbucks to change their ingredients, the company didn't bite. In fact, Starbucks practically ignored Ms. Hari's query about the timeline for phasing out caramel coloring. At least they were tactful and kind enough to respond as follows:

> *"We actually don't have anything else to share at this time, but thanks for checking!"*

Although caramel coloring is considered safe, [2] this hasn't stopped [3] the tenacious Food Babe.

Next in her arsenal is the *Monsanto milk* in Starbucks' beverages. On October 5th, Food Babe's "army" along with Moms Across America and

---

1   http://foodbabe.com/2014/09/02/drink-starbucks-wake-up-and-smell-the-chemicals/

2   http://www.fda.gov/Food/IngredientsPackagingLabeling/FoodAdditivesIngredients/ucm364184.htm

3   https://www.facebook.com/thefoodbabe/photos/a.208386335862752.56063.132535093447877/830361756998537/?type=1&theater

other anti-GMO activists [4] will be calling on Starbucks to exclusively serve organic milk. According to GMO Inside, "Since March 2014, Starbucks CEO Howard Schultz has received over 120,000 petitions asking for organic milk. Despite the overwhelming feedback, Starbucks has remained completely silent. It's time to turn the campaign volume up a notch."

This is because the entire movement against Starbucks serving conventional milk is pointless at best. Readers—I have no qualms in saying organic milk is no safer [5] or more nutritious than its conventional counterparts. Vani does this because she is an attention-seeker with a financial incentive. These ploys get her devotees riled up, in turn leading to a larger following. This larger following will convert to extra clicks on her sponsor links, increasing her sponsor income.

I've said it once, [6] and many times more, [7] and don't mind sounding like a broken record. Genetic Modification is a toolbox and not a product.

Publicity-seeking schemes like this anti-Starbucks crusade are not only pointless but misleading and must be combated by scientifically-savvy media and public, a science-based army if you will. These ploys would best be ignored by corporations like Starbucks.

I'm happy to report that my comrade Chow Babe wrote a petition [8] entitled, "Starbucks, please ignore the organic extremists. We love your coffee and don't want the price to go up because you bowed to a small number of self-centered people."

I couldn't have titled it better myself.

Kavin

Adapted from Grounded Parents [9]

---

4 http://gmoinside.org/starbucks-national-day-action-organicmilknext/

5 http://www.forbes.com/sites/jonentine/2013/12/19/got-healthier-milk-how-activist-scientists-and-journalists-bungled-a-report-on-organic-foods/

6 http://groundedparents.com/2014/06/20/choosy-moms-choose-gmos/

7 http://groundedparents.com/2014/07/09/good-parents-with-good-hearts-are-pro-gmo/

8 https://www.change.org/p/starbucks-starbucks-please-ignore-the-organic-extremists-we-love-your-coffee-and-don-t-want-the-price-to-go-up-because-you-bowed-to-a-small-number-of-self-centered-people

9 http://groundedparents.com/2014/10/01/food-babe-moms-across-america-stop-drinking-starbucks/

Wisconsin, November 6, 2014

Dear Reader,

I was going through old notes and came across a disturbing tidbit. Vani has not only promulgated inaccurate information on food; she's also doling out cancer advice. While I'm no expert on cancer, my assertions are based in solid science. I have a high-level understanding of how cancers work, which is leagues more than Vani can claim. Furthermore, arguing for consensus requires far less expertise than spouting fabricated misinformation does. Extraordinary claims require extraordinary evidence.

Food Babe   👍 Like Page

May 15, 2013 · Charlotte, NC · ✎

If you got tested positive for the BRCA gene (a gene responsible for cancer) - would you remove your breasts? or testicles for that matter even if they found NO cancer in your body? Or would eat the best foods on the planet, avoid as many environmental toxins as possible and try to prevent cancer naturally? The story in the news about Angelina Jolie has me puzzled and concerned.

Share

👍 1,317 people like this

Figure: 11.1 Seriously Vani? Do you even science? O wait... you don't do you. (Food Babe/Facebook.com)

Vani made this sweeping, non-evidence based claim on BRCA mutations in 2013 (Figure: 11.1).

I'm having difficulty scraping the remnants of my jaw off the floor. I responded as follows on my Facebook fan page[1]:

> *"This is why ignorance from people like Food Babe makes me so angry. Spouting so called "puzzlement" and "concern" about cancer while you obviously have no idea what you're talking about is deplorable. First of all, one doesn't test "positive for the BRCA gene." *Everyone* has BRCA1 and BRCA2 genes. Both of these genes code*

---

1   https://www.facebook.com/Ksenapathy

for tumor suppressor proteins. When there is a defective mutant allele in a certain region of these genes, the tumor suppressor proteins aren't produced, or don't function correctly. Still, everyone has a copy of these genes inherited from each parent, so the un-mutated copy produces the proper proteins, thus compensating for the deleterious mutation on the other copy. The problem is it's much more likely, almost certain that a mutation will occur in one cell on the "good" version, so now both copies are messed up eventually leading to cancer. For someone without one of these inherited mutations, a somatic mutation would have to occur on *both* copies of the gene in the same cell. Statistically, it's very unlikely that this will happen, so this specific, nasty form of breast cancer will not occur in a person without a mutation inherited from mom or dad. So statistically, a person that has inherited one of these problem alleles is pretty much screwed. (This is a very simplified explanation.) Sorry Food Babe, all the organic kale and healthy smoothies in the world don't change that. Shame on you. Stick with what you know. And no, you don't "know" anything about agriculture, chemistry, or biology worth the sugar in my toxic morning coffee."

To put it simply, there are two main types of genes associated with cancer: Proto-oncogenes and tumor suppressor genes. Proto-oncogenes code for proteins that regulate cell growth. When these proteins are synthesized properly, some tell cells when they should grow (e.g. during fetal development). Other proto-oncogenes help synthesize proteins that tell cells when to take one for the team and die. Certain mutations in these genes can lead to cells growing out of control, AKA cancer.

BRCA genes are tumor suppressor genes. The relevant deleterious mutations in BRCA1 and BRCA2 demonstrate the "two-hit" tumor suppressor carcinogenesis model, also known as the Knudson Hypothesis [2]. We each get two copies of all twenty-two somatic chromosomes, one from each parent, plus one sex chromosome from each parent, an X from mom, and an X or Y from dad. We inherit two copies of every gene, including BRCA1 and BRCA2. These genes produce proteins that help repair a specific type of

---

2   http://link.springer.com/article/10.1007/BF01366952

DNA damage. The likelihood of both copies sustaining deleterious mutations in the same cell (two somatic hits) is relatively low.

Let's say one of the copies you got from either parent is mutated in a way that makes this protein either not work (along with other complex events I won't describe today) or not get synthesized at all. (A mutation you get from a parent is called a "germline" mutation; germ cells make sperm and egg cells. Mutations that happen in your body after you're conceived are called "somatic.") In this case, you're born with one hit in every single cell already. All it takes is for the second copy to get mutated anywhere (along with other complex events I won't describe today), and you're well on your way to cancer. Thus, when someone is born with one of these BRCA mutations, s/he is far more likely [3] to develop breast or ovarian cancer—up to a

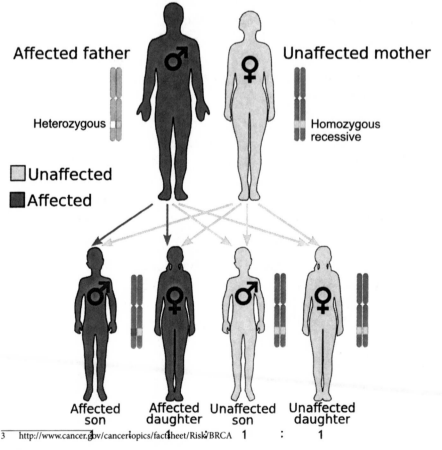

3   http://www.cancer.gov/cancertopics/factsheet/Risk/BRCA

65% or more lifetime chance of breast cancer. In addition, a parent with an inherited mutation has a 50% chance of passing it to each offspring.

Imagine a situation in which most people get to roll two dice, and rolling two 3s means a likely cancer sentence. People born with these mutations have two dice, but one of them has 3s on all sides.

There is much that scientists have to learn about cancer. But there is much that science already knows. While my explanation is extremely abridged, it is embarrassingly obvious that Vani never understood any of this. It's painfully clear that she is "puzzled." Not for the snarky reason she implies, but because she doesn't understand even the basics of carcinogenesis. If she did, she would realize that eating the "best foods" or avoiding so-called toxins won't "prevent cancer naturally."

Yes, cancers are immeasurably more complex than I've described them here. Yes, healthy diet and lifestyle are important. But what Vani deems "healthy" and what experts deem healthy are vastly different. Environmental factors that cause cancer include smoking, obesity, certain viral infections, and radon gas. [4] Factors that don't cause cancer [5] include GMO foods, vaccines, sugar, and caramel coloring in lattes. Things that don't prevent or treat cancer include organic foods, herbal remedies, or green juice.

Anyhow, I'm off to commiserate with the other science advocates. I'm almost certain that Vani will delete her post well before you lay eyes on this letter. We've learned to preserve her statements for posterity.

More soon,

Kavin

Adapted from Grounded Parents: [6]

---

4   http://www.cancer.gov/cancertopics/factsheet/Risk/radon
5   http://www.cancer.gov/cancertopics/myths
6   http://groundedparents.com/2014/11/06/food-babe-stop-giving-cancer-advice/

The Fear Babe

Dear Reader,

NPR did an exposé on Food Babe and her army, and Vani is retaliating big time. As you know, I'm a mother and science writer, and I've been critical [1] of Hari's work over the last several months. I am not a scientist by the traditional definition. I don't have a Ph.D, nor have I authored peer-reviewed research publications. Still, I have a unique perspective afforded by the intersection of a sound working knowledge of genomics, genetics, and bioinformatics. I've garnered this knowledge being raised by a molecular biologist, working for a small private-sector genomics R&D company, and via course work and extensive reading on the subject.

In addition to writing on the subjects of feminism, atheism, and biotechnology in agriculture and medicine, I took the position of spokesperson for Chow Babe, [2] an open social media critic of Food Babe. While Chow Babe is a parody of Food Babe, she has gained thousands of followers sharing one common notion—that Vani Hari is a charlatan without evidence for her propaganda.

Maria Godoy of NPR's *The Salt* took notice and contacted me and a few scientists to discuss scientific backlash against Food Babe. Considering that NPR is a renowned and reputable organization, I gladly obliged. Over the weekend–shortly after the piece [3] was published and after declining to be interviewed for NPR–Food Babe lashed out at her critics.

Vani refers to me as follows (and yes, I'll explain why I know she's talking about me specifically):

> Seemingly reputable news organizations like NPR (in a blog post titled "Is The Food Babe A Fearmonger? Scientists Are Speaking Out") even linked to the hate groups—quoting one of their spokespeople and repeated their ridiculous and biased messages as if they have any merit. [4]

---

1   http://groundedparents.com/2014/10/01/food-babe-moms-across-america-stop-drinking-starbucks/

2   https://www.facebook.com/thechowbabe

3   http://www.npr.org/blogs/thesalt/2014/12/04/364745790/food-babe-or-fear-babe-as-activist-s-profile-grows-so-do-her-critics

4   http://www.geneticliteracyproject.org/2014/12/08/gmo-opponent-vani-hari-food-babe-responds-to-criticisms/

I am the only one quoted in the NPR piece with the title of "spokesperson." (For more information, see this [5] post describing how I became spokesperson for a public figure known as Chow Babe in late October.) Therefore, it's obvious that Food Babe is referring to me. As with all of the individuals she criticizes in her response, she is too cowardly to call me by name for fear of having to engage in extensive discourse. Also, it's likely that she's been advised to refrain from naming her foes to avoid liability.

Although this isn't the first letter [6] I've written to Food Babe, here is the response I've penned:

Dear Vani,

Scientists, skeptics, farmers, and science writers like me have given you ample occasions to have civil debates. Not once have you taken the opportunity to do so. Nevertheless, I will continue to reach out with the hope that you'll agree to a direct dialog.

Yes, I happen to be Chow Babe's spokesperson, but first and foremost I'm an outspoken writer [7] challenging unscientific and misleading propaganda. Early on in my criticism of scientific misinformation, I noticed you perhaps unintentionally misleading your followers on the subject of cancer. For example, you once asked your readers whether eating the "best foods on the planet" and avoiding environmental toxins would prevent cancer in an individual with a BRCA 1 or 2 mutation. In short, this notion is completely erroneous. The likelihood of breast or ovarian cancer is very high with these specific hereditary mutations, and your suggestions to avoid a cancer diagnosis are mere wishful thinking. Here is my piece [8] criticizing your stance on BRCA mutations in detail.

In addition, you frequently demonize so-called carcinogens without scientific basis. For instance, you demonize group 2b carcinogens like carrageenan. Carrageenan is categorized as "possibly carcinogenic to humans," yet you happily post selfies drinking alcoholic beverages. You must know that wine, beer, and spirits are classified by the IARC as

---

5   http://chowbabearmy.com/?p=20

6   https://www.facebook.com/Ksenapathy/photos
     /a.1488948321372476.1073741830.1488134174787224/1491477724452869/

7   http://www.geneticliteracyproject.org/contributor/ksenapathy

8   http://groundedparents.com/2014/11/06/food-babe-stop-giving-cancer-advice/

group 1 carcinogens, meaning they are known to cause cancer in humans. You discuss cancer often on your blog, yet it's painfully clear that you don't understand how carcinogenesis works even at the most basic level.

This brings me to my next point. You state in your response that one doesn't need a Ph.D to be a consumer advocate or food investigator, and that "just because you have a degree, doesn't make you right."

Indeed, I wholeheartedly agree that one doesn't need a Ph.D to discourse about food and food-related science. Nevertheless, I always believe that it's critical to draw from mainstream experts. Claims need to be supported by the broad weight of empirically based studies and not just reflect someone's opinion or a one-off study that fits preconceived notions. To blithely abandon the scientific consensus to embrace views considered unscientific by the most reputable science bodies in the United States and world suggests ideology and activism for its own sake, and not science. At minimum, one needs a solid grasp of the science behind claims in order to be credible.

You do not appear to understand what a "science experiment" means as distinct from pure opinion; what you deem "personal experience." You state the following:

> I know with my own body, that eliminating food additives was one of the best decisions I ever made—before that I was on several prescription drugs, felt and looked awful. I have more energy now than I did 10 years ago, 10 years older!—How is that possible if there isn't something to all of this healthy eating? Or more directly, to eliminating the chemicals that major food companies have yet to justify to us with any explanation.
>
> Others without a Ph.D have also conducted the same experiments, using their bodies and personal experience and have come to a similar conclusion.
>
> I use a variety of published scientific papers, interviews with experts, studies and opinions from noteworthy and respected public interest groups in my writings (they are usually blue hyperlinked throughout my posts). We are still learning the impacts of the food we eat—much of it hasn't even been studied—

thousands of chemicals in our food supply remain untested. So much new information is being discovered every single day.

Vani, using one's body and personal experience does not a science experiment make, no matter what the self-proclaimed "conclusion." A valid experiment must be conducted under controlled conditions with a clear hypothesis, and confounding factors must be minimized. For the results to be compelling, they must be reproducible. In other words, you need confirming independent studies by reputable scientists.

As Carl Sagan once said, "Extraordinary claims require extraordinary evidence." The evidence you cite to corroborate your extraordinary claims is far from extraordinary; indeed it's dicey and weak. The so-called credentialed experts you cite may have Ph.Ds, yet this makes them no less wrong. There is no body of evidence to support their claims, and they are not primary researchers in these fields. You take dubious or totally fabricated findings, almost always unscientific and often anecdotal, and tout them as alarming, scary truth. If this isn't unscientific fear mongering, I don't know what is.

I was shocked and heartbroken to see you conflating my message and those of my comrades with the hateful, and violently misogynistic messages you've received. You call me the spokesperson for a "hate group," yet I'm a feminist, a skeptic and, above all else, compassionate. Many women have been targets of misogyny online. Internet misogyny is a scourge that we all should continue to combat together. I too have been targeted, told that I'm "poisoning" my children and that it will be my fault if they ever suffer a terminal illness. In addition, I'm Indian-American just like you and have always defended [9] you against ignorant racist remarks, in part because I know how it feels.

While these attacks are deplorable, they are irrelevant to the majority of sensible, scientific and civil backlash against your work. Conflating misogyny with relevant opposition is underhanded. You are using this in an attempt to derail the entire conversation–a public conversation in which you've never even been willing to engage. You're throwing yourself a pity party and inviting your entire army.

---

9   https://www.facebook.com/Ksenapathy/posts/1494891477444827

The fact is you have refused to engage with reasonable critics of your writings–the misinformation, sometimes dangerous, that you spread so carelessly. Being critical of your campaigns does not make someone hateful. I'll repeat, it's hurtful and offensive to paint all of your opponents with a "hate group" brush. Peruse the 9000+ members of the Banned by Food Babe group [10] and read the comments. These are not the comments of a hate group.

Vani, you exemplify the most condemnable misogynistic attacks as representative of your opponents. None of the people or organizations you lambast in your post condone these awful attacks. You are personally responsible for unsubstantiated, utterly fabricated ad hominem attacks against many of us, and to which I've been subjected [11] all too often–the shill gambit.

Not everyone who is critical of you is automatically a shill for Big Ag or Big Biotech. The unfounded accusation of shilling is based in ignorance and disingenuousness. This is an empty tactic. If any of us truly has a "financial incentive" to oppose you, please, produce tangible evidence, don't just spew rhetoric.

How is Dr. Kevin Folta, department chair of Horticultural Sciences at the University of Florida, one of the most independent of scientists in the world with no industry connections making money from the biotech industry and Monsanto? How are Chow Babe, Science Babe, Food Hunk or I profiting from criticizing your views? Produce evidence.

Vani, I implore you to stop name-calling and throwing tantrums, and to respond to the relevant questions posed to you. And if you disagree, rather than retreat into your echo chamber [12] of support, venture out and engage with critics. We're all willing and eager for dialog, in public, and in any forum of your choosing.

Sincerely,
Mother, Feminist and Science Advocate,
Kavin Senapathy

---

10   https://www.facebook.com/groups/BannedByFoodBabeOpen/
11   http://groundedparents.com/2014/07/21/monsanto-shill-mom/
12   https://www.facebook.com/groups/foodbabearmy

Do you think she'll respond? I doubt it, but it was worth a shot.

Yours truly,

Kavin

As of the publication of this letter, Senapathy and Chow Babe have parted ways professionally but remain friends.

Adapted from Genetic Literacy Project [13]

---

13   http://geneticliteracyproject.org/2014/12/evolution-of-food-babe-from-misguided-consumer-advocate-to-crude-bully/

The Fear Babe

Dear Reader,

Now and then when I'm exposing charlatans' shenanigans, I find that I "can't even." You know the feeling, when you're so flabbergasted you're nearly at a loss for words. Luckily, I'm an articulate gal. I was reading Vani Hari's book and noticed a common theme: The *appeal to India*. Here's what I have to say to her:

Dear Vani,

Your exotification [1] of India, and simultaneous painting of the nation as full of people who can only afford cheap food is offensive. As an Indian-American, I'm appalled and disgusted by your frequent "appeals to India" in your new book "The Food Babe Way." There is so much this-is-how-my-ancestors did it, this-is-how-all-Indians live and eat rhetoric. This is no better than a ploy to make your "way" seem exotic, Eastern, and therefore, good. For example in chapter four you state,

> For thousands of years, my ancestors in India had one cow that they shared with the rest of the villagers. [2]

Oh, how charming. Gag me with a finger (Indians don't use spoons, don't you know?). Vani, you're generalizing and fallaciously homogenizing a vast country populated by over a billion diverse people. You go on to blather,

> Indian immigrants and other immigrants from raw-milk-producing countries are being duped by the US dairy industry and don't even know it. I'd really like to see my family recipes passed down from generation to generation, but I'm not sure we can do this safely for our future children and grandchildren unless we can all get access to real raw milk. [3]

Are you really trying to tell me that Indian recipes call only for raw milk? Purely anecdotal here, but my mom makes perfectly delicious and authentic Indian dishes with regular, pasteurized American yogurt,

---

1 http://mediadiversified.org/category/exotification-notyourfetish/
2 The Food Babe Way, p. 110
3 The Food Babe Way, p. 113

milk, and buttermilk and no, she doesn't buy organic milk. But I'm sure your sad little lament about not being able to pass your family's traditions to your descendants is moving to the average, unsuspecting American.

Further, you claim to give credence to your heritage and culture, yet can't be bothered to know that India is a vast, diverse nation with many languages. Case in point:

> Dad and Mom had my brother first and then, seven years later, me. They named me Vani, a name I hated as a child because my schoolmates made fun of it and no one could pronounce it. But in Indian, it means "voice"–how prophetic, because I've definitely developed one. [4]

Vani, you must be aware that there is no language called "Indian." India has a rich and varied culture, where over a hundred [5] officially recognized languages are spoken. More accurately, "Vani" can mean "voice" or "expression of thoughts" in Hindi; the word originated from Sanskrit. If you were aware of this fact, did you doubt that your audience is savvy enough to know or look up the word "Hindi?"

You repeatedly make these "appeals to India." Here, you either grossly exaggerate or lie about your father:

> My dad has always liked fast food because it's cheap, and that's why he fed us at fast food restaurants when we were kids... Growing up in India, he was brought up to believe that food's sole purpose was to keep you alive, and you never wasted food. Buying food cheap was the only way to get it. After moving to the United States, he mostly subsisted on fast food because it was a good buy. Sadly, this reasoning meant that my dad never paid attention to the nutritional value of good food. Over time, he developed type 2 diabetes. [6]

Guess what? Not everyone "growing up in India" is brought up the same way. Not everyone who grew up in India is naïve enough to think it's a good idea to subsist on fast food because "it's a good buy." A typical In-

---

4   The Food Babe Way. p. 7

5   http://blogs.reuters.com/india/2013/09/07/india-speaks-780-languages-220-lost-in-last-50-years-survey/

6   The Food Babe Way. p. 151

dian diet isn't significantly more expensive to cook than buying fast food every meal. Indian non-vegetarians tend to only eat meat once or twice a week and consume a diet high in vegetables and lentils. I assure you, my mom fed her whole family a nutritious Indian meal every night on a low grocery budget.

Here's where your story doesn't add up. In your Experience Life interview, you state:

> Actually, my dad wanted us to fit into the American lifestyle, so my brother and I were never required to eat the Indian food my mom cooked. She would cook one meal for herself and my dad— gourmet, Indian, from scratch, full of spices and vegetables from her garden—which to me looked weird and gross. And for us kids, she relied on processed foods: microwavable Salisbury steak, mozzarella sticks, chicken tenders, and all that stuff that came in a box from the frozen section. McDonald's and Burger King and Wendy's. Really, we were allowed to eat whatever we wanted, to fit in with the world around us. [7]

So what was it, did your dad subsist primarily on fast food or eat home-made, fresh Indian meals? It seems that you weren't quite honest one of these two times. If I'm wrong, please explain how.

Additionally, you clearly have no idea about the complexity of type 2 diabetes, especially among the Indian population. Would you know what I mean if I said that the genotype [8] of type 2 diabetes is believed by scientists to be different [9] from that of the western population despite similar phenotype/clinical presentation? That non-overweight Indians are more prone to developing type 2 diabetes despite healthy diets and active lifestyles than their western counterparts? I think not. But I digress. I can't imagine what other drivel the rest of your book spouts about India. I've only read five chapters of Food Babe Way, and I'm not sure how much more I can take….

Incredulously,

Kavin Senapathy

---

7   https://experiencelife.com/article/the-voice-vani-hari/
8   http://www.ncbi.nlm.nih.gov/pubmed/17496355
9   http://diabetes.diabetesjournals.org/content/62/5/1369

By the way, my name "Kavin," [10] is pronounced exactly like the word, "coven."
Growing up, almost nobody pronounced it correctly. It means "beauty" in
Tamil, my parents' native language. Apparently they had high hopes for their
daughter to be beautiful, or to bring beauty to the world? I love my name
though I didn't appreciate it until adulthood.

Sincerely,

Kavin

Adapted from Skepchick [11]

---

10 The team on this book call Kavin, "Sir!" (As you should. Now stand up straight, soldier!—Kavin)
11 http://skepchick.org/2015/02/kavin-cant-even-food-babe-way-exotifies-india-lies-about-her-dad/

Dear Reader, Or shall I say, friend? Our ongoing correspondence has certainly brought us closer.

I feel compelled to address this upsetting statement. I'm going to do this as quickly as possible because I'd rather spend my time debunking scientific misinformation. Yesterday, on the evening of the release of her book "The *Food Babe Way*," Vani Hari decided to have a Twitter "party." It appears that she decided to pre-emptively defend herself from opponents. I may be wrong, but as her most outspoken Indian-American, feminist critic, I think I'm uniquely qualified to address this. I hope you agree.

 Food Babe @thefoodbabe · Feb 11

Twitter party at 9pm EST to celebrate The #FoodBabeWay I refuse to be intimidated by racists, sexists, shills & haters. Keep your voice loud

While it's admirable to stand your ground, most of the people Food Babe refers to here are actually experts who did nothing more than critique her misrepresentation of science. (Food Babe/Twitter)

Hari has previously referred to her critics as misogynist, sexist, industry shills, to which I responded in detail here. [1] To borrow a quote from myself:

> "*Many women have been targets of misogyny online. Internet misogyny is a scourge that we all should continue to combat together. I too have been targeted, told that I'm "poisoning" my children and that it will be my fault if they ever suffer a terminal illness. In addition, I'm Indian-American just like you, and have always defended [2] you against ignorant racist remarks, in part because I know how it feels…Conflating misogyny with relevant opposition is*

---

1   http://geneticliteracyproject.org/2014/12/10/evolution-of-food-babe-from-misguided-consumer-advocate-to-crude-bully/

2   https://www.facebook.com/Ksenapathy/posts/1494891477444827

underhanded. You are using this in an attempt to derail the entire conversation–a public conversation in which you've never even been willing to engage. You're throwing yourself a pity party and inviting your entire army."

If you're not with her, you're against her: evil, sexist racists—you name it.

From the above passage, my readers should glean that I have been tactful, eloquent, and civil with Food Babe in the past. Here's what I need to say to Vani:

Girl, please. Calling your opponents racist is no minor allegation. You don't get to pull the race card from your Deck of Deflection without looking naïve at best, and like a bona fide sociopath at worst. Included in your Deck of Deflection are the Sexist Card, Shill Card, Hater Card, and now the Racist Card. Like I've said, I'm a woman, I'm an ethnic minority, and as such I'm extremely careful about calling anyone racist or sexist. If and when one claims racism or sexism, s/he should be ready to show some evidence. I'll make it easy for you by naming some of your critics. Then, you can go ahead and show us instances of their being racist or sexist. This is not an all-inclusive list:

Dr. Kevin Folta [3]

Dr. Steven Novella

Dr. John Coupland

Dr. David Gorski

Kavin Senapathy [4]

Yvette d'Entremont [5]

Amanda, The Farmer's Daughter USA [6]

Your move, Vani. Where is the racism? Where is the sexism? Like many others, I've been a target [7] of both of these "isms," yet I would never deign

---

3   https://www.facebook.com/pages/Kevin-M-Folta/712124122199236
4   https://www.facebook.com/ksenapathy
5   http://scibabe.com/
6   http://www.thefarmersdaughterusa.com/
7   http://groundedparents.com/2014/03/20/go-home-little-terrorist/

to slap those labels on people without warrant. To do so is deplorably un-ethical. These allegations are highly offensive, and your detractors deserve to know where they're coming from. I can only speak for myself, but if you can point out any legitimate instances of my being sexist or racist, I will apologize.

As for calling us shills, I won't address that here because it's a cheap trick you pull far too often. See my post with a tongue-in-cheek title, "Monsanto Shill Mom [8]"

You say in your recent Alex Jones interview (and believe me, I didn't watch that entire train wreck. One of my followers brought this to my attention):

> It is about making sure we stand up for the truth no matter what... The information that I am going to share...are meant to help the world, meant to bring a healthier world, and also help reduce the amount of disease rates in this country. What I want to ask my detractors is this: Why do you spend all day attacking me? Why don't you spend some of your time finding something healthy to bring to the world? [9]

Puh-lease. You have got to be kidding. Nobody is spending all day attacking you. You seem to have delusions of grandeur, or you're disingenuous as usual. Many of your critics are doctors, scientists, and science commu-nicators. By their very nature, these people's lives are all about making the world a healthier and better place. Others like me are doing just what you claim to be doing, standing up for the truth no matter what. I spend most of my time keeping my kids healthy, participating in science activism and advocacy, and communicating science to a lay audience.

Why do we "spend all day attacking" you? Unlike your claim in the Alex Jones interview that most of your critics' work is about you, I write about you very little, as is demonstrable by my body of work. I believe the same is true of your other critics. Still, your pre-emptive contention that your crit-ics are somehow obsessed with you is brilliant. This way, whenever anyone tries and refutes your claims, you can pull the "Obsessed with Food Babe" card. Indeed, Vani Hari's Deck of Deflection keeps growing and growing.

---

8   http://groundedparents.com/2014/07/21/monsanto-shill-mom/
9   https://www.youtube.com/watch?v=RAXgZ8IG84Q

Nevertheless, your non-evidence-based fear mongering needs refutation, and this is why we spend our valuable time addressing your blunders. When you arbitrarily demonize beneficial and inherently benign tools like biotech, promote chemophobia, and conflate consuming conventionally grown foods with eating "processed" junk, you contribute to the hindrance of progress. You contribute to the perpetuation of American scientific illiteracy. [10] You contribute to irrational conspiracy theories.

Now, you've called a group of hard working writers, scientists, and doctors sexist, racist, shills. Either you should be ashamed of yourself or you'll explain why you continuously make these allegations. As I've borrowed from Carl Sagan countless times—extraordinary claims require extraordinary evidence.

So put up or shut up.

Thanks for letting me get that off my chest.

Sincerely,

Kavin

Adapted from Grounded Parents [11]

---

10   https://www.youtube.com/watch?v=RAXgZ8IG84Q

11   http://groundedparents.com/2015/02/12/no-food-babe-your-detractors-arent-racists-sexists-haters-or-shills/

12

Confessions of a Shopaholic

*"Profit is sweet, even if it comes from deception."—Sophocles,
Ancient Greek playright*

Food Babe seems to take great joy in pointing out alleged double standards and hypocrisy in corporate product labeling. We must admit we enjoy doing the same with the items she sells. It's so easy. You'd be hard pressed to find any product sold on FoodBabe.com that doesn't somehow run afoul of at least one claim in one of her "sky is falling" blog pieces.

To date, we've counted over six hundred ingredients/brands/"chemkillz" upon which she's swung her infamous Ban Hammer. Finding the same additives in products she recommends–for profit–is as simple as reading the labels of her wares.

A handful of science advocates frequently write about Food Babe's hypocrisy (or lazy/poor research) and this small selection of articles highlights her double standards. These pieces originally appeared on the web. We believe they translate to other formats well. Please keep in mind as you read that all of the products being discussed have sterling safety records. If we use the word dangerous, it's always done sarcastically, because the Food Babe is saying an ingredient is dangerous while simultaneously selling it.

In the first piece, we'll look at Food Babe's oft-repeated warnings about certain supposed endocrine system disruptors in beauty products–even though nearly every beauty product she sells contains the same "disruptors."

Things heat up in the second article: Vani is infamous for calling out Kraft and other companies over the use of certain dyes, even though, as we'll see, she sells a lip stain that contains the same dyes. In fact, she fronts for no less than three companies that use these dyes. To up the ante, the same product discussed in this article contains aluminum, which Food Babe links to Alzheimer's, and saccharine, which she links to cancer, and… well, just wait and see!

Speaking of aluminum, Food Babe's hypocrisy is on full display in the expose on her deodorant blog. In one fell swoop, she manages to condemn all antiperspirants that contain aluminum, while at the same time selling her followers a deodorant that contains that same element–and none of them ever notice.

From there, we move on to one of a series of articles that briefly put Food Babe in the cross hairs of the national media. In the midst of her petition drive against Kellogg's and General Mills for the removal of the preservative BHT from their products, we pointed out that Food Babe had been selling an item laced with BHT for nearly three years. A reporter picked up on the BHT revelation and questioned her, but apparently, let her slip away without checking her story. As you'll discover, her claims about not knowing what was in the body scrub she claimed to have personally used and sold for all those years just don't add up.

The final piece illustrates Food Babe's lack of investigative skills and transparency. For many years, she's warned about the dangers of the additive cellulose, even though she's sold cellulose-laden products intended for human ingestion. When pointed out in the story you'll be reading, she quietly pulled all of these products from her shopping pages without comment, despite a very public promise for full transparency and admission of mistakes in light of previous, similar gaffes.

And so it goes…

Mark Alsip, Lexington, Kentucky

Kentucky, December 30, 2014

In her article "Throw This Out of Your Bathroom Cabinet Immediately" [1,] Food Babe slams modern deodorants because they contain aluminum.

One of the alternative products Food Babe recommends is *Naturally Fresh Crystal Roll-On Deodorant (Fragrance Free)*. She says this is the best deodorant she's tried. Food Babe likes it so much she's encoded her Amazon.com affiliate ID in a link (amzn.to/1ghktrO) so that when you buy a bottle, she earns a commission.

- *Vermont Soap Organics ($13)– This "sage lime" scented stuff is awesome. One of my personal favorites and the scent is neutral enough for all genders.*
- *Naturally Fresh ($6)– This one works the best to keep me actually dry out of all the ones I tried, and other family members agree!*
- *Primal Pit Paste ($11)– It works great for some people like my husband, but didn't work for me because it made my underarms red—which wasn't pretty! Many people love it, but it's hit or miss.*
- *Nourish ($5- $8)—They have the best scents, but you need to re-apply! The Almond Vanilla and Lavender Mint smell so good!*

Let's take a look at the ingredients of *Naturally Fresh*, according to the manufacturer's page on Amazon.com: [2]

Indications

Our newest underarm deodorant Extremely Effective with soothing Chamomile for after shaving. Fragrance Free. Hypoallergenic.

Ingredients

Ammonium alum, potassium alum

Figure: 12.1 Naturally Fresh Deodorant. Something strange reveals itself in the ingredients list.

---

1   http://foodbabe.com/2013/04/10/throw-this-out-of-your-bathroom-cabinet-immediately/
2   http://www.amazon.com/Naturally-Fresh-Crystal-Deodorant-Fragrance/dp/B005P0WRLU/

Hmm… Ammonium alum and potassium alum. Keeping in mind Food Babes's hatred of all leading deodorants because they contain aluminum, let's look more closely these two ingredients:

Ammonium alum, $(NH_4)Al(SO_4)2 \cdot 12H_2O$ is better known as Aluminum ammonium disulfate dodecahydrate.

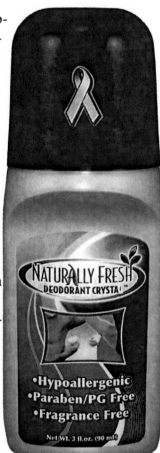

Can you see the enormous hypocrisy in Food Babe's article?

Let that sink in for a moment.

Food Babe has written an article telling you to throw out all the deodorants in your bathroom because they contain supposed Alzheimer's-inducing aluminum. In the next breath, she refers you to a website that sells a deodorant containing aluminum and earns a commission when you buy it.

The only significant difference between the aluminum in the deodorants that Food Babe hates and the aluminum in Naturally Fresh is that Food Babe LLC pockets money on purchases of the latter. (We could get into a discussion on how the aluminum is bound, but that's out of scope. Remember, Food Babe's flawed argument is that the mere presence of aluminum means you're in danger of cancer and Alzheimer's. Read her article if you don't believe me.)

In *Flu Vaccine: The Aluminum Lining* [3] I mentioned that aluminum–the most common metal in the earth's crust–is an unavoidable part of our diets, and is easily processed by the bodies of healthy people, so I won't go into that again. I'd like to concentrate on deodorants here.

The other ingredient in *Naturally Fresh*, Potassium alum, is better known as *aluminum potassium sulfate*, $Al(SO_4)2 \cdot 12H_2O$. Yes, you guessed it, there's that pesky aluminum again.

---

3   https://badscidebunked.wordpress.com/2014/10/07/flu-vaccine-the-aluminum-lining/

The Fear Babe

Ironically, one of Food Babe's fellow pseudoscientists, Dr. Mercola, warns against using natural deodorants that contain alum. [4] Food Babe often quotes Dr. Mercola, so to see her peddling *Naturally Fresh* while he's warning it can kill you is amusing.

So Food Babe

- Scares you to death with false information about aluminum
- Tells you your deodorants contain aluminum (throw 'em out!)
- Points you to an alternative deodorant that contains aluminum
- Earns a sales commission on the alternative deodorant

Ka-ching!

What Food Babe doesn't tell you is that the bodies of healthy humans process aluminum without any problems. Foods near and dear to Food Babe's heart–such as spinach [5, 6] are rich in aluminum.

It's no wonder that out of all the alternative deodorants Food Babe's tried, *Naturally Fresh* works the best. It's the only one that definitely contains aluminum!

Buyers should be wary of the other three deodorants she recommends, because of a cryptic legal disclaimer to the effect that the materials you receive may be different than the packaging.

But, unless you're suffering from a problem such as kidney disease where aluminum can't be removed from your body efficiently, there's nothing wrong with *Naturally Fresh* deodorant. I encourage you to buy it (or any other leading brand) containing aluminum because it works.

Just please don't buy by clicking on a link on a Food Babe web page.

---

4   http://articles.mercola.com/sites/articles/archive/2010/02/16/aluminum-lurks-in-crystal-deodorants.aspx
5   http://foodbabe.com/2014/01/27/creamy-kale-and-artichoke-dip-with-homemade-chips/
6   http://www.who.int/water_sanitation_health/dwq/chemicals/en/aluminium.pdf

Kentucky, February 5, 2015

As luck would have it, I've got some extra spending money this week, so I thought I'd go shopping at FoodBabe.com. I want to be extra careful though, and not buy anything that might harm my body. So I'm going to use Food Babe's excellent article, "Be a Drug Store Beauty Dropout" [1] as a reference, and closely examine the ingredients of any product I might buy.

Come with me, won't you? It'll be fun!

One warning that particularly stands out in Food Babe's thought-provoking piece is the following, where she says we must avoid:

> Siloxanes. Look for ingredients ending in "–siloxane" or "–methicone." Used in a variety of cosmetics to soften, smooth and moisten. Suspected endocrine disruptor and reproductive toxicant (cyclotetrasiloxane). Harmful to fish and other wildlife. [2]

OK. Avoid anything ending in "-siloxane" or "-methicone." Got it. Let's go shopping!

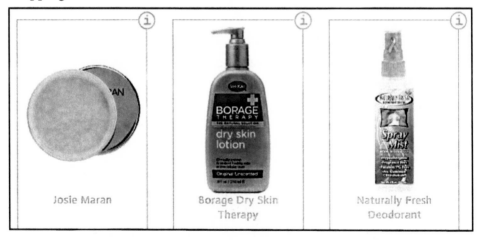

Josie Maran	Borage Dry Skin Therapy	Naturally Fresh Deodorant

Figure: 12.2 Borage Dry Skin Therapy on FoodBabe.com's shopping page, complete with an encrypted Amazon.com affiliate ID. (Food Babe LLC)

Mmmm… that Borage Dry Skin Therapy lotion looks wonderful. The cold winter weather does have me feeling a bit chapped in the old nether regions.

---

1   http://foodbabe.com/2011/07/31/how-to-find-safe-beauty-products/
2   http://foodbabe.com/2011/07/31/how-to-find-safe-beauty-products/

And the highlighted Amazon.com affiliate ID tells me that Food Babe earns a sales commission from every purchase. This means I'm helping further this woman's vitally important work. What's not to love?

But wait… don't click the buy button just yet!

Following the sage advice of Food Babe, we need to take a close look at the ingredients in this skin therapy lotion. We wouldn't want to find anything harmful in there! Thankfully Borage gives us a nice ingredient list on Amazon:

> *Purified water, aloe vera gel*, safflower seed oil, glyceryl stearate, glycerin, jojoba seed oil, borage seed oil, cetyl alcohol (vegetable wax), vitamin E acetate, dimethicone, shea butter, sodium ascorbyl phosphate (vitamin C), phenoxyethanol, L-ergothioneine, ethylhexyl glycerin.*
>
> **Certified organic.*

Figure: 12.3 The ingredients in Borage's Dry Skin Therapy

Uh oh. Help me out here: Food Babe said that we're supposed to avoid ingredients ending in -siloxane or -methicone! Damn my eyes: doesn't dimethicone end in -methicone?

Maybe Food Babe just made a mistake. She's an investigator, but she's also human, after all! This could just be a case of mistaken identity. Let's see if we can find a more commonly used name for dimethicone by heading over to the US. National Library of Medicine's PubChem database*

> *"Also known as: Trisiloxane, octamethyl-, DIMETHICONE, 107-51-7, Dimethicones, Dimeticone, dimeticonum"*

Out of the frying pan and into the fire: dimethicone is also known as octamethyltrisiloxane–which ends in Food Babe's banned "-siloxane."

This isn't going very well. I'd better pull up that Food Babe reference again and make sure I read what she wrote correctly because she clearly told me to avoid:

> Siloxanes. Look for ingredients ending in "–siloxane" or "–methicone." Used in a variety of cosmetics to soften, smooth

and moisten. Suspected endocrine disruptor and reproductive toxicant (cyclotetrasiloxane). Harmful to fish and other wildlife. [3]

What the hell? Is Food Babe also trying to sell me a skin care product that's going to mess with my endocrine system, screw up my reproductive organs, and–as an afterthought–kill my pet fish?

I want my money back!

If you've read any of the other articles in this series, [4] you know that this is where I usually debunk Food Babe's claims that the ingredient in question (in this case, octamethyltrisiloxane) is really dangerous.

It's getting old. I've written about a dozen of these pieces now, and have already once shot down the -siloxane/-methicone garbage. [5] I just don't have the energy to do it all again. Why reinforce the negative impact of Food Babe's ridiculous claims by going on and on about the safety? Psychiatrists call this the "Backfire Effect", and I'm loathed to do it.

Borage Dry Skin Lotion is completely safe.

However, if you're curious and would like to hear what experts say about octamethyltrisiloxane (dimethicone, the ingredient in the skin lotion), you're welcome to read the toxicity summary at PubChem [6] and see Food Babe's been pulling the wool over your eyes.

On the other hand, if you believe Food Babe and think that octamethyltrisiloxane (dimethicone) is toxic, then head over to her Facebook page and ask her why she's selling a product laced with it. I can, more or less, guarantee your comment will be deleted and you'll be banned… never allowed to comment again.

I'm out of here. I'm going to go buy some Borage skin lotion. I'm just not going to buy it from Food Babe.

---

3   http://foodbabe.com/2011/07/31/how-to-find-safe-beauty-products/

4   https://badscidebunked.wordpress.com/2015/02/05/food-babe-pushing-dangerous-items-borage-therapy-dry-skin-lotion/#Others

5   https://badscidebunked.wordpress.com/2015/01/14/food-babe-pushing-dangerous-items-tarte-lights-camera-action-mascara/

6   http://pubchem.ncbi.nlm.nih.gov/compound/24705

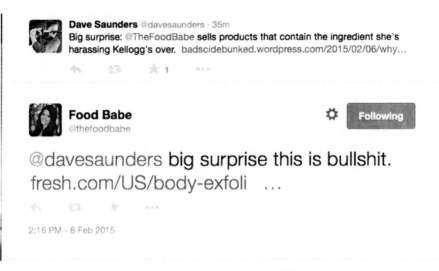

Figure: 12.4 *This tweet wasn't well received—with Food Babe crying foul after being called out for doing what she does best. Note the date this one appears. (Mark Alsip/ twitter.com)*

Kentucky
February 16, 2015

All of her denials aside [1], a product being sold by Food Babe contains BHT, and she has apparently been associated with a company selling at least a dozen such products since the summer of 2012. This despite the fact that she's gone on record saying BHT should be avoided in all beauty products, due to supposed toxicity. Because Food Babe claims to personally use each and every product she sells, it's troubling that she feigned ignorance [2] of the product contents in a Chicago Business Journal interview yesterday, during which she offered a rebuttal of the article you're now reading.

In a tweet (Figure: 12.4), Food Babe called my proof of BHT in her product bullshit and said the ingredients listed on the manufacturer's website (no BHT) were correct–despite being confronted with photos of product labels clearly showing the additive.

I wrote to the manufacturer and received the following response today:

---

1 https://badscidebunked.wordpress.com/2015/02/06/why-is-food-babe-selling-a-product-with-bht/

2 http://www.bizjournals.com/chicago/news/2015/02/11/the-food-babe-under-attack-explains-herself-and.html

INGREDIENTS: Sucrose, Prunus Amygdalus Dulcis (Sweet Almond) Oil, Prunus Armeniaca (Apricot) Kernel Oil, Simmondsia Chinensis (Jojoba) Seed Oil, Oenothera Biennis (Evening Primrose) Oil, Citrus Limon (Lemon) Peel Oil, Passiflora Incarnata Seed Oil, Citrus Grandis (Grapefruit) Peel Oil, Heiianthus Annuus (Sunflower) Seed Oil, Litsea Cubeba Fruit Oil, Citrus Aurantium Bergamia (Bergamot) Fruit Oil, Citrus Aurantium Dulcis (Orange) Oil, Cymbopogon Schoenanthus Oil, Panax Ginseng Root Extract, Tocopherol, Limonene, Citral, Linalool, BHT, Triethyl Citrate <06338/A>

Figure: 12..5 The ingredient list in Borage Brown Sugar (Mark Alsip/BadScienceDebunked)

Dear Mark,

Thank you for contacting us!

Our apologies that our website incorrectly does not list BHT as an ingredient in Brown Sugar Body Polish. The packaging picture you attached lists the correct ingredients included in the product.

Fresh uses BHT as an antioxidant to protect the ingredients against the risk of oxidation. Our toxicologists certify that this use of BHT may be incorporated in our products according to the recommendation of the joint FAO/WHO expert committee on food additives and the Cosmetic Ingredient Review expert panel which confirm that the use of BHT in cosmetics is safe.

Fresh is correct–and according to experts, BHT is safe. I appreciate the honesty of this company. What I want to concentrate on here is the hypocrisy of Food Babe. How is it possible that she has been selling this product for 2½ years without ever reading the label (Figure: 12.5)?

To be certain of my claims, I placed an order for Fresh Brown Sugar Body Polish via the FoodBabe.com shopping page on Friday, February 6. Food Babe earned an affiliate sales commission from this purchase.

The order arrived February 9—but something has changed over at Foodbabe.com. When I placed this order (February 6, 2015), Fresh Brown Sugar

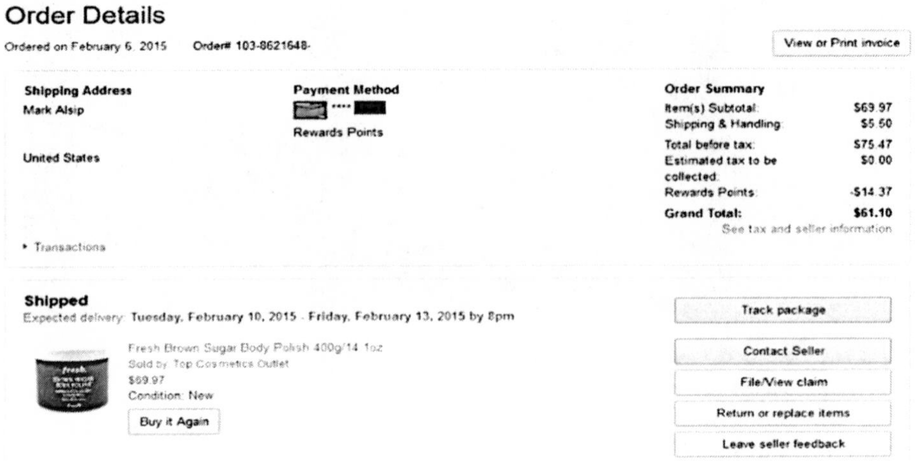

Order Details

Ordered on February 6, 2015   Order# 103-8621648-

View or Print invoice

Shipping Address
Mark Alsip

United States

Payment Method
[card] **** [card]
Rewards Points

Order Summary

Item(s) Subtotal:	$69.97
Shipping & Handling:	$5.50
Total before tax:	$75.47
Estimated tax to be collected:	$0.00
Rewards Points:	-$14.37
Grand Total:	**$61.10**

See tax and seller information

▸ Transactions

Shipped
Expected delivery: Tuesday, February 10, 2015 - Friday, February 13, 2015 by 8pm

Fresh Brown Sugar Body Polish 400g/14.1oz
Sold by: Top Cosmetics Outlet
$69.97
Condition: New

Buy it Again

Track package

Contact Seller

File/View claim

Return or replace items

Leave seller feedback

Figure: 12.6 Mark's proof of order—Feb 6 2015 (Mark Alsip/Amazon.com)

is listed. Now, compare the image of her shopping page just three days later (Figure: 12.8). The Fresh brown sugar body polish has disappeared.

Based on simple forensic work on her website, it's apparent that Food Babe has been associated with Fresh since July, 2012. The date of her association can easily be determined by examining the source code of her shopping page, which I saved before she had a chance to delete it:

```
data-src="http://media.foodbabe.com/wp-content/up-
loads/2012/07/BrownSugarBodyPolish.jpg" alt="This is
quite an
```

Figure: 12.7 Sample HTML mark-up from FoodBabe.com shopping page.

The year and month that Food Babe uploaded each product image is included as part of the URL (Uniform Resource Locator). In this case, she uploaded the brown sugar body polish content in July, 2012. (Similarly, she got started with Josie Maran "Eye Love You" in December 2013, and John Masters' Shampoo in December, 2011.)

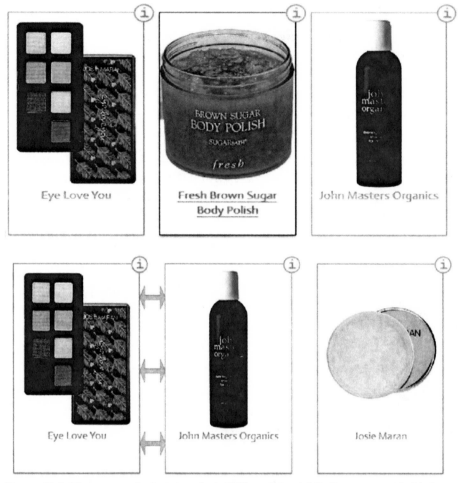

Figure: 12.8: Now you see it, then you don't. Will you hear it? Perhaps you won't. It's the meaning of survival in a very nasty world. (Mark Alsip/Terry Jones/Amazon.com)

I think the Food Babe Army deserves an explanation as to how their leader could have been using this product for 2½ years and not seen the BHT on the label. Here's what Food Babe said about the body polish in 2012:

> This is quite an amazing scrub. I could use it everyday. Makes my skin baby smooth and the smell is so nice." [3]

---

3   Archived here: https://www.pinterest.com/gingerlynn63/food-babe/

FoodBabe.com specifically states (our emphasis):

> *"Posts may contain affiliate links for products Food Babe has*
> *approved and researched herself. If you purchase a product through*
> *an affiliate link, your cost will be the same (or at a discount if a*
> *special code is offered) and Food Babe will automatically receive a*
> *small referral fee. Your support is crucial because it helps fund this*
> *blog and helps us continue to spread the word. Thank you."*

Really? Apparently, everyone else has known about the BHT all along. Sephora's Question and Answer page [4] listed it as far back as 2011–a full year before FoodBabe.com put it on sale. Amazon.com, the fulfillment source for Food Babe, lists BHT. The product label lists BHT.

Does Food Babe actually use this product, or has she just been quoting the Fresh.com web site?

Fresh sells over a dozen products containing BHT. Isn't it hypocritical for a blogger to criticize companies for selling a product with a certain additive and yet have a commercial affiliation with one that does the same? In July, 2011, she specifically said (using a list copied from David Suzuki [5, 6]) BHT in beauty products should be avoided. [7]

> BHA and BHT. Used mainly in moisturizers and makeup as preservatives. Suspected endocrine disruptors and may cause cancer (BHA). Harmful to fish and other wildlife.

As the *Chicago Business Journal* article [8] notes, Hari claimed her BHT wasn't as dangerous as the General Mills/Kellogg's BHT. A clever dodge, as the charge made against her is much simpler: she told her readers not to buy any beauty product with BHT, but sold that very thing for over two years and claimed to use it personally.

It's important to stress yet again that Fresh is not the villain here. Like Kellogg's and General Mills, they are selling a product with an additive that is recognized as safe by experts. On a personal note, my wife and I like Fresh products. I hope they won't be punished for this.

---

4   http://answers.sephora.com/answers/8723/product/P7844/questions.htm

5   Dr. Suzuki is a zoologist and environmental campaigner.

6   http://www.davidsuzuki.org/issues/health/science/toxics/dirty-dozen-cosmetic-chemicals/

7   http://foodbabe.com/2011/07/31/how-to-find-safe-beauty-products/

8   http://www.bizjournals.com/chicago/news/2015/02/11/the-food-babe-under-attack-explains-herself-and.html

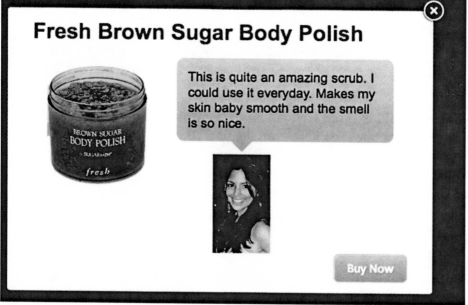

Figure: 12.9: Product sold by Hari via FoodBabe.com. She could use it every day!

What saddens me is the willingness of some news outlets to promote Food Babe as a hero campaigning against giants. The fact that Food Babe has been *in bed with BHT* since 2012 has been made known to these publications and is now public knowledge. Thankfully the Chicago Business Journal (and sister publications) did present my BHT charges to her. Sadly, she sidestepped the issues.

Kentucky, February 16, 2015

Despite a very vocal campaign against Kraft over the use of the dyes Blue #1, Yellow #5, and Yellow #6 in their products [1, 2] Food Babe sells items containing a form of these same dyes via her shopping page, and has apparently been doing so since December, 2013.

The items sold by Kraft are food products while those sold by Food Babe are cosmetics intended for use on the lips. The only difference in the dyes is the addition of a metallic salt in the cosmetics to prevent the dyes from becoming water soluble. Unfortunately for Food Babe, the metal in question is aluminum, which she falsely links to Alzheimer's disease and breast cancer. [3, 4] It must be pointed out that experts in food/product safety strongly disagree with Food Babe over her claims about the dyes in question–and the aluminum.

Not only did Food Babe miss the presence of the dyes in an item that she claims to use personally–also escaping her attention were four compounds she specifically warns should be avoided in beauty products because of alleged endocrine system disruption, [5] saccharine (which she says is toxic), [6] and retinyl palmitate (which she falsely links to skin cancer when used in the presence of the sun). [7]

I am not writing as an expert in food and product safety–only to point out Food Babe's double standards. [8] The products being discussed in this writing all have a solid safety record. Please keep that in mind as you read.

Food Babe earns an Amazon.com sales commission via click-throughs on a Tarte Cosmetics link on her shopping page, where she features that company's Lipsurgence Lip Stain [9] Figure: 12.10 & Figure: 12.11:

---

1   http://foodbabe.com/2013/03/25/kraft-acknowledged-petition-but-didnt-address-concerns-of-over-a-quarter-million-people/
2   tttp://foodbabe.com/2014/05/21/this-childhood-favorite-has-a-warning-label-in-europe-why-not-here/
3   http://foodbabe.com/2013/04/10/throw-this-out-of-your-bathroom-cabinet-immediately/
4   http://foodbabe.com/2013/07/27/how-to-find-the-best-natural-mascara-that-actually-works/
5   http://foodbabe.com/2011/07/31/how-to-find-safe-beauty-products/
6   http://foodbabe.com/tag/refined/
7   http://foodbabe.com/2013/05/05/what-you-need-to-know-before-you-ever-buy-sunscreen-again/
8   https://badscidebunked.wordpress.com/2015/02/09/bht-product-purchased-from-foodbabe-com-hari-incorrect-about-ingredients
9   http://foodbabe.com/shop/for-your-beauty/

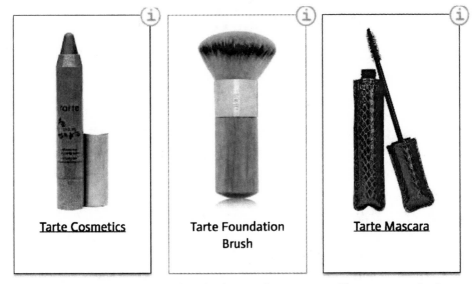

Tarte Cosmetics | Tarte Foundation Brush | Tarte Mascara

Figure: 12.10 :Screen capture of FoodBabe.com shopping page. There are several color options available.

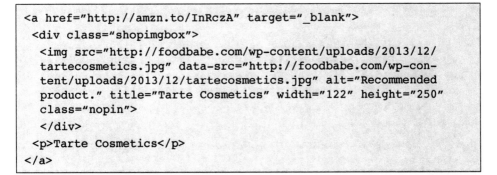

```
<a href="http://amzn.to/InRczA" target="_blank">
<div class="shopimgbox">
  <img src="http://foodbabe.com/wp-content/uploads/2013/12/
  tartecosmetics.jpg" data-src="http://foodbabe.com/wp-con-
  tent/uploads/2013/12/tartecosmetics.jpg" alt="Recommended
  product." title="Tarte Cosmetics" width="122" height="250"
  class="nopin">
  </div>
  <p>Tarte Cosmetics</p>
</a>
```

Figure: 12.11: Every product in Food Babe's online shop has an encoded (hidden) referral link. Above is an example for the Tarte Cosmetics Lip Stains. The link uniquely identifies Food Babe LLC as being the referrer--perhaps without your knowledge despite the disclaimers (see page 298.)

Let's have a look at the full list of ingredients, according to the Tarte web site. [10] [This is edited for space, but the complete list appears in the appendix "Tarte Cosmetics" on page 384]

- ***lucky***: Octyldodecanol [...] iron oxides (CI 77491, CI 77492, CI

---

10   http://tartecosmetics.com/tarte-item-lipsurgence-natural-matte-lip-tint

77499), red 7 lake (CI 15850), yellow 6 lake (CI 15985), red 40 *lake* (CI 16035).

- *hope*: Octyldodecanol [...]iron oxides (CI 77491, CI 77492, CI 77499), red 7 lake (CI 15850), red 40 lake (CI 16035), blue 1 lake (CI 42090).
- *lively*: Octyldodecanol [...] red 7 lake (CI 15850), red 40 lake (CI 16035), iron oxides (CI 77492, CI 77499), red 27 lake (CI 45410).
- *envy*: Octyldodecanol [...] iron oxides (CI 77491, CI 77492, CI 77499), red 7 lake (CI 15850), red 40 lake (CI 16035), blue 1 lake (CI 42090).
- *exposed*: Octyldodecanol [...] iron oxides (CI 77491, CI 77492, CI 77499), red 7 lake (CI 15850), red 40 lake (CI 16035), yellow 5 lake (CI 19140), red 6 lake (CI 15850).
- *fiery*: Octyldodecanol[...]iron oxides (CI 77491, CI 77492, CI 77499), red 7 lake (CI 15850), yellow 6 lake (CI 15985), red 40 lake (CI 16035).

Ingredients for the full-color array of Tarte Lipsurgence lip stains.

A bit of explanation is in order here. You'll notice the word lake after each of the dyes. According to the FDA, approved dyes become lakes when a salt is added to make them non-water soluble. [11]

Simply put, in some products (such as cosmetics or potato chips) you don't want the colors to run. According to both the FDA and the manufacturer, the salt in this case is an aluminum compound (e.g., aluminum hydroxide).

Does making the dyes into lakes change their toxicity? That is, would you expect them to behave in a different manner than Food Babe's gloom and doom cherry picked "research" would indicate? I'm not a chemistry expert, but I found three scholarly resources all of which cite the FDA. These sources state that for toxicological purposes, the dyes and their lake forms are identical [12, 13, 14]

---

11 http://www.fda.gov/ForIndustry/Color Additives/ColorAdditiveInventories/ucm106626.htm
12 Food Additive Toxicology Maga, CRC Press, Sep 13, 1994. p. 185
13 Handbook of Food Toxicology Deshpande S.S., CRC Press, Aug 29, 2002. ISBN 0-8247-0760-5. p. 228.
14 Food Safety Handbook Schmidt R, Roderick G, Wiley, Mar 10, 2003. ISBN 0-471-21064-1. p. 254

Of course, if Food Babe wants to argue this point, she's left in the awkward position of explaining how the addition of an element she claims to be toxic (aluminum) to a dye she claims is toxic suddenly makes both safe.

So how long has Food Babe been selling Blue #1 lake, Yellow #5 lake, and Yellow #6 lake? A quick look at the source code of her shopping page at FoodBabe.com [15] suggests that she's been doing this since December, 2013. By convention, uploaded content (such as product images) is stored in folders tagged with the month and year the con-

	Calories	2,000	2,500
Total Fat	Less than	65g	80g
Sat Fat	Less than	20g	25g
Cholesterol	Less than	300mg	300mg
Sodium	Less than	2,400mg	2,400mg
Total Carbohydrate		300g	375g
Dietary Fiber		25g	30g

Ingredients: Sunflower Oil, Whole Wheat, Wheat Flour, Wheat Starch, Corn Flour, Rice Flour, Sugar, Whole Barley Flour, Whole Oat Flour. Contains 2% or less of: Salt, Whey, Maltodextrin, Onion Powder, Potassium Chlorid Garlic Powder, Monosodium Glutamate, Reduc Lactose Whey, Dried Jalapeno Peppers, Tomat Powder, Spices, Dried Cheddar Cheese (milk, cheese cultures, salt, enzymes), Dried Blue Cheese (milk, cheese cultures, salt, enzymes), Citric Acid, Natural and Artificial Flavor, Canola Oil, Colored with (artificial color, yellow 6, yellow 5, yellow 6 lake, yellow 5 lake), Freshness Preserved by Citric Acid, Sodium Caseinate.

Figure: 12.11: The FDA says lakes are used when you don't want colors to run–like in this bag of potato chips we borrowed from the editor's lunch box. (Mark Alsip)

tent was stored on the web site. Looking at the screen capture Figure: 12.10 and code Figure 12.11, the association is readily apparent.

But, as I said in the introduction, the food coloring is only the tip of the iceberg. In *Be a Drug Store Beauty Dropout*, Food Babe warns her readers to avoid the following in all beauty products:

Siloxanes. Look for ingredients ending in "-siloxane" or "-methicone." Used in a variety of cosmetics to soften, smooth and moisten. Suspected endocrine disruptor and reproductive toxicant (cyclotetrasiloxane). Harmful to fish and other wildlife. [16]

The product she sells and claims to use personally includes:

- Cyclopenta**siloxane**
- Phenyl Tri**methicone**
- Di**methicone**
- Castor Oil Bis-hydroxypropyl di**methicone** esters

15   http://foodbabe.com/shop/for-your-beauty/
16   http://foodbabe.com/2011/07/31/how-to-find-safe-beauty-products/

These are the very -methicones and -siloxanes Food Babe told us to avoid.

I'd like to pause here and remind the reader that all of these ingredients have been studied by experts who, unlike Food Babe and myself, are qualified to pass judgment on them. Tarte is a reputable company with a superb safety record, and I hope that Food Babe's lack of research doesn't reflect negatively on them. When caught in this situation before, [17] Food Babe's response has been to blame the manufacturer for her own mistakes. [18]

I've contacted Tarte customer service several times with questions about their ingredients and have always received swift replies with references to scientific literature and government safety regulations. Just like Kraft, Tarte is selling products that experts overwhelmingly agree are safe.

Please do not punish an honest company for Food Babe's mistakes.

Having said that: Food Babe's lip stain also contains saccharin, which she links to unspecified diseases, [19] retinyl palmitate (vitamin A), which she falsely links to cancer, [20] and even an IARC group 2B carcinogen (titanium dioxide)–significant because it's on the very same list as 4-MeI, a compound found in the caramel coloring over which she previously lambasted Starbucks. [21]

Of course all of these additives are recognized as safe. It's just that Food Babe cherry picks literature to make them sound dangerous. Rather than debate the safety issue with her, however, why not just ask her: if these additives are so dangerous, why does she sell so many products that contain them? It's hard to find an item on the Food Babe shopping page that doesn't contain something she says is harmful. And yet she accuses other companies of hypocrisy and double standards? Food Babe says all these additives are dangerous. They're not. But why is she selling products that contain them?

Additionally, in the first quarter of 2015, the FTC issued new and clearer (some might say, hard line) guidance for bloggers like Food Babe. These

---

17   https://badscidebunked.wordpress.com/2015/02/09/bht-product-purchased-from-foodbabe-com-hari-incorrect-about-ingredients/
18   https://badscidebunked.wordpress.com/2015/02/16/food-babes-bht-denial-doesnt-hold-water/
19   http://foodbabe.com/tag/refined/
20   http://foodbabe.com/2013/05/05/what-you-need-to-know-before-you-ever-buy-sunscreen-again/
21   http://foodbabe.com/2014/09/02/drink-starbucks-wake-up-and-smell-the-chemicals/

may seem harsh, but it helps to level the playing field for hobbyist bloggers and those who run a highly profitable business.

We believe Food Babe LLC is already in direct contravention of many of the new rules (as of this writing) because her afflilate links are so deeply embedded in the site, and she fails to disclose this front and center.

> "... there are several hyperlinks before that disclosure that could distract readers and cause them to click away before they get to the end of the post. Given these distractions, the disclosure likely is not clear and conspicuous." [22]

For example, an August update "*Love Your Skin With This Simple Treatment. You'll Be Amazed At The Results!*", contains a short passage of just two paragraphs containing no fewer than eight different affiliate links.

Although the example we're quoting is for a different type of required disclosure, it's clear that having a disclosure at the bottom of each page is no longer enough. Affiliate Marketing specialist Tricia Meyer told us:

> "*Unless she [Vani Hari] can somehow make an argument that the link above is not an affiliate link, even though it has affiliate link tracking in it, she is clearly violating the FTC Act's prohibition on 'unfair or deceptive acts or practices.'* "

■

22   https://www.ftc.gov/sites/default/files/attachments/press-releases/ftc-staff-revises-online-advertising-disclosure-guidelin es/130312dotcomdisclosures.pdf

Kentucky, March 2, 2015

Food Babe's hypocrisy and double standards reached new heights (lows?) this week. While Food Babe is openly selling products that contain cellulose, she's angry that companies such as Kraft, Taco Bell, and Jimmy Dean use the same additive (which she refers to as a "wood filler") in their wares. According to her, not only are they cheating customers by offering less of a real product, they're also doing great harm to their digestive systems [1, 2]

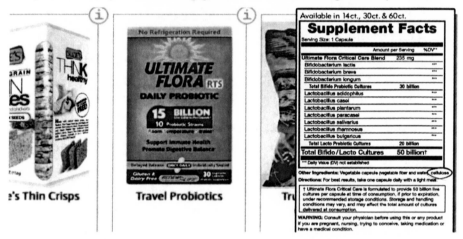

Figure: 12.12: Ultimate Flora as it originally appeared on Food Babe's site—with the ingredients list overlayed. The cellulose is highlighted for the sake of illustration. (Mark Alsip/ ReNew Life Formulas, Inc.)

The problem is, as always, that Food Babe is selling products that contain the same ingredient. [3, 4] In the wake of the revelation that she's doing the same with no less than three companies [5] using dyes she dubiously links to a myriad health problems, [6] you've got to wonder how her "Army" can continue to trust her.

1   http://foodbabe.com/tag/cellulose/

2   https://www.facebook.com/thefoodbabe

3   http://foodbabe.com/shop/for-your-belly/

4   http://www.amazon.com/gp/product/B007VGBSLG

5   https://badscidebunked.wordpress.com/2015/02/27/she-did-it-again-food-babe-linked-to-another-company-using-same-dyes-she-forbids/

6   https://badscidebunked.wordpress.com/2015/02/27/she-did-it-again-food-babe-linked-to-another-company-using-same-dyes-she-forbids/

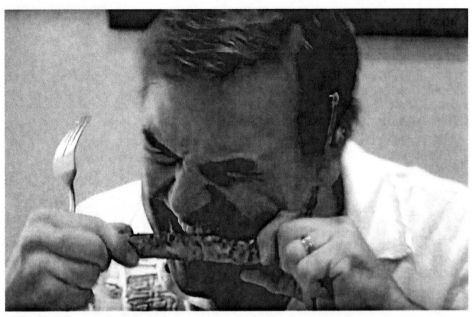

Figure: 12.13: "Do you eat wood? Well do ya, punk?" In classically disingenuous fashion from 2013, Food Babe wrongly conflates cellulose with trees in order to create fear and distrust. (Food Babe LLC/YouTube)

Ultimate Flora, Food Babe's Amazon.com affiliate, uses cellulose in their probiotics line. [7] She proudly features Ultimate Flora products on the FoodBabe.com shopping page. [8]

The ingredients in Ultimate Flora [9] are shown in Figure: 12. along with a screen capture of the original page. Keep in mind that Food Babe claims to personally use each and every product sold on her website and reads the labels of these products. In a February 27 Facebook post (an old article, resurrected to boost sagging book sales?), Food Babe says she doesn't know whether to be "scared to death for the millions still eating cellulose," or grateful that she stopped buying it long ago.

Did she really stop buying it long ago? If so, why does she say this on the web page where she's selling the cellulose-containing Ultimate Flora?

---

7 http://www.renewlife.com/ultimate-flora-probiotics/ultimate-flora-critical-care-50-billion.html

8 http://foodbabe.com/shop/for-your-belly/

9 http://www.renewlife.com/ultimate-flora-probiotics/ultimate-flora-critical-care-50-billion.html

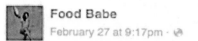

Food Babe
February 27 at 9:17pm ·

I don't know whether to be scared to death for the millions eating this substance or grateful that I stopped buying this food ingredient a long time ago. I always thought, even after my research that it was kinda safe but I still had my suspicions. When I originally brought this subject to light a few years ago, I got a lot of flack for it because there wasn't any major data showing that it could be harmful but regardless I wanted you to know what's in your food and that's wh... See More

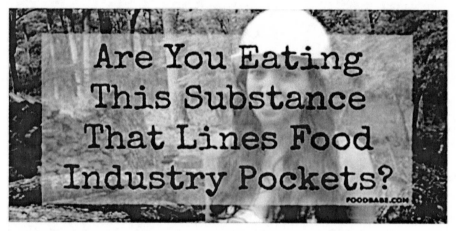

Are You Eating This Substance That Lines Food Industry Pockets?

Are You Eating This Substance That Lines Food Industry Pockets?

Figure: 12.14: Food Babe's Facebook post (the page has subsequently been updated but the misleading information remains). (Food Babe LLC/Facebook)

> Thanks for stopping by the Food Babe shop! Below are items that I enjoy using on a daily basis. Click the info icon for additional information. Click the item to purchase

On the web page where Food Babe says she uses every product sold on a daily basis, we find products containing cellulose. Yet she tells us she stopped eating this "additive" long ago.

You choose: does she really use every item on her shopping page (such as the cellulose-ridden Ultimate Flora probiotics)? If Food Babe is "scared to death," perhaps it should be because she's been caught in yet another lie. She's selling products containing cellulose in the "For Your Belly" section of her FoodBabe.com shopping site, all the while telling people that it (which she calls "fake fiber") will harm their digestive systems.

Cellulose is present in all plants—not just wood. There's nothing magical, mysterious or dangerous about it and we get it from all fruits and vegetables. It's not fake fiber—it IS the very definition of fiber! In Food Babe's cellulose video [10], she employs a time lapse of an apple molding—not admitting the decay is attracted to the fruit's sugars and thinner cell walls. Nature designed fruit to decay rapidly and protects the living trunk with a thick layer of dry bark.

It's difficult to find a product sold by Food Babe that does not contain an ingredient that she says is dangerous. When will her adoring fans and the media wake up to this fact? All you have to do is exactly what she encourages: read the labels of the products she's selling.

Update 19 March 2015

Despite her promises of transparency in dealing with errors, Food Babe quietly pulled all cellulose-containing products from her web site approximately two weeks after this piece was originally published. She offered no explanation for her actions.

■

---

10   https://www.youtube.com/watch?v=4Keh9AmtKJU

13

Food Babe in Florida

Kevin Folta describes the events when a prestigious university fell for a charismatic sales pitch.

It was 6:30 pm in the lab and I was just thinking about the last things I'd need to get done before I could go home. Typical night. Usually I'm riding home about 7 pm, but an email popped up asking me if I was going to go watch the Food Babe. A click on a link would take me to the note on a UF Dean for Students Good Food Revolution Events website. Vani Hari would be spreading her corrupt message of bogus science and abject food terrorism here at the University of Florida. Oh joy.

There's something that dies inside when you are a faculty member that works hard to teach about food, farming and science, and your own university brings in a crackpot to unravel all of the information you have brought to students.

She might have started from honest roots. Her story says she was duped by an organic yogurt stand (join the club) into buying taro toppings that were filled with artificial, non-organic colors. She realized that she could use social media to coalesce affluent consumers in a formation to cyber-slander change from businesses. Shove this dookie through a conduit of the science illiterate and...

An entrepreneur was born!

She found that a popular social media site was more powerful than science itself, more powerful than reason, more powerful than actually knowing what you're talking about. Her discussion was a narcissistic, self-appointed attack on food science and human nutrition. There is a vein in my head that pulses when I hear someone deliberately misrepresent science for personal celebrity, and it was pounding.

She went on about her exploits against Chik-fil-A, forcing them to change their formulation. She spoke about how she and her army of online vandals slammed Subway into removing a safe and useful food chemical from their bread. She spoke of her "5 million person army" with a sly and knowing smile. Vani likes Vani.

Fallacy and deception

She went on about labeling GMO, making the argument ad populum that 64 countries label them so why don't we get the same rights?"

She explained transgenic crops (of course not using that language) as dangerous, and untested. There were claims about how the crops were linked to cancer and autism. She also claimed that "GMO crops cause an increase in pesticides" which is completely false—and she knows it. Her words were cleverly chosen, carefully stated, so if someone holds her accountable she can weasel out.

Food Terrorism.

Hari then went on to talk about her successes in strong-arming Chick-fil-A, Budweiser and Subway into reformulating their foods and beverages. She's proud that she was invited to corporate headquarters to force change, proud that a know-nothing with a following can affect change simply by propagating false information via the Internet.

That's not healthy activism or change based on science. That's coercion, fear mongering and (yes) terrorism to achieve short-sighted political non-victories in the name of profit and self-promotion, ironically the same thing she accuses the companies of.

Luckily, Starbucks didn't fold. They refused her assault on Pumpkin Spiced Lattes and the demand for organic milk. Unfortunately it was not corporate cojones- it was likely simple economics. There's no way that they could source that much organic milk. Otherwise, Hari would have blackmailed them too.

The UF Audience Reaction

There was a silver lining on that cloud. I was really proud to see that the student audience was not buying it. Throughout her presentation that was about Hari in the spotlight and "me-me-me", students got up and left. She left gaping pregnant pauses where previous performances got applause- only to hear nothing. Not even crickets. This audience was not buying it, at least as a whole it was not excited by it. Maybe they just wanted a Chick-fil-A and Starbucks.

No Question and Answer Session

While microphones stood ready in the audience to answer questions, there was no public Q&A period where a scientist that knows the research could publicly challenge her false assertions. The audience filed out of the building, and apparently she may have stuck around to meet with individuals. However, I wanted her answers in a way students could hear, helping them to critically assess the arguments of scholars vs. self-appointed celebrities.

Questions like:

- Why am I blocked for posting hard science facts to your websites?
- How do you feel about transgenic solutions to citrus greening?
- What is your evidence for higher pesticide rates?

… and a dozen others.

Overall

It was disappointing. If this is a charismatic leader of a new food movement it is quite a disaster. She's uninformed, uneducated, trite and illogical. She's afraid of science and intellectual engagement. She's Oz candy at best.

I guess I'm just angry because I didn't get to lock science horns with The Food Babe. I would have liked to have asked a few questions that she could never answer. Moreover, the funds my university spent to bring her here would have bought a lot of seeds for school gardens county wide, field trips to real farms, and the opportunity to visit functioning labs and ask questions of actual scientists.

But who needs actual scientists in lab coats with lifetime dedication to science, when you can have a fly-by-night activist profiting from ignorance? After all, she is a (self-described) babe…

I have to put a lid on this post. I have an undergrad spending her first morning in the lab tomorrow and I need to meet her at 7 AM. If I teach her well, maybe she'll get to stand up and hold the Food Babe accountable for her junk science someday. That would make me remarkably happy. ■

14

Rich Man, Poor Man, Poultryman

If I had a quarter for every time I was asked what we put into laying hens to make them lay so many eggs....I would NOT be setting my alarm early so I could shovel my driveway out for the 4th time this week. I can't keep track of the number of times or ways I have been told about the constant flow of antibiotics, hormones and additives that go into laying hens. It has stopped being a surprise, but it used to be...

I always wondered what I was doing wrong as a vet! If everyone else was using all these good drugs on their hens, what was I missing? Then I figured it out....what I was missing was immersion in the Internet. The amount of misinformation out there is staggering. I'm sure it's true when I do a quick search on nuclear energy, or free trade coffee, or Beyoncé's plastic surgery history (not that I would... honest).

The difference is, in this case, I know how much is misinformation....on other subjects, I can be convinced by a smooth argument and repetition.

I can only swear to the truth about the birds I look after, here in Ontario. As the vet on record for over half of the laying hens in Ontario, I can state that it is much more common for flocks to never see antibiotics than to be treated. I use antibiotics if a flock needs them to fight off a disease, but that is rare....I used antibiotics less than 20 times last year in the more than 300 flocks I am in charge of.

Professional laying hen farmers spend a lot of time, effort and money in prevention of disease. This includes extensive vaccine programs, strict biosecurity programs, excellent control of the environment the hens are in, clean barns, high quality feed and water, and protection from wild animals (this is especially important right now, when waterfowl are shedding Avian Influenza in many areas of North America).

That and the fact that laying hens are mostly in cages, separated from their manure, means that it is uncommon for laying hens to get diseases that require treatment with antibiotics.

I think it is crucial for animal welfare to allow for the treatment of sick flocks when medically necessary. I also think it is crucial for

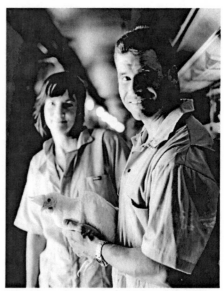

Would you buy a used chicken from this man? Mike is a dedicated veterinarian and knows chickens inside out. Literally. (mikethechickenvet.wordpress.com)

farmers to take disease prevention and prudent use of antibiotics very seriously… and, in my experience, they do. We manage flocks so we don't have to treat, but will treat if it becomes necessary.

I still wondered if I was running a different practice than my colleagues though. I know the vast majority of the laying hen vets in North America, but they don't tell me what they are doing on a day-to-day basis. I was in an international poultry expo in Atlanta last month….a who's-who of the poultry world, and about 30 of us laying hen vets got together for a meeting (we are not a big group….there are more pro sports teams in the US than laying hen vets). The subject of antibiotic resistance came up, as it does in every vet meeting I've attended in the past 5 years. One of the most distinguished vets in our group said he thought our industry was doing well in antibiotic usage….his quote:

> *"I belong to a group called AA… Antibiotic Anonymous… whenever I feel the urge to try to solve a problem with antibiotics, I phone another vet, and they talk me out of it."*

That made me feel that we were all pushing in the same direction.

As for hormones, the last time I saw commercial laying hens administered hormones, they were given by a unicorn, and brought onto the farm by one of the giant alligators from the sewers.

It's an urban myth and, in reality: *It. Doesn't. Happen. Ever.*

If I could say it more clearly, I would. There is no hormone product for sale for poultry, there is not a farmer who would want it, there is no way it would make economic sense, and there is absolutely no reason to use such a product. Our hens have been genetically selected so well that they almost lay an egg every day….that is all they can produce! There would be no way to feed a hen enough nutrients to allow her to produce more than that! Besides…many of you readers have backyard hens, who also lay close to an egg a day… where are you getting your hormone supplements from?

As for all the additives we use in laying hen feed, there is some truth to that. We add vitamins, lutein, Omega 3 fatty acids and other nutrient enrichments that are passed on to the people who eat the eggs. We also add things to improve the health of the birds….electrolytes (think Gatorade, without the sugar), calcium for bone strength, probiotics (similar to yogurt, but not as gross), and organic acids (similar to vinegar), to help with digestion and keep the gut healthy (actually this is one of the more recent focuses of disease prevention…gut health).

I hope this makes some sense to readers who are unfamiliar with professional egg production….at first glance, it might make sense for us to use a lot of drugs or even hormones. But once you look a little deeper, disease prevention and good management do more good than either of those strategies.

Mike the Chicken Vet

Ontario
February 12, 2015

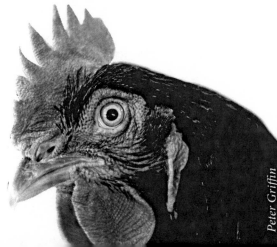

Peter Griffin

15
E for Ingredients

E numbers are the universal food additive numbering system in the UK and Europe; the USA uses an entirely different system but the chemicals are the same and the most important ones are referenced both by their E number and their FD&C number where known.

The Southampton Six

What we now call ADD/ADHD is not a new phenomenon. Its discovery predates much of what we now recognize as fast food. It was first clinically recorded in the early part of the 20th century by the British pediatrician Sir George Still (1868-1941). [1] Still observed that while some children were of normal intelligence, they were otherwise unable to control their behavior. In 1923 Dr. Franklin Ebaugh Sr. further noted ADHD could be brought on by certain types of brain injury.

Still's findings didn't have a name at the time. It was not until 1936 when the anti-asthma medication Benzedrine sulfate (black market tablet form: "bennies") became available that someone noted an unusual side effect. Careful studies by psychiatrist Dr. Charles Bradley resulted in this observation published in the 1937 American Journal of Psychiatry:

> *"The most striking change in behavior occurred in the school activities of many of these patients. There appeared a definite "drive" to accomplish as much as possible. Fifteen of the 30 children responded to Benzedrine by becoming distinctly subdued in their emotional responses. Clinically in all cases, this was an improvement from the social viewpoint."* [2]

1   Lange KW, Reichl S, Lange KM, Tucha L, Tucha O. The history of attention deficit hyperactivity disorder. Attention Deficit and Hyperactivity Disorders. 2010;2(4):241-255. doi:10.1007/s12402-010-0045-8.

2   Strohl, M.P. Bradley's Benzedrine Studies on Children with Behavioral Disorders. Yale J Biol Med. 2011 Mar; 84(1): 27–33.

Later treatments for ADHD included other *methamphetamines* such as *desooxyl* and *biphetamine*. The best known is probably Ritalin, with new products being researched all the time. Perhaps ironically, all these early medications are better known as stimulants: "speed," or "billy whiz" deriving from the larger doses they used to prevent sleep (clinically for the sleep disorder, narcolepsy) and to heighten awareness. Caffeine has a similar effect, even though few people would consider it a drug.

Dr. Benjamin Feingold (1899-1992) was an American physician who, during the 1970s, proposed that certain chemicals: *salicylates* (e.g. aspirin), certain artificial food colors [AFCs] and additives such as BHA and BHT could cause hyperactivity in children. Although popular, the Feingold Diet is not thought to be effective, with a 1983 meta-analysis of 23 studies published in the Journal of Learning Disabilities saying:

"It is concluded that extant research has not validated the Feingold hypothesis and that diet modification should be questioned as an efficacious treatment for hyperactivity." [3]

The FDA reviewed the available data again in 1986 and concluded there was still insufficient evidence to assume additives (including Yellow 5/Tartrazine) were implicated in childhood disorders.

A further meta-analysis appeared in the *Journal of Developmental and Behavioral Pediatrics* and although it found what appeared to be a causative link between some additives and ADHD, the authors did add the cautionary note:

"Improvement in the identification of responders is required before strong clinical recommendations can be made." [4]

and further observed:

"On the other hand, the restrictiveness of an AFC-free diet may burden hyperactive children, who are already at risk for poor psycho social outcomes. Therefore, imposition of the diet should be done

---

3   Kavale KA, Forness SR. Hyperactivity and Diet Treatment A Meta-Analysis of the Feingold Hypothesis. J Learn Disabil. 1983 Jun-Jul;16(6):324-30. doi: 10.1177/002221948301600604

4   Schab DW1, Trinh NH. Do artificial food colors promote hyperactivity in children with hyperactive syndromes? A meta-analysis of double-blind placebo-controlled trials. J Dev Behav Pediatr. 2004 December;25(6):423–434.

reluctantly until more certain methods have been developed to identify who is AFC-responsive." [5]

In 2007, the UK's Food Standards Agency, responding to public disquiet over food additives, commissioned a study by the University of Southampton to determine if there was any evidence to suggest that AFCs triggered hyperactivity in children. The study ran for six weeks, including ages 3 and 8-9 years. For this reason, the study is often referred to as the Southampton Six, although journals reference it from McCann et al. after the study's authors.

The study looked at the following:

1. E102: Tartrazine/Yellow #5
2. E104: Quinoline Yellow/Yellow #10
3. E110: Sunset Yellow/Yellow #6
4. E124: Ponceau 4R
5. E129: Allura Red
6. E122: Azorubine (carmoisine)
7. E211: Sodium Benzoate

American readers might be interested to note the following:

Azorubine & Ponceau 4R have never been approved by the FDA for any food use. Azorubine was used briefly in the 1960s for cosmetics.

Yellow #10 is approved for use in drugs, cosmetics, and contact lenses but has never been approved for use in food.

Yellow #5 is approved for use in food, but it must be declared, as it is known to cause mild allergic reactions (hives) in a small number of people.

Red #40 and Yellow #6 are both approved by the FDA for use in food drugs and cosmetics.

Sodium Benzoate is a preservative generally regarded as safe (GRAS) by the FDA but must not exceed 0.1% of the total content of any food. It is used to inhibit the growth of bacteria, yeasts and molds that are known to be harmful to health.

---

5   Schab DW1, Trinh NH. Do artificial food colors promote hyperactivity in children with hyperactive syndromes? A meta-analysis of double-blind placebo-controlled trials. J Dev Behav Pediatr. 2004 December;25(6):423–434.

This means only four of the seven additives tested in the Southampton study are even relevant to food and should be easy to spot.

Upon completion the study's authors conclude:

> *"Artificial colors or a sodium benzoate preservative (or both) in the diet result in increased hyperactivity in 3-year-old and 8/9-year-old children in the general population."* [6]

Which is a pretty damning indictment and an example of tabloid science: the sort of scaremongering journalists lap up like hungry cats around a bowl of milk. Stories like this result in exciting headlines, often creating a mass panic.

Patience rarely brings rewards in newspaper publishing.

As science has shown us, time after time, a single study is just that: it might be wrong, it might not—the essence of science is repeatability. It's essential that when scientists publish their results, other scientists are:

- Able to reach the same conclusions from their data and
- Are able to repeat the experiment and either reproduce the same results -or- repeat and invalidate them.

This idea, at the very core of science, takes time—sometimes years or even decades.

The Committee on Toxicity, an independent group of scientists advising the FDA, concluded that there was a possible link between these additives and hyperactivity in children. [7] However, it cautioned that due to the limitations (sample size, observational methodology) the results could not be applied to the wider population and recommended that further studies be performed.

The Southampton study was analayzed twice more in 2008 & 2009 by the European Food Safety Authority (EFSA). Press releases from 2008/2009

---

6   McCann, D. et al. Food additives and hyperactive behaviour in 3-year-old and 8/9-year-old children in the community: a randomised, double-blinded, placebo-controlled trial. The Lancet, Volume 370, Issue 9598, 1560-1567. DOI: http://dx.doi.org/10.1016/S0140-6736(07)61306-3

7   http://www.fda.gov/downloads/AdvisoryCommittees/CommitteesMeetingMaterials/FoodAdvisoryCommittee/UCM248549.pdf

appear at the end of this chapter. (Science is often a process of continuous re-evaluation and the EFSA is currently conducting even more tests, and is scheduled to report back at the end of 2015.)

Crucially, to the dismay of the FDA and despite there being lack of support from the weight of scientific evidence, in 2010 the EU (bending to considerable political pressure) began requiring manufacturers to include warning labels on foods that contain any of the seven substances from the Southampton study. The FDA already requires manufacturers to label artificial colors by name: FD&C (Food Drugs and Cosmetics Act) Yellow #5 (tartrazine) and FD&C Red #40 (allura red) where they are used. A 2011 document published online by the FDA and based on a further meta-analysis of the data concludes:

"Based on our review of the data from published literature, FDA concludes that a causal relationship between exposure to color additives and hyperactivity in children in the general population has not been established. For certain susceptible children with Attention Deficit/Hyperactivity Disorder and other problem behaviors, however, the data suggest that their condition may be exacerbated by exposure to a number of substances in food, including, but not limited to, synthetic color additives. Findings from relevant clinical trials indicate that the effects on their behavior appear to be due to a unique intolerance to these substances and not to any inherent neurotoxic properties." [8]

As recently as 2013, EFSA has not revised its position on most of the sulfonated mono azo dyes: Amaranth (E 123), Ponceau 4R (E 124), Sunset Yellow FCF (E 110), Tartrazine (E 102) and Azorubine/Carmoisine (E 122), and that only children who consume excessive amounts (not specified) are likely to exceed the current recommended maximum exposure.

It's worth noting that a human's acceptable daily allowance (ADI) represents a significant safety margin—the level considered safe in experimental animals is divided (usually by 100) to arrive at the ADI. The ADI applies daily over the course of a lifetime to ensure that acute and cumulative toxic effects are accounted for.

---

8   http://www.fda.gov/downloads/AdvisoryCommittees/CommitteesMeetingMaterials/FoodAdvisoryCommittee/
     UCM248549.pdf

EFSA did, however, recommend that further testing should be carried out on these colors to determine if there is any evidence of genotoxicity (DNA damage). While this question remains unanswered, the current evidence supports the hypothesis that they are not genotoxic.

It's interesting to note here that some colors are not tested because they are derived from natural sources.

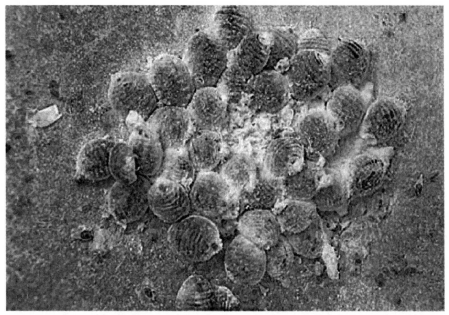

Dactylopius coccus. This tasty-looking scale insect is harvested, crushed and processed into a popular red food dye and lake. Don't worry though, it's 100% organic and natural. Bon Appétit! (Frank Vincentz/Wikipedia)

- E100: Turmeric. Curcuminoids;
- E120: Cochineal/Carmine a red dye derived from the cochineal insect... *yum!
- E140: Chlorophyllin a green dye extracted from chlorella algae;
- E150a-d: Caramel coloring made from caramelized sugar;
- E160a: Saffron. Carotenoids;
- E160b: Annatto. Extracted from achiote seeds;

- E160c: Paprika;
- E160d: Lycopene;
- E162: Betanin. From beets.

How these colors are derived from their sources is likely to make Food Babe's head explode, because efficient industrial processing requires "toxic" compounds such as hexane to be used as a solvent.

This is no different from the processing of Stevia glycosides (even Food Babe herself used ethanol). We'd love to be a bunch of flies on the wall when she hears about this: small amounts of solvent are likely to remain in the final product but do not need to be declared because they are seen as "carry over" compounds and are only present in small, but detectable amounts.

Further, although rare, the UK's FSA has found that carmine, cochineal and carminic acid (all processed from the scale insects) have caused mild to severe allergic reactions, including a 19 year-old volunteer who experienced anaphylactic shock (a severe allergic reaction) so severe his blood pressure could not be recorded. [9]

Dyes & Lakes

Manufacturers get their food colors in one of two forms: dyes and lake pigments (commonly called lakes). Lakes tend to be used in smaller amounts to color things like candies, cosmetics, and drugs; dyes are used in much larger quantities because they have to color the entire product—typically drinks such as sodas and beers. It's difficult or impossible to avoid synthetic colors in our modern diet (even natural colors are still colors) but it's worth remembering that if you're looking to avoid artificial colorings, you need to start looking closely at what you drink—and that includes some processed dairy products such as chocolate milk.

■

EFSA PRESS RELEASE—12 November 2009

After reviewing all the available evidence, the European Food Safety Authority's scientific panel on additives, the ANS Panel, has lowered the Acceptable Daily Intakes (ADIs) for the artificial food colors Quinoline Yellow (E104), Sunset Yellow FCF (E110) and Ponceau 4R (E124). [1] As a result, the Panel concluded that exposure to these colors could exceed the new ADIs for both adults and children.

The Panel found that the currently available data did not require a change to the existing ADIs for the three other colors evaluated—Tartrazine (E102), Azorubine/Carmoisine (E122) and Allura Red AC (E129). According to the Panel, only some children who consume large amounts of food and drink containing Azorubine/Carmoisine or Allura Red AC could exceed the ADIs for these colors.

John Larsen, the Chair of the ANS Panel, said: "Many food colors have been in use for decades since their initial approval and so after such a long period of use we are now looking at the overall data available, including any new evidence on their safety, to help protect European consumers. We are doing this work systematically for all food additives, and have started with these colors for which some concerns have been raised."

The six colors re-evaluated by the Panel can be used in a range of foodstuffs including soft drinks, bakery products and desserts. The Panel concluded that one of the colors, Tartrazine, may bring about intolerance reactions—such as irritations to the skin—in a small part of the population. For the remaining five colors (Quinoline Yellow, Sunset Yellow FCF, Ponceau 4R, Azorubine/Carmoisine and Allura Red AC), no firm conclusion could be drawn on a possible link with intolerance reactions from the limited scientific evidence available.

EFSA is currently assessing the safety of all individual food additives which are approved for use in the EU, starting with food colors. The European Commission asked EFSA to consider these six colors as a priority after a study was published by Southampton University (McCann et al) in 2007—the so-called "Southampton study"—linking certain mixtures of these colors and the preservative sodium benzoate with hyperactivity in children.

The Fear Babe

John Larsen added: "We have now reduced the ADIs for three of the six colors we assessed, but for different reasons in each case as different data were available on each individual compound. The data which are currently available—including the Southampton study itself—did not substantiate a causal link between the individual colors and possible behavioral effects."

EFSA's scientific advice will help to inform any follow-up action to be taken by the European Commission and the EU Member States.

EFSA opinions on six food colors—FAQ [12]

Scientific Opinion [13] on the re-evaluation of Allura Red AC (E 129) as a food additive

Scientific Opinion [14] on the re-evaluation of Ponceau 4R (E 124) as a food additive

Scientific Opinion [15] on the re-evaluation of Quinoline Yellow (E 104) as a food additive

Scientific Opinion [16] on the re-evaluation of Sunset Yellow FCF (E 110) as a food additive

Scientific Opinion [17] on the re-evaluation Tartrazine (E 102)

Scientific Opinion [18] on the re-evaluation of Azorubine/ Carmoisine (E 122) as a food additive

Topics A-Z [19]: Food additives

For media enquiries please contact:

EFSA Media Relations Office

Tel. +39 0521 036 149

E-mail: Press@efsa.europa.eu

E for Ingredients

EFSA PRESS RELEASE—14 March 2008

EFSA evaluates Southampton study on food additives and child behavior

Scientists at Europe's food safety watchdog have completed an assessment of a recent study [1] on the effect of two mixtures of certain food colors and the preservative sodium benzoate [2] on children's behavior. The study, published last year by researchers at Southampton University in the United Kingdom (McCann et al, 2007), suggested a link between these mixtures and hyperactivity in children.

The European Food Safety Authority's (EFSA) AFC Panel[3], with the help of experts in behavior, child psychiatry, allergy and statistics, concluded that this study provided limited evidence that the mixtures of additives tested had a small effect on the activity and attention of some children. However, the effects observed were not consistent for the two age groups and for the two mixtures used in the study.

Considering the overall weight of evidence and in view of the considerable uncertainties [4], such as the lack of consistency and relative weakness of the effect and the absence of information on the clinical significance of the behavioral changes observed, the Panel concluded that the findings of the McCann et al study could not be used as a basis for altering the ADI [5] of the respective food colors or sodium benzoate.

Among the limitations of the new study was the inability to pinpoint which additives may have been responsible for the effects observed in the children given that mixtures and not individual additives were tested.

Although the findings from the study could be relevant for specific individuals showing sensitivity to food additives in general or to food colors in particular, it is not possible at present to assess how widespread such sensitivity may be in the general population.

The Panel, assisted by behavioral experts, considered that the significance of the effects on the behavior of the children was unclear since it was not known if the small changes in attention and activity observed would interfere with schoolwork or other intellectual functioning.

The Fear Babe

Based on surveys conducted from 2002 to 2005 in sweets and soft drinks [6], the colors were shown to be frequently used. Sodium benzoate is also often present in soft drinks. The AFC Panel concluded that children who consume brightly colored sweets and soft drinks could reach intake levels for some of the additives tested in the study that would be similar to the daily amounts given in that study.

The Panel evaluated the McCann et al study against the background of previous studies, going back to the 1970s, on the effect of food additives on behavior and acknowledged that it is the largest study carried out on a suggested link between food additives and hyperactivity in the general population. The Panel noted that the majority of the previous studies used children described as hyperactive and these were therefore not representative of the general population.

The AFC Panel is currently re-evaluating the safety of all food colors authorized in the European Union on a case-by-case basis and the colors used in the McCann et al study are included in EFSA's review. Opinions on some of the colors concerned, such as Allura Red, are expected to be adopted by the end of the year.

For media enquiries please contact:

EFSA Media Relations Office

Tel. +39 0521 036 149

E-mail: Press@efsa.europa.eu

[1] The study conducted by McCann et al (2007), commissioned by the UK Food Standards Agency, involved 153 children aged 3 years old and 144 children aged 8-9 years old from the general population, including children with normal to high level activity, but not children medicated for Attention Deficit Hyperactivity Disorder (ADHD). The study is published in The Lancet [10].

The UK's Committee on Toxicology evaluated the study and issued a comprehensive statement (PDF [11])

[2] The additives included in the two mixtures given to the children were Tartrazine (E102), Quinoline Yellow (E104), Sunset Yellow FCF (E110), Ponceau 4R (E124), Allura Red AC (E129), Carmoisine (E122) and sodium benzoate (E211).

[3] The Panel on Food Additives, Flavorings, Processing Aids and Materials in Contact with Food.

[4] Lack of consistency in the results with respect to age and gender of the children; the effects of the two mixtures of additives tested and the type of observer (parent, teacher, independent assessor); the unknown clinical relevance of the effects measured; lack of information on dose-response; unknown relevance of the small effect size; the fact that mixtures were used and it is not possible to identify the effects of individual additives; the lack of a plausible biological mechanism that might explain the possible link between the consumption of colors and behavior.

[5] ADI, or Acceptable Daily Intake, is a measure of the amount of a substance, such as a food additive, which can be consumed over a lifetime without an appreciable health risk. ADIs are expressed by milligrams (of the substance) per kilograms of body weight per day.

[6] UK Food Standards Agency (FSA) (2002); unpublished survey by the Food Safety Authority of Ireland (FSAI) (2005); Union of European Beverage Associations (UNESDA) (2005).

16

Logically Speaking

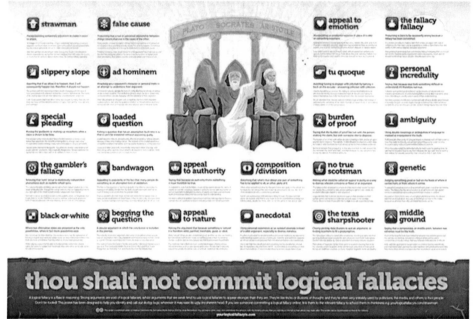

In this chapter we're going to list a few of the more common fallacies—which are all errors in reasoning or argument—and explain how to spot them. The website "***Your Logical Fallacy Is***" [1] has a free PDF and low-cost wall poster to help everyone understand these better and we highly recommend it. Logic and reasoning are complex subjects, and this primer barely scratches the surface. It's intended to show some examples of how the devious and invested play to our fears and ignorance to undermine science and technology for their own gain.

---

1   https://yourlogicalfallacyis.com/

Ad Hominem

> These Hired "Experts" Are Infiltrating The Media To Confuse You About Food... [2]

A variation on the *ad hominem* fallacy as played by Food Babe. The ad hominem itself is caused by placing the word experts in quotes—suggesting these people are not experts in the field being discussed. This example is dicussed further under "Poisoning the Well." Note that name calling ("you're an idiot and a troll") does not even satisfy an ad hominem and is the lowest form of fallacy possible.

Anecdotal Evidence

> One of the ongoing treatments I am doing with my regular needle Acupuncture, is figuring out all of my allergies and then using laser acupuncture to eliminate them. I found out I was incredibly allergic to refined sugar. About 3 months ago I was treated for this—it doesn't mean I can eat all the refined sugar I want now, rather it means that my body can tolerate it better. [3]

Anecdotal evidence is powerful but that doesn't make it right and more often that not, it's plain wrong. When someone relates something that happened to them, they're relating an event—a story. Without hard evidence—a record of the before and after compared against many other similar cases, there is nothing to prove the story is likely to hold true. Charismatic people often produce outrageous claims that many of us take at face value despite them being anecdotes. The authors usually abide by the well-known adage, "the plural of anecdote is not evidence".

Appeal to Authority

> According to Dr. Stephanie Seneff, a senior research scientist at MIT, glyphosate is largely responsible for the escalating incidence of autoimmune and other neurological disorders that we are experiencing. [4]

---

2 http://foodbabe.com/2015/07/27/who-are-the-experts-hired-to-downplay-public-concerns-about-food/
3 [http://foodbabe.com/2011/09/22/seize-your-sugar-cravings/
4 http://foodbabe.com/2015/02/26/difference-between-organic-non-gmo-labels/

Although a simple fallacy in nature: *"So and so is an expert and she agrees with me so that means I'm right"* this isn't always false so this one can be tricky to spot.

For example, *"**Dr Folta says that chlorophyll uses light to perform photosynthesis—so it can't operate inside our body**"* is a correct (albeit simplified) use of the application of the appeal to authority, because Dr. Folta holds a Ph.D in biology and this is his specialist field.

The true fallacy occurs when someone references an authority or an academic paper that has either (a) been written outside the person's area of expertise (e.g. computer AI specialist Dr. Stephanie Seneff writing about autism) or (b) has been shown to be completely wrong (the Seralini paper). [5, 6] These fallacies are difficult to unravel for most of us because we're not experts in the many diverse fields required. It's important to note here that Food Babe does not flag the fact that Dr. Seneff is not an expert in this field but plays to her employer (MIT Computer Science and Artificial Intelligence Laboratory) .

Food Babe's most egregious use of this fallacy is her impressively named advisory council, [7] which appears to consist of some highly qualified doctors, but is not independent and consists of people who share the same views — and may be working outside of their own highly specialized fields. It's particularly questionable that this advisory council, which consists of several medical doctors, a few of which are known to promote fringe advice, has allowed Food Babe's advice on sunscreens and even vaccination to stand. Not one of them is a practicing food scientist, a fact that should raise serious concerns.

Appeal to Belief

"Many people believe that genetic modification is creating novel proteins we don't fully understand so we should take a stand against it."

See also the *Appeal to Common Practice*. This is one of simpler fallacies to spot because it's so cliched. Just because a lot of people believe something

---

5   http://www.sciencedirect.com/science/article/pii/S0278691512005637

6   http://www.sciencedirect.com/science/article/pii/S0278691514000052

7   http://foodbabe.com/advisorycouncil/

to be true does not automatically make it so. Mass beliefs change over time and history is replete with examples where common knowledge developed in a quaint footnote. For instance, many people believe that Sushi is raw fish, where in fact the term relates to the rice. While most sushi dishes contain raw fish, a significant number do not. The "Weasel Word" variation of this fallacy employs the phrase "Many scientists believe." The problem here is the identities of the scientists are not defined. Science writers tend to avoid this citing scientific consensus and/or naming a world-respected authority or study.

Appeal to Common Practice

"We don't need GMOs, we've been farming the natural way for years!"

Variations of this argument are littered throughout the the organic food movement's pages. The appeal to common practice relies on our reluctance to embrace change and is widely witnessed in political debates in the USA over everything from GM organisms to gun control.

Appeal to Emotion

First Lady Michelle Obama's endorsement of Subway as a "healthy choice" for kids saddens me. [8]

Food Babe relies on this fallacy so often it's hard to find examples where she isn't doing so. Also known as argumentum ad passions, this logical fallacy manipulates emotions to win an argument, especially when there is little factual evidence to corroborate a claim. And after all, invoking sadness to conjure protectiveness over our nation's children is a powerful way to demonize an innocuous chemical (remember azodicarbonamide?) in an innocuous sandwich chain's bread.

Here's another one which leverages the tendency for overweight people to feel bad about themselves.

Organic foods prohibit many of the chemicals known as "obesogens" that trigger our bodies to store fat. [9]

---

8   The Food Babe Way, p. 33
9   http://foodbabe.com/2015/02/26/difference-between-organic-non-gmo-labels/#more-20384

For this example, see also *Anecdotal Evidence,* because it relies on the unproven thesis and buzzword: **obesegens**. The idea that certain chemicals can upset our hormonal balance (primarily the hormones *leptin* and *ghrelin* but also *thyroxin* and *triiodothyronine*) is not new. Antibiotics, for example, interfere with the action of many contraceptive pills. However, applying this very crude measure to food where these chemicals, if present at all, occur in such small amounts they have no measurable effect, is intended to create fear. See *Red Herring* for more specific *appeal to emotion,* where the intent is to create a camaraderie in the peer group in order to manipulate it more easily.

Appeal to Ignorance

○ Starbucks Vanilla Syrup: (Sugar, Water, **Natural Flavors,** Potassium Sorbate (Preservative), Citric Acid)

Natural flavors. "I don't know what these are ergo they must be bad." This is both a **non sequitur** *and an* **argument from ignorance** *in one. (Foodbabe.com)*

Latinized as the *argumentum ad ignorantiam,* this is a propostion based on lack of knowledge. The arguer often relies on the fact that the listener is equally or more ignorant. Note that ignorance denotes a lack of understanding, not necessarily lack of intelligence. By highlightling Natural Flavors here, the implication is that these colors must automatically be bad. Here's another:

> I could spend days discussing each ingredient, but one synthetic ingredient that jumped out at me is cellulose – otherwise known as wood pulp. [10]

Although this is also a *red herring* (wood pulp only *contains* cellulose in the same way as all plants contain it) it relies on the reader's ignorance of the fact to make the point. Further, cellulose is an entirely natural product. Food Babe continues her appeal to ignorance with an *appeal to emotion:*

> I don't know about you, but I certainly don't want to eat things that my system can't process. I can't believe companies are allowed to sell food we can't even digest as humans! [11]

---

10   http://foodbabe.com/2012/05/24/full-list-of-non-organic-ingredients-allowed-in-organic-food/
11   http://foodbabe.com/2012/05/24/full-list-of-non-organic-ingredients-allowed-in-organic-food/

Rather strange considering that without cellulose (fiber) our digestive transport functions very poorly indeed, giving rise to real health problems.

Appeal to Nature

> These high-tech genetically engineered crops can include genes from several species—a phenomenon that almost never occurs in nature. [12]

The Appeal to Nature is one of Food Babe's most often used logical fallacies. At the simplest level this states that if something is found in nature then it must be safe. This is clearly untrue as the most potent toxins known to science, ricin and the botulinum toxin, are derived from natural sources; as are many, many others.

Milk (aka Monsanto Milk?!)

Pumpkin Spice Flavored Sauce: (Sugar, Condensed Skim Milk **(Monsanto Milk?!)**, Pumpkin Puree, Contains 2% or Less of Fruit and Vegetable Juice for Color, Natural Flavors, Annatto (Color), Potassium Sorbate (Preservative), Salt)

Whipped Cream: (Light Whipping Cream [Cream **(Monsanto Milk?!)**, Mono and Diglycerides, Carrageenan])

Monstano milk, used here against Starbucks Pumpkin Spice Latte, is a complete fabrication, as gentically modified cows are still the preserve of experiemtnal science. (Foodbabe. com)

Argumentum Ad Monsantium

"Milk (aka Monstano Milk?!)" [13]

Also called the *Reductio Ad Monsantium,* this is one of the most clichéd *ad hominems* used against scientists working in genetics and food and their science loving supporters. By using an evil person or hated corporation

12 The Food Babe Way, p. 217
13 http://foodbabe.com/2015/08/17/youll-never-guess-starbucks-just-announced-hint-made-happen/

(see *Reductio Ad Hitlerium*) this poisons the well by creating a fog of hatred or mistrust around what may otherwise be a sound argument.

It's an a*d hominem, non-sequitur, straw man* and *red herring* all rolled into one. As such, you can bet that the instant someone pulls this out of their hat, they've lost the argument. But *beware that anyone watching the argument may be just as ignorant as the person making the claims!*

Bandwagon

"I want a cup of coffee, but I don't want a GMO. I'd like to start my day off, without helping Monsanto" [14]

Celebrities love jumping on the Bandwagon—usually front and center—because it puts them in the public spotlight. Gwyneth Paltrow's "gluten free" diets, Neil Young is anti-GMO, Jim Carey conflates MMR vaccine with autism, and so on; and many of us follow in a way, confusing our love of these celebrities with their personal hangups. Food Babe has become a leader herself—an internet celebrity of the most pernicious variety; she rides every "orthorexic" bandwagon that comes along. A further bandwagon fallacy in Mr. Young's lyric is the **Argumentum ad Monsantium,** which is so commonplace now it should not need further description.

Begging the Question

"Dear Friend, a man who has studied law to its highest degree is a brilliant lawyer, for a brilliant lawyer has studied law to its highest degree." Oscar Wilde, "De Profundis"

One of those fallacies that can tie you in knots, because it's circular, and might not be as obvious as Wilde's example. Here's a rather deliciously devious version from a scientific journal. [15]

"The elemental composition of Jupiter is known to be similar to the sun... The core would be composed mainly of iron and silicates, the materials that make up most of the earth's bulk.

14   http://www.dailymail.co.uk/news/article-3105964/I-want-cup-coffee-don-t-want-GMO-Neil-Young-s-blasts-Starbucks-relationship-Monsanto-new-protest-song.html

15   http://philosophy.lander.edu/logic/circular.html

Such a core is expected for cosmogonic reasons: If Jupiter's composition is similar to the sun's, then the planet should contain a small portion of those elements." J. Wolfe, "Jupiter," Scientific American (Vol. 230 No. 1), 119.

Black-or-White

Give up fast food for the rest of your life—if you value that life. [16]

This fallacy frames an argument between two diametrically opposed viewpoints, as if there is no middle ground. In this example, we've used a fairly emotional statement and it's not always this clear—this statement also embodies the *appeal to emotion*. Food Babe frequently frames entire essays using precisely this tactic though, so while an individual statement might be valid, the argument taken as a whole is fallacious.

Burden of Proof

Chewing gum messes with your body's ability to produce digestive enzymes, a critical substance that helps you get all the nutrition from food you need into your bloodstream. [17]

As the late Christopher Hitchens notes, "that which can be said without evidence, can be dismissed without evidence." In latin: *Quod gratis asseritur, gratis negatur* (what is asserted gratuitously may be denied gratuitously). The burden of proof lies with the person making the claim, not the person hearing it. When Vani Hari claims aspartame is bad for us or that chewing gum interferes with digestion, the onus is on her to prove that position. She does this using nests of other fallacies (often the *Appeal to Authority*) which makes her arguments particularly difficult to deconstruct for the unprepared.

Exclusionary Detailing

Named as one of the most influential people on the internet by Time Magazine, Vani Hari started FoodBabe.com in April 2011 to spread information about what is really in the American food

---

16 The Food Babe Way, p. 151

17 http://foodbabe.com/2011/12/09/wanna-a-piece-of-gum/

supply. [18]

A common practice in public relations and political spin (also called *lying by omission*), the idea is to take something that could be viewed as damaging and turning it on its end, simply by omitting critical, negative, details. This is a form of quote mining. Time did name Food Babe in its 2015 list but it was far from complimentary, opening as follows:

> *"The former management consultant, 35, commands an army of amateur nutritionists who look to her blog, Food Babe, to see which "unsafe" ingredients they should protest next. She bills herself as an investigator, posting exposés under headlines like 'General Mills or Generally Toxic?'"* [19]

Clearly, Time Magazine's Mandy Oaklander wasn't fooled. Nevertheless

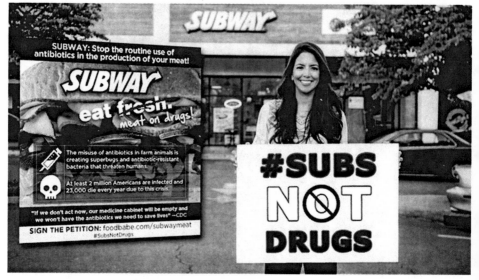

Figure 15.1: Vani launches another petition, but moves to remove antibiotics from food animals have already been underway since at least 2013.

Food Babe ran the entire piece herself. Opening with:

> Time Magazine has named me as one of "The 30 Most Influential

18   http://foodbabe.com/about-me/
19   http://time.com/3732203/the-30-most-influential-people-on-the-internet/

People On The Internet." This honor is not just for me. It's for all of us. Our movement is getting recognized in big ways. [20]

The majority of uncritical commentaries are from her army of fans blinded into congratulation. Although it's possible these fans didn't catch on to Time's sarcasm, it's equally possible they just didn't read the article, and based their view on the headline. This form of lazy reasoning is becoming more common as we are swamped with so much information that we unconsciously filter out what we don't want to see. In science this very real problem is referred to as researcher bias.

In late August 2015 Food Babe launched another petition - implying (using exclusionary detailing) that she was the primary driver. In fact a total of 60 separate groups co-signed the letter (including FoodBabe.com) leading Subway's head of PR, Kevin Kane, to make the following statement.

"Our commitment to serve high quality, affordable food to our customers has always been a cornerstone of the Subway brand. We support the elimination of sub-therapeutic use of antibiotics. This will take time and we continue to work with our suppliers to reach that goal." [21]

Fallacy Fallacy

"Your position sounds like baloney, therefore it is baloney"

Recall that Vani Hari, The Food Babe, was once a nationally ranked debater. The essence of good debate is to not so much to prove your opponent's position wrong, but to make a better case for your own side. This puts good science at a severe disadvantage simply because science is often difficult to grasp and requires considerable understanding of concepts that may themselves be counter-intuitive. Just because an expert makes a *faux pas* while trying to explain something doesn't change the facts they are trying to portray. Make such a mistake on the Internet and your words will follow you until long after you die.

20   http://foodbabe.com/2015/03/06/what-it-means-to-be-one-of-the-30-most-influential-people-on-the-internet/
21   http://www.takepart.com/article/2015/06/23/will-subway-do-right-thing-and-help-save-antibiotics

False Cause

> There's another big reason to eat organic... It can help you stay thin! [22]

The quote above frames a perfect example of *false cause* because it equates organic foodstuff with weight loss. Obesity is a major crisis facing the developed world so claims like this carry amazing weight (no pun intended). It's just a shame they're also completely wrong.

Eating healthy food does not mean spending huge amounts on fancy foods, it just means understanding what your body needs. Conversely, you could easily gorge on organic food all day and end up massively overweight. (See Dr. Seneff's laundry list of claims against glyphosate on page 164 for a further example of this.) Food Babe bases this claim entirely on *anecdotal evidence.*

Flummery & Prattle

> Thank you for standing by me and for your determination to improve our food supply. I know that it is taking time and these changes can't be made overnight, but it's happening. Keep sharing and keep spreading the word – together we are changing the food system.
>
> It's really happening! I love you so much. [23]

Strictly speaking this isn't a fallacy because it's not an error in logic (although when employed as a defense, you can bet there will be fallacies in there). Flummery is a variation of the *red herring* because the intention is to divert attention from the argument. (Food Babe employs it, deliberately or not, widely in communication with her followers who lap it up and fall under her thrall.)

Prattle (Brit. slang *waffle*) is a verbal smokescreen where the speaker (or writer) argues at length without ever coming to any conclusion or defending the central point of the argument made against them. Many people, particularly nervous speakers, will prattle at length without ever getting anywhere; often accidentally employing other fallacies along the way. The

---

22   http://foodbabe.com/2015/02/26/difference-between-organic-non-gmo-labels/#more-20384
23   http://foodbabe.com/2015/08/17/youll-never-guess-starbucks-just-announced-hint-made-happen/

idea is to confuse the listener or reader into a false sense that something has been said when in fact the discourse has barely moved forward.

American biochemist *Duane Gish* was a proponent of this technique and his version became known as the *Gish Gallop*. Formerly known as *spreading* in spoken debate, Food Babe is a master of this technique of producing huge amounts of information which are difficult to deconstruct. By the time critics have gotten through analyzing one set of claims, she will have produced several more, often returning to posts claims and removing the most specious arguments.

Genetic Fallacy

I didn't need to search far to learn how to include dairy nutritiously in my diet; I just listened to the stories of my parents. For thousands of years, my ancestors in India had one cow that they shared with the rest of the villagers. [24]

The genetic fallacy, sometimes known as the "fallacy of origins", relies on the often non-existent merit of something's history instead of its current value or meaning within present context. In the case of Food Babe invoking her ancestral village we are, therefore, led by the nose into believing this information is accurate or meaningful because it's inherited from some prior source. She even goes on to say that because her ancestors supposedly consumed raw milk, and claims (wrongly) that raw milk is imperative to Indian tradition, therefore raw milk is beneficial and necessary to carry on that tradition. Truly fallacious reasoning indeed.

Honor/Dishonor by Association

"I work with a leading cardiac surgeon so what I say about heart health must be true"

This can be a tricky one to unravel. One of the best live examples is of Betty Martini, one of the people behind the aspartame scare. It's not clear from public record what Ms. Martini's academic qualifications are, but she touts her work with a hematologist as if it endows some medical expertise. It's

---

24   The Food Babe Way, p 115

the veracity of the claim itself that counts. This fallacy might also be touted against an employer in these alternate forms:

"You're biased because you work for Monsanto"

or

"What do you know? I work at the CDC!"

In both cases—association is with the employer, not the person making the argument. (The first example might be more dishonor by assocation and would be an *ad hominem, argumentum ad monsantium* and *poisoning the well*.)

Loaded Question

What Is Trader Joe's Hiding? [25]

A more common example is *"When did you stop taking money from the till?"* You won't usually find it in a essay because the idea is to undermine your opponent's position by asking a question that is going to blow up in their face. In defending yourself against a rabid woo monger, you are likely to find yourself faced with something like this sooner or later, which is why we're including it.

Name Dropping

See *Honor by Assocation*. Food Babe associates herself with Charlotte Gerson in the an interview with *Food Integrity Now*. [26] To her supporters that would probably seem honorable, à la "wow you've met a celebrity." The reality is that the elderly Gerson still fronts an organization that promotes a failed cancer treatment that is directly responsible for loss of life and suffering.

No True Scotsman

Is Subway Real Food? [27]

---

25 http://foodbabe.com/2013/08/07/what-is-trader-joes-hiding/
26 http://foodbabe.com/2013/06/13/listen-how-i-became-the-food-babe-on-food-integrity-now/
27 http://foodbabe.com/2012/06/12/is-subway-real-food/

This headine (and the article that goes with it) is a wonderful example of this fallacy — a form of special pleading. The argument goes like this:

Jock: *"All scotsmen put salt on their porridge!"*

Dave: *"Not true. I know several scotsmen who put sugar on theirs."*

Jock: *"In that case, they're not true scotsmen!"*

Suggesting, as Food Babe does in this inflammatory headline, that Subway is serving something other than real food is confusing. The Oxford dictionary [28] describes food as:

Food: noun

> *any nutritious substance that people or animals eat or drink or that plants absorb in order to maintain life and growth.*

Therefore, by this argument, if Subway were not serving real food, then their customers would be complaining rather loudly; and this is where we come up to against No True Scotsman. Food Babe complains that the Subway foods are not "real" because:

> To top it off, the majority of foods at Subway have been conventionally sourced and probably include pesticides, antibiotics, and/or growth hormones. In my research, I didn't find one single organic ingredient or menu item available at over 36,000 stores. Even the lemon juice comes in a pre-packaged squirt pack filled with preservatives. Because of this I haven't consciously ever considered going to a Subway in the last 7 years. [29]

In other words, because it's not organic (by Food Babe's standards) it's not real food. Quite how she expects a chain the size of Subway to operate without using preservatives isn't mentioned. Recall that we've been preserving our food for centuries and, when left unprotected, fresh produce and meats are potential vectors for a laundry list of deadly pathogens.

Non Sequitur

"If you're pro-biotechnology, then you must be a Big Agra apologist"

---

28 http://www.oxforddictionaries.com/definition/english/food
29 http://foodbabe.com/2012/06/12/is-subway-real-food/

This Latin phrase simply means "it does not follow." Arguments based in logic must follow just as numbers in a sequence:

1, 3 , 5, 7, 9, 11, 13, 15, 17, 21

Most of us will be able to answer the next number in this simple progression is 19—not 21. The same applies here in this fallacy: just because someone works for a company it does not follow that they automatically support everything that company does.

> Processed sugar makes your skin dull, causes weight gain, and creates an inflammatory response in your body. When your body is inflamed, you can start to develop all sorts of ailments like asthma, arthritis, or even cancer. [30]

This statement is a **non sequitur** because people who develop the condition, through confirmation bias ,assume that sugar, in this case, was to blame. (cf. *Slippery Slope*).

Personal Incredulity

"I don't understand you, therefore you are wrong."

Even scientists often strive for elegant answers. The universe is quite beautiful, and the mathematics that describe it are often equally wonderful. Take $e=MC^2$ for example. This simple equation describes the amount of energy contained in a piece of matter (assuming that matter could be completely converted into energy). The same level of certainty does not apply in many biological concepts. We used to believe that inheritance of traits, or Mendelian heredity, was simple and easily traceable. Now we've started to realize that it's not so simple. Even the wording can be enough to make many of us stumble over the pile of dictionaries as we retreat for something lighter, say *War and Peace* or *The Iliad.*

This argument is used again and again by charismatic personalities like Gwyneth Paltrow, Jim Carrey and self-styled evangelists like David Wolfe and, of course, Vani Hari. (Behind closed doors, scientists and skeptics alike refer to this as the "WTF?" fallacy.)

---

30 [http://foodbabe.com/2011/05/07/fro-yo-craze-is-just-well-crazy/

Poisoning the Well

> You'll Never Guess What's In A Starbucks Pumpkin Spice Latte (Hint: You Won't Be Happy) [31]

This is a fallacy that has become so hackneyed in recent years it's amazing that people still fail to recognize it for what it is. Poisoning the well means to bias the argument in your favor before your opponent even has chance to speak. In the example above, Food Babe uses a loaded statement "(Hint: you won't be happy.)" to prime the reader into indignation before they even begin to read the piece. Here's another example (also a group ad hominem):

> These Hired "Experts" Are Infiltrating The Media To Confuse You About Food... [32]

Note how the word experts is quoted? This poisons the well by implying that the persons mentioned are not experts in their field. Ironic coming from a person who actually admits to not being an expert in food additives. Note also in this quote the weasel word "inflitrating" - another *appeal to emotion* meant to get the reader fired up and angry. Finally another bucket of botulinum into the drinking water in:

> Most GMO crops were genetically engineered to either be (1) pesticide-resistant or (2) herbicide-resistant (or both), and not to be more healthy for us. [33]

Using *Exclusionary Detailing* this statement is true but ignores the point that the aforementioned crops are cheaper for the farmer, more efficient and cost effective, and save the consumers money. GM crops that confer health benefits for people in developing countries (such as golden rice) are not mentioned.

---

31   http://foodbabe.com/2014/08/25/starbucks-pumpkin-spice-latte/
32   http://foodbabe.com/2015/07/27/who-are-the-experts-hired-to-downplay-public-concerns-about-food/
33

Red Herring

The most basic form of this is changing the subject, but done well, the listener or reader should be sufficiently distracted so as to not notice. (Magicians refer to this technique "the steal" because they distract the audience's attention to something else—often the attractive assistant—while they pull some trick or sleight of hand.) So called "click bait" is, perhaps, the most obvious example of the red herring and Food Babe isn't above using that either. See the tweet about flu vaccines on page 1 for a truly egregious example, but here's another:

> The truth is (as many of you have seen through my campaigns) there are plenty of scientists and consumer organizations [34] (including my advisory council [35]) that back my work and there is a mountain of evidence that synthetic, carcinogenic and neurotoxic insecticides are bad for human health and the environment. [36]

Red herring fallacies are rarely as obvious as the example above and often take place over many sentences. There are actually two red herrings in this particular quote. The first—a link to Maxwell Goldberg's personal page—is quite weak and contains a few examples of the usual suspects and fallacious claims that Food Babe herself is so frequently guilty of. This is hardly the long list of scientists implied in the quote. The second is more subtle because it's true: "… there is a mountain of evidence that synthetic, carcinogenic and neurotoxic insecticides are bad for human health and the environment." There are a lot of chemicals out there, some natural, some man made, that are amazingly toxic: what's missing here is the fact that few of us are subject to the exposures required.

Reductio Ad Hitlerium

Put simply, this is a name calling exercise where one person becomes so lost for competing arguments they liken their adversary to a Nazi. Hitlerium is a Latinized version of Aldof Hitler. Godwin's law, is an informal propostion stating that, over time, all Internet discussions must eventually end up at this point. Ironically, many do.

---

34 http://livingmaxwell.com/what-the-media-food-industry-wont-tell-you

35 http://foodbabe.com/advisorycouncil/

36 http://foodbabe.com/2015/07/27/who-are-the-experts-hired-to-downplay-public-concerns-about-food/

Slippery Slope

"If you allow one or two immigrants into the country, pretty soon

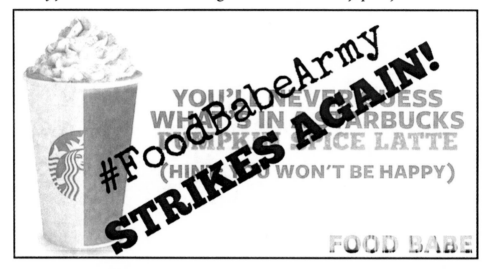

By taking credit for everyday product development, Food Babe uses a variation of the Texas Sharpshooter fallacy. See also Non Sequitur, Flummery & Prattle. (Foodbabe.com)

we'll be overrun and there will be no jobs left for the rest of us!"

The general form of this fallacy predicts that if we do allow a thing to happen then something else must surely follow (even when there is no evidence to support that assertion). Here's Food Babe using this fallacy to great effect (implying a spiralling problem):

> The biotech industry is contributing to a "pesticide-treadmill", by creating an environment that fosters the growth of pesticide-resistant weeds and pests. This allows them to sell more of their toxic chemicals along with their GMO seeds, to further increase their bottom line – and it's escalating fast. [37]

Sophism

"This man is a peripatetic pedagogue and an admitted sapiophile!

---

[37] http://foodbabe.com/2015/02/12/dirty-pr-campaign/

If you're thinking, "What does that mean?" you're not alone. There's something oddly sexual in there. Although originally employed to describe reasoned, intellectual debate, sophism now applies to the act of "baffling them with bullsh*t." Let's break that down.

peripatetic: adjective

> *travelling from place to place, in particular working or based in various places for relatively short periods: the peripatetic nature of military life.*

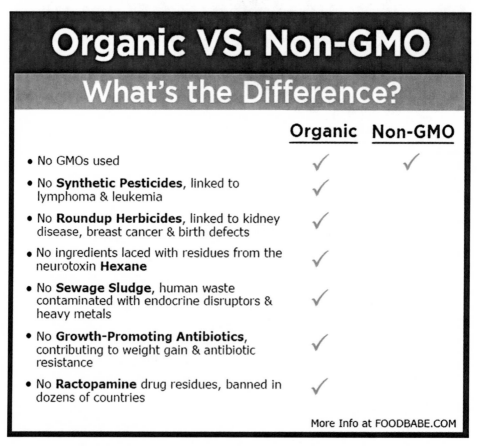

Now that's what I'm talking about! This laundry list of comparisons contains a number of fallacious arguments and poor science. See how many you can spot. (Foodbabe.com)

pedagogue: noun formal or humorous

a teacher, especially a strict or pedantic one.

Sapiophile (noun) is a neoligism - a new word that is just starting to enter common use but it means someone who is atracted to intelligence.

When employed in this way (as the speaker above might have) this isn't an ad hominem because the person being described is a relief teacher who is attracted to intelligent people.

Spoken with conviction and faux abhorrence—such a quote would fly right over the heads of the majority of people. Although strictly an ad hominem (the quote is directed at the person) this isn't the usual form, which is little more than calling someone a name.

Special Pleading

"Ah but [your argument here] doesn't apply in this case because..."

This is one of the simpler fallacies to spot, because the retort invariably relies on some unknown case that hasn't previously been made clear. This is a diversionary tactic because it also requires the opponent to evaluate the new evidence to decide if it is valid or invalid reasoning. Typically, when special pleading is employed, the reasoning is invalid, but this takes time to prove. Food Babe uses this fallacy to argue against anything she sees as unhealthy: for example because something contains a tiny percentage of a preservative. See "No True Scotsman" for an example of how she applies this to Subway's claim its food is fresh.

The Texas Sharpshooter

Blue 1 is used to color candy, beverages and baked goods and may cause cancer. Blue 2, found in pet food, candy and beverages, has caused brain tumors in mice. [38]

Food Babe might not rely on this one directly, but you can be sure she relies on it aplenty by proxying studies that have employed it. The sharp-shooter takes its name from the reversal of cause and effect. Imagine you have a six-shooter, blindfold yourself in a some remote building, and then take all six shots at random waving the gun around like a loose firehose.

---

38   http://foodbabe.com/2011/05/07/fro-yo-craze-is-just-well-crazy/

Now, go to each bullet hole and paint a neat target around each one. Of course it's cheating—but it's easy to do when you have enough data with some random clumps and something to prove. Suggestions that 4-MeI, some food colors and other chemicals cause cancer often rely on this rather dark, if colorfully named fallacy.

Tu quoque

> I never thought in a million years I would be subjected to this disgusting PR game. [39]

When SciBabe (Yvette d'Entremont) skewered Food Babe quite brilliantly in her Gawker article, Food Babe's response [40] was a classic example of this fallacy. The idea of *tu quoque* (literally, "you too") is to turn the criticism back on the critic in order to divert attention from the real issue at hand. Food Babe went after d'Entremont personally and professionally rather than address the issues she had raised. An expert in misleading the public, Food Babe cries *tu quoue* when others critique her work.

■

---

39   http://foodbabe.com/2015/02/12/dirty-pr-campaign/
40   http://foodbabe.com/response-to-gawker-the-food-babe-blogger-is-full-of-shit/

17

A for Aspartame

Email hoaxes spread far faster than the correct information and create mass panic. If you've ever wondered why Food Babe detests aspartame so much, we're going to share the most popular version of the hoax targeting this artificial sweetener. The article is attributed to one Nancy Markle, but it's thought to be the work of "Dr." Betty Martini. [1]

For completeness we should mention this claim is contested by Dorway, [2] a website devoted to giving aspartame a bad name in the interests of... well, who knows. Although not conclusive in and of itself we should note that many of these sites promote Stevia as a natural alternative to aspartame – including Food Babe.

Food Babe frequently references both Mercola.com and the Center for Science in the Public Interest but presumably, since she promotes Stevia, she isn't aware of this gem on mercola.com

> "There is some concern about Stevia. "Just because it's natural doesn't mean that it's safe," says Michael Jacobson, executive director of the Center for Science in the Public Interest. "That's why tests should be done." Stevia may be linked to genetic mutations in lab animals." [3]

Anyone who speaks out for aspartame (and against these interests) is accused of being part of some global conspiracy and yet, so far, no one has ever been able to show such a thing exists. Still, that doesn't stop the rumor mill from churning out misinformation:

---

1   http://urbanlegends.about.com/library/blasp2.htm
2   http://www.dorway.com/nomarkle.html
3   http://articles.mercola.com/sites/articles/archive/2008/12/16/stevia-the-holy-grail-of-sweeteners.aspx

"At one time the FDA actually embargoed Stevia and the rumor is Monsanto wants to add a molecule so they can patent it, and sell it themselves." [4]

Stevia is widely used today and not a whiff of a Monsanto scientist anywhere.

Ms. Martini is the founder of the impressively named Mission Possible World Health Organization—which is just a front for another anti-aspartame lobby. She has no published medical qualifications and her doctorate in humanities is purely honorific. Dorway excuses her lack of medical qualifications like this:

"Betty had three children instead of a doctor's degree but spent 22 years in the medical field." [5]

While raising children is no picnic, there are many medical doctors who are also mothers in their own right. Motherhood is no substitute for relevant credentials when making extraordinary claims. It's particularly damning when she creates falsehoods like this:

"Worst of all," Betty says, "It's not a diet product. Aspartame defeats the brain's ability to detect serotonin so you crave carbohydrates. It makes most people fat! This entire travesty, this horrible atrocity against our poor human race is driven only by greed! greed! greed! And because of the damage to the hypothalamus some consumers suddenly drop dead (see Dr. Blaylock's paper on Aspartame, MSG and Other Excitotoxins And the Hypothalamus). This may be associated with recent sudden death of athletes." [6]

"Detect serotonin," you say? That's an interesting phrase, and a clear indication of someone with zero medical knowledge, but a Dunning-Kruger style self-belief in her own misunderstanding. Serotonin is a neurotransmitter involved in mood and, therefore, is widely targeted by antidepressant drugs. Too much serotonin is highly toxic, leading to the potentially life-threatening condition serotonin syndrome. [7]

---

4 http://dorway.com/whistleblowers/what-is-mission-possible/mission-possible/

5 http://dorway.com/whistleblowers/what-is-mission-possible/mission-possible/

6 http://dorway.com/whistleblowers/what-is-mission-possible/mission-possible/

7 http://www.mayoclinic.org/diseases-conditions/serotonin-syndrome/basics/definition/con-20028946

Based upon Martini's claim, if aspartame was somehow blocking the brain's ability to detect this chemical, our mood would be seriously affected or we would suffer a rapid onset of seratonin syndrome. There is no evidence to support her rather ludicrous assertion. There never has been and we can confidently say there isn't ever likely to be either.

Regardless of who created this email—it was patently written with the singular mission to disparage aspartame. As of March 2015, Mission Possible World Health Organization remains engaged in a search for "victims" of the sweetener. A strong rebuttal from a qualified scientist appears at the end of the Markle email.

If you've ever heard a bad word spoken about aspartame, then it probably orginated from this one viral and sensationalist email from someone with absolutely no relevant qualifications at all: just a bellyful of misplaced hate.■

The Fear Babe

Subject: FW: Health information on ASPARTAME

WORLD ENVIRONMENTAL CONFERENCE and the MULTIPLE SCLEROSIS FOUNDATION

F.D.A. ISSUING FOR COLLUSION WITH MONSANTO

Article written by Nancy Markle (1120197)

I have spent several days lecturing at the WORLD ENVIRON-MENTAL CONFERENCE on "ASPARTAME marketed as 'NutraSweet', 'Equal', and 'Spoonful"'. In the keynote address by the EPA, they announced that there was an epidemic of multiple sclerosis and systemic lupus, and they did not understand what toxin was causing this to be rampant across the United States.

I explained that I was there to lecture on exactly that subject. When the temperature of Aspartame exceeds 86 degrees F, the wood alcohol in ASPARTAME coverts to formaldehyde and then to formic acid, which in turn causes metabolic acidosis. (Formic acid is the poison found in the sting of fire ants). The methanol toxicity mimics multiple sclerosis; thus people were being diagnosed with having multiple sclerosis in error. The multiple sclerosis is not a death sentence, where methanol toxicity is.

In the case of systemic lupus, we are finding it has become almost as rampant as multiple sclerosis, especially Diet Coke and Diet Pepsi drinkers. Also, with methanol toxicity, the victims usually drink three to four 12 oz. Cans of them per day, some even more. In the cases of systemic lupus, which is triggered by ASPARTAME, the victim usually does not know that the aspartame is the culprit. The victim continues its use aggravating the lupus to such a degree, that sometimes it becomes life-threatening.

When we get people off the aspartame, those with systemic lupus usually become asymptomatic. Unfortunately, we cannot reverse this disease. On the other hand, in the case of those diagnosed with Multiple Sclerosis, (when in reality, the disease is methanol toxicity), most of the symptoms disappear. We have seen cases where their vision has returned and even their hearing has returned. This also applies to cases of tinnitus. During a lecture I said "If you are using ASPARTAME (NutraSweet, Equal, Spoonful, etc.) and you suffer from fibromyalgia symptoms, spasms, shooting pains, numbness in your legs, cramps, vertigo, dizziness, headaches, tinnitus, joint pain, depression, anxiety attacks, slurred speech, blurred vision, or memory loss-you probably have ASPARTAME DISEASE!" People were jumping up during the lecture saying, "I've got this, is it reversible?"

It is rampant. Some of the speakers at my lecture even were suffering from these symptoms. In one lecture attended by the Ambassador of Uganda, he told us that their sugar industry is adding aspartame! He continued by saying that one of the industry leader's son could no longer walk—due in part by product usage!

We have a very serious problem. Even a stranger came up to Dr. Espisto (one of my speakers) and myself and said, "Could you tell me why so many people seem to be coming down with MS?" During a visit to a hospice, a nurse said that six of her friends, who were heavy Diet Coke addicts, had all been diagnosed with MS. This is beyond coincidence.

Here is the problem. There were Congressional Hearings when aspartame was included in 100 different products. Since this initial hearing, there have been two subsequent hearings, but to no avail. Nothing has been done. The drug and chemical lobbies have very deep pockets. Now there are over 5,000 products containing this chemical, and the PATENT HAS EXPIRED!!!!! At the time of this first hearing, people were going blind. The methanol in the aspartame converts to formaldehyde in the retina of the eye. Formaldehyde is grouped in the same class as cyanide and arsenic- DEADLY POISONS!!! Unfortunately, it just takes longer to quietly kill, but it is killing people and causing all kinds of neurological problems.> Aspartame changes the brain's chemistry. It is the reason for severe seizures. This drug changes the dopamine level in the brain. Imagine what this drug does to patients suffering from Parkinson's Disease. This drug also causes Birth Defects.

There is absolutely no reason to take this product. It is NOT A DIET PRODUCT!!!! The Congressional record said, "It makes you crave carbohydrates and will make you FAT." Dr. Roberts stated that when he got patients off aspartame, their average weight loss was 19 pounds per person. The formaldehyde stores in the fat cells, particularly in the hips and thighs.

Aspartame is especially deadly for diabetics. All physicians know what wood alcohol will do to a diabetic. We find that physicians believe that they have patients with retinopathy, when in fact, it is caused by the aspartame. The aspartame keeps the blood sugar level out of control, causing many patients to go into a coma. Unfortunately, many have died. People were telling us at the Conference of the American College of Physicians, that they had relatives that switched from saccharin to an aspartame product and how that relative had eventually gone into a coma. Their physicians could not get the blood sugar levels under control. Thus, the patients suffered acute memory loss and eventually coma and death.

Memory loss is due to the fact that aspartic acid and phenylalanine are neurotoxic without the other amino acids found in protein. Thus it goes past the blood brain barrier and deteriorates the neurons of the brain. Dr. Russell Blaylock, neurosurgeon, said, "The ingredients stimulates the neurons of the brain to death, causing brain damage of varying degrees. Dr. Blaylock has written a book entitled "EXCITOTOXINS: THE TASTE THAT KILLS" (Health Press 1-800-643-2665). Dr. H.J. Roberts, diabetic specialist and world expert on aspartame poisoning, has also written a book entitled "DEFENSE AGAINST ALZHEIMER'S DISEASE" (1-800-814-9800). Dr. Roberts tells how aspartame poisoning is escalating Alzheimer's Disease, and indeed it is. As the hospice nurse told me, women are being admitted at 30 years of age with Alzheimer's Disease. Dr. Blaylock and Dr. Roberts will be writing a position paper with some case histories and will post it on the Internet. According to the Conference of the American College of Physicians, 'We are talking about a plague of neurological diseases caused by this deadly poison."

Dr. Roberts realized what was happening when aspartame was first marketed. He said "his diabetic patients presented memory loss, confusion, and severe vision loss." At the

Conference of the American College of Physicians, doctors admitted that they did not know. They had wondered why seizures were rampant (the phenylalanine in aspartame breaks down the seizure threshold and depletes serotonin, which causes manic depression, panic attacks, rage and violence).

Just before the Conference, I received a FAX from Norway, asking for a possible antidote for this poison because they are experiencing so many problems in their country. This "poison" is now available in 90 PLUS countries worldwide. Fortunately, we had speakers and ambassadors at the Conference from different nations who have pledged their help. We ask that you help too.

Print this article out and warn everyone you know. Take anything that contains aspartame black to the store. Take the "NO ASPARTAME TEST" and send us your case history.

I assure you that MONSANTO, the creator of aspartame, knows how deadly it is. They fund the American Diabetes Association, American Dietetic Association, Congress, and the Conference of the American College of Physicians. The New York Times, on November 15, 1996, ran an article on how the American Dietetic Association takes money from the food industry to endorse their products. Therefore, they cannot criticize any additives or tell about their link to MONSANTO. How bad is this? We told a mother who had a child on NutraSweet to get off the product. The child was having grand mal seizures every day. The mother called her physician, who called the ADA, who told the doctor not to take the child off the NutraSweet. We are still trying to convince the mother that the aspartame is causing the seizures. Every time we get someone off of aspartame, the seizures stop. If the baby dies, you know whose fault it is, and what we are up against. There are 92 documented symptoms of aspartame, from coma to death. The majority of them are all neurological, because the aspartame destroys the nervous system.

Aspartame Disease is partially the cause to what is behind some of the mystery of the Dessert Storm health problems. The burning tongue and other problems discussed in over 60 cases can be directly related to the consumption of an aspartame product. Several thousand pallets of diet drinks were shipped to the Dessert Storm troops. (Remember heat can liberate the methanol from the aspartame at 86 degrees F). Diet drinks sat in the 120 degree F. Arabian sun for weeks at a time on pallets. The service men and women drank them all day long. All of their symptoms are identical to aspartame poisoning. Dr. Roberts says "consuming aspartame at the time of conception can cause birth defects." The phenylalanine concentrates in the placenta, causing mental retardation, according to Dr. Louis Elsas, Pediatrician Professor—Genetics, at Emory University in his testimony before Congress.

In the original lab tests, animals developed brain tumors (phenylalanine breaks down into DXP, a brain tumor agent). When Dr. Espisto was lecturing on aspartame me, one physician in the audience, a neurosurgeon, said, "When they remove brain tumors, they have found high levels of aspartame in them."

Stevia, a sweet food, NOT AN ADDITIVE, which helps in the metabolism of sugar, which would be ideal for diabetics, has now been approved as a dietary supplement by the F.D.A. For years, the F.D.A. has outlawed this sweet food because of their loyalty to MONSANTO.

If it says "SUGAR FREE" on the label-DO NOT EVEN THINK ABOUT IT! Senator Howard Hetzenbaum wrote a bill that would have warned all infants, pregnant mothers and children of the dangers of aspartame. The bill would have also instituted independent studies on the problems existing in the population (seizures, changes in brain chemistry, changes in neurological and behavioral symptoms). It was killed by the powerful drug and chemical lobbies, letting loose the hounds of disease and death on an unsuspecting public. Since the Conference of the American College of Physicians, we hope to have the help of some world leaders. Again, please help us too.

There are a lot of people out there who must be warned, *please* let them know this information.

We've said many times in this book that aspartame is safe but given the rancid piece of fearmongering and misinformation that you might have just had to sift through, we present the official rebuttal from Dr. David Hattan.

Unlike Mrs. Martini, Dr. Hattan is a qualified and practicing scientist.

I have been requested by the FDA Center for Drug Evaluation and Research to respond to your request for an evaluation of the article written by Nancy Markle received via an e-mail message on the alleged toxicities of the artificial sweetener, aspartame.

My name is David Hattan and I am currently Acting Director of the Division of Health Effects Evaluation in the United States Food & Drug Administration (USFDA) Center for Food Safety and Applied Nutrition. I have worked on questions relating to the safety of aspartame repeatedly since 1978 and am familiar with the safety studies that have been conducted to support the safety of this food additive. There were well over 100 separate toxicological and clinical studies conducted to establish the safety of aspartame before it was approved for regulatory acceptance. Since its approval in 1981 by the USFDA, there have been many additional studies performed to follow up on some of the more creditable reports of aspartame- mediated adverse effects. Below I have tried to succinctly respond to certain of the allegations of toxicity proposed by Nancy Markle.

First, reports of the ingestion of aspartame in patients who later have suffered multiple sclerosis or systemic lupus is obviously not scientifically sustainable evidence that aspartame is responsible for the occurrence of either disease. Both of these disorders are subject to spontaneous remissions and exacerbations so it is entirely possible that when patients stopped using aspartame they might have also coincidentally have had remission of their symptoms. There is no credible evidence that I am aware of that suggests that aspartame elicits multiple sclerosis or systemic lupus.

Second, the claim that aspartame ingestion results in the production of methanol, formaldehyde and formate: These claims are factual. In the gastrointestinal tract aspar-

---

tame is hydrolyzed to one of its component materials, methanol, as well as the two amino acids, phenylalanine and aspartic acid. This methanol is taken up by the cells of the body and metabolized first to formaldehyde and then to formate. The key information that is missing in the description by Ms. Markle is that the levels of ingestion are very modest. In fact, there are other foodstuffs that we ingest that supply as much and sometimes even more methanol; e.g., citrus fruits and juices, and tomatoes or tomato juice. There are even higher quantities of methanol ingested when ethanol is consumed. Thus, in the final analysis this methanol is the same as from other sources and in the quantities consumed from aspartame, it is readily and naturally metabolized via the one-carbon biochemical cycle to entirely innocuous and natural body components.

Third, the claim that the two amino acids, phenylalanine and aspartic acid have neurotoxic effects. This is true in certain individuals and in high enough doses. The only subpopulation of individuals potentially susceptible to adverse effects from phenylalanine is homozygous phenylketonurics and in this case, food itself with much higher levels of phenylalanine from the protein in the diets contributes much higher toxicity for these unfortunate individuals. For those individual phenylketonurics that want to carefully control their intake levels of phenylalanine, they can do that by simply taking into consideration the amount of phenylalanine supplied by the aspartame product or, even more likely, simply refraining from use of these products. The USFDA requires that the aspartame product be labeled specially for phenylketonurics patients so that they will be aware of its presence in these products. As for the other amino acid in aspartame, the levels of aspartic acid ingested with aspartame use are many fold less than those levels responsible for causing adverse effects on the brain of animals and/or man. In fact, it is not clear that the experimentally derived data from animals is relevant to man. In any case, the levels of aspartic acid intake from aspartame are many fold below those needed to mediate neurologic effects.

Fourth, there have been numerous animal and human studies done to evaluate the possibility that aspartame causes seizures or enhances the susceptibility to seizures. In clinical studies done in adults and children with pre-existing seizures, there was no evidence of contributing to the frequency of occurrence or severity of seizures in seizure-prone individuals. There were additional studies done on seizure-prone experimental animal models to assess the possible influence of aspartame on their seizuring activity. Again, the result was the same and no influence was demonstrated on the frequency or severity of seizures.

Fifth, aspartame was comprehensively evaluated for its potential to mediate reproductive effects and birth defects. In all cases of animal testing, there was no evidence of aspartame-mediated effects on the experimental animals at doses many times higher than those to which the human population is exposed.

Sixth, more recent allegations about aspartame mediating an increase in the incidence of brain tumors in the human population has been thoroughly refuted by both government and academic scientists.

The Internet provides a convenient means of communicating information of all kinds in a potentially widespread manner. Unfortunately, the recipient of that information has no way of assessing the strength and reality of that information. There are a number of Internet web sites that regularly distribute information adverse reactions supposedly mediated by aspartame that is based on anecdotal reports that cannot be confirmed. The legitimate attempts that have been made to confirm and replicate these allegations of adverse reactions from aspartame ingestion have not been successful and the USFDA continues to consider this to be among the most thoroughly tested of food additives and that this information continues to confirm the safety of aspartame.

David G. Hattan, Ph.D.

Acting Director, Division of Health Effects Evaluation

Appendix A
Patently Obvious

The following claims are reproduced from the public record of patent US20070292582 A1, the Coca-Cola Company's method for purifying rebaudioside A from the unrefined product.

```
Purifying Rebaudioside
```

A method for purifying rebaudioside A comprising the steps of:

1. combining crude rebaudioside A and an aqueous organic solvent to form a rebaudioside A solution, the aqueous organic solution comprising water in an amount from about 10% to about 25% by weight;

   and crystallizing from the rebaudioside A solution in a single step a substantially pure rebaudioside A composition comprising rebaudioside A in a purity greater than about 95% by weight on a dry basis.

2. The method of claim 1, further comprising the step of heating the rebaudioside A solution.

3. The method of claim 2, further comprising the step of cooling the rebaudioside A solution.

4. The method of claim 1, wherein rebaudioside A solution in the single crystallization step is stirred or unstirred.

5. The method of claim 1, further comprising the step of seeding (optional) the rebaudioside A solution at an appropriate temperature with an amount of rebaudioside A sufficient to promote crystallization of rebaudioside A.

6. The method of claim 1, further comprising the steps of separating and washing the substantially pure rebaudioside A composition.

7. The method of claim 6, further comprising the step of drying the substantially pure rebaudioside A composition.

8. The method of claim 1, wherein the crude rebaudioside A comprises substantially no rebaudioside D impurity, and the method further comprises slurrying the substantially pure re-

baudioside A composition in an aqueous organic solvent or in an organic solvent.

9. The method of claim 8, further comprising the steps of separating and washing the substantially pure rebaudioside A composition.

10. The method of claim 9, further comprising the step of drying the composition of a substantially pure rebaudioside A.

11. The method of claim 1, wherein the aqueous organic solvent comprises a mixture of at least one organic solvent and water.

12. The method of claim 11, wherein at least one organic solvent comprises an alcohol.

13. The method of claim 12, wherein the alcohol comprises ethanol.

14. The method of claim 12, wherein the alcohol comprises methanol.

15. The method of claim 12, wherein the alcohol comprises a mixture of ethanol and methanol.

16. The method of claim 15, wherein the ethanol and methanol are present in the aqueous organic solution in a weight ratio from about 20 parts to about 1 parts ethanol to about 1 part methanol.

17. The method of claim 15, wherein the ethanol and methanol are present in the aqueous organic solution in a weight ratio from about 3 parts to about 1 part ethanol to about 1 part methanol.

18. The method of claim 1, wherein the at least one aqueous organic solvent comprises an organic solvent selected from the group consisting of acetone, acetonitrile, methanol, ethanol, 1-propanol, isopropanol, 1-butanol, 2-butanol, tert-butanol, and mixtures thereof.

19. The method of claim 1, wherein the aqueous organic solvent and the crude rebaudioside A are present in the rebaudioside A solution in a weight ratio from about 4 to about 10 parts aqueous organic solvent to about 1 part crude rebaudioside A.

20. The method of claim 1, wherein the aqueous organic solvent and the crude rebaudioside A are present in the rebaudioside A solution in a weight ratio from about 3 to about 5 parts aqueous organic solvent to about 1 part crude rebaudioside A.

21. The method of claim 1, wherein aqueous organic solvent com-

prises water in an amount from about 10% to about 25% by weight.

22. The method of claim 1, wherein the crude rebaudioside A mixture comprises rebaudioside A in a purity from about 40% to about 95% by weight.

23. The method of claim 1, wherein the crude rebaudioside A mixture comprises rebaudioside A in a purity from about 60% to about 85% by weight.

24. The method of claim 1, wherein the crude rebaudioside A mixture comprises rebaudioside A in a purity from about 70% to about 85% by weight.

25. The method of claim 1, wherein the method is carried out at approximately room temperature.

26. The method of claim 2, wherein the step of heating the rebaudioside A solution comprises heating the rebaudioside A solution to a temperature in a range from about 20° C. to about 40° C.

27. The method of claim 2, wherein the step of heating the rebaudioside A solution comprises heating the rebaudioside A solution to a temperature in a range from about 40° C. to about 60° C.

28. The method of claim 2, wherein the step of heating the rebaudioside A solution comprises heating the rebaudioside A solution to about a reflux temperature.

29. The method of claim 3, wherein the step of cooling the rebaudioside A solution comprises cooling the rebaudioside A solution to a temperature in a range from about 4° C. to about 25° C.

30. The method of claim 3, wherein the step of cooling the rebaudioside A solution comprises cooling the rebaudioside A solution for about 0.5 hours to about 24 hours.

31. The method of claim 1, wherein the substantially pure rebaudioside A product comprises rebaudioside A in a purity greater than about 97% rebaudioside A by weight on a dry basis.

32. The method of claim 1, wherein the substantially pure rebaudioside A product comprises rebaudioside A in a purity greater than about 98% rebaudioside A by weight on a dry basis.

33. The method of claim 1, wherein the substantially pure rebaudioside A product comprises rebaudioside A in a purity greater than about 99% rebaudioside A by weight on a dry basis.

34. The method of claim 1, further comprising the steps of

    heating the rebaudioside A aqueous organic solvent mixture;

    cooling the rebaudioside A solution;

    separating and washing a substantially pure rebaudioside A composition;

    and drying the substantially pure rebaudioside A composition.

35. A substantially pure rebaudioside A composition made according to the method of claim 1, wherein the substantially pure rebaudioside A composition comprises a polymorph having an X-ray diffraction pattern substantially similar to FIG. 7.

36. A substantially pure rebaudioside A composition made according to the method of claim 1, wherein the substantially pure rebaudioside A composition comprises a polymorph having an X-ray diffraction pattern substantially similar to FIG. 8.

37. A substantially pure rebaudioside A composition made according to the method of claim 1, wherein the substantially pure rebaudioside A composition comprises a polymorph having an X-ray diffraction pattern substantially similar to FIG. 9.

38. A substantially pure rebaudioside A composition made according to the method of claim 1, wherein the substantially pure rebaudioside A composition comprises a polymorph having an X-ray diffraction pattern substantially similar to FIG. 10.

39. A substantially pure rebaudioside A composition made according to the method of claim 1, wherein the substantially pure rebaudioside A composition comprises an amorphous form having an X-ray diffraction pattern substantially similar to FIG. 11.

40. The method of claim 1, further comprising the step of forming an amorphous form of the substantially pure rebaudioside A composition.

41. The method of claim 38, wherein the step of forming an amorphous form of the substantially pure rebaudioside A composition comprises a method selected from the group consisting of ball milling, precipitation, lyophilization, cryogrinding, and spray-drying

42. A substantially pure rebaudioside A composition made according to the method of claim 1.

Appendix B
IARC Group 1

The IARC (International Agency for Research on Cancer) provides these reference lists for specialists in risk assessment and management. The IARC website, *www.iarc.fr*, should always be used as the primary reference.

☆ Acetaldehyde associated with consumption of alcoholic beverages
☆ Acheson process, occupational exposure associated with acid mists
☆ Aflatoxins
☆ Alcoholic beverages
☆ Aluminium production
☆ 4-Aminobiphenyl
☆ Areca nut
☆ Aristolochic acid
☆ Aristolochic acid, plants containing
☆ Arsenic and inorganic arsenic compounds
☆ Asbestos (all forms, including actinolite, amosite, anthophyllite, chrysotile, crocidolite, tremolite should also be regarded as carcinogenic to humans.)
☆ Auramine production
☆ Azathioprine
☆ Benzene
☆ Benzidine
☆ Benzidine, dyes metabolized to
☆ Benzo[a]pyrene
☆ Beryllium and beryllium compounds
☆ Beryllium and beryllium compounds
☆ Betel quid with tobacco
☆ Betel quid without tobacco
☆ Bis(chloromethyl)ether; chloromethyl methyl ether (technical-grade)
☆ Busulfan
☆ 1,3-Butadiene
☆ Cadmium and cadmium compounds
☆ Chlorambucil
☆ Chlornaphazine

☆ Chromium (VI) compounds
☆ Clonorchis sinensis (infection with)
☆ Coal, indoor emissions from household combustion of
☆ Coal gasification
☆ Coal-tar distillation
☆ Coal-tar pitch
☆ Coke production
☆ Cyclophosphamide
☆ Cyclosporine (see ciclosporin)
☆ 1,2-Dichloropropane
☆ Diethylstilbestrol
☆ Engine exhaust, diesel
☆ Epstein-Barr virus
☆ Erionite
☆ Estrogen-only menopausal therapy
☆ Estrogen therapy, postmenopausal (see Estrogen-only menopausal therapy)
☆ Estrogen-progestogen menopausal therapy (combined)
☆ Estrogen-progestogen oral contraceptives (combined)
☆ Ethanol in alcoholic beverages
☆ Ethylene oxide
☆ Etoposide
☆ Etoposide in combination with cisplatin and bleomycin
☆ Fission products, including strontium-90
☆ Fluoro-edenite fibrous amphibole
☆ Formaldehyde
☆ Haematite mining (underground)
☆ Helicobacter pylori (infection with)
☆ Hepatitis B virus (chronic infection with)
☆ Hepatitis B virus (chronic infection with)
☆ Human immunodeficiency virus type 1 (infection with)
☆ Human papillomavirus types 16, 18, 31, 33, 35, 39, 45, 51, 52, 56, 58, 59
(The HPV types that have been classified as carcinogenic to humans can
differ by an order of magnitude in risk for cervical cancer)
☆ Human T-cell lymphotropic virus type I
☆ Ionizing radiation (all types)
☆ Iron and steel founding (occupational exposure during)
☆ Isopropyl alcohol manufacture using strong acids
☆ Kaposi sarcoma herpes virus
☆ Leather dust
☆ Magenta production

- ☆ Melphalan
- ☆ Methoxsalen (8-methoxypsoralen) plus ultraviolet A radiation
- ☆ Methyl-CCNU
- ☆ 4,4'-Methylenebis(2-chloroaniline) (MOCA)
- ☆ Mineral oils, untreated or mildly treated
- ☆ MOPP and other combined chemotherapy including alkylating agents
- ☆ 2-Naphthylamine
- ☆ Neutron radiation
- ☆ Nickel compounds
- ☆ N'-Nitrosonornicotine (NNN)
- ☆ 4-(N- Nitrosomethylamino)-1-(3-pyridyl)-1-butanone (NNK)
- ☆ Opisthorchis viverrini (infection with)
- ☆ Outdoor air pollution
- ☆ Outdoor air pollution, particulate matter in
- ☆ Painter (occupational exposure as a)
- ☆ Particulate matter in outdoor air pollution
- ☆ 3,4,5,3',4'-Pentachlorobiphenyl (PCB-126) (see Polychlorinated biphenyls, dioxin-like, with a TEF according to WHO)
- ☆ 2,3,4,7,8-Pentachlorodibenzofuran
- ☆ Phenacetin
- ☆ Phenacetin, analgesic mixtures containing
- ☆ Phosphorus-32, as phosphate
- ☆ Plutonium
- ☆ Polychlorinated biphenyls
- ☆ Polychlorinated biphenyls, dioxin-like, with a Toxicity Equivalency Factor (TEF) according to WHO (PCBs 77, 81, 105, 114, 118, 123, 126, 156, 157, 167, 169, 189)
- ☆ Radioiodines, including iodine-131
- ☆ Radionuclides, alpha-particle-emitting, internally deposited
- ☆ Radionuclides, beta-particle-emitting, internally deposited
- ☆ Radium-224 and its decay products
- ☆ Radium-226 and its decay products
- ☆ Radium-228 and its decay products
- ☆ Radon-222 and its decay products
- ☆ Rubber manufacturing industry
- ☆ Salted fish, Chinese-style
- ☆ Schistosoma haematobium (infection with)
- ☆ Semustine (see Methyl-CCNU)
- ☆ Shale oils
- ☆ Silica dust, crystalline, in the form of quartz or cristobalite

☆ Solar radiation
☆ Soot (as found in occupational exposure of chimney sweeps)
☆ Sulfur mustard
☆ Tamoxifen
☆ 2,3,7,8-Tetrachlorodibenzo-para-dioxin
☆ Thiotepa
☆ Thorium-232 and its decay products
☆ Tobacco, smokeless
☆ Tobacco smoke, second-hand
☆ Tobacco smoking
☆ ortho-Toluidine
☆ Treosulfan
☆ Trichloroethylene
☆ Trichloroethylene
☆ Ultraviolet radiation (wavelengths 100-400 nm, encompassing UVA, UVB, and UVC)
☆ Ultraviolet-emitting tanning devices
☆ Vinyl chloride
☆ Wood dust
☆ X- and Gamma-Radiation

Appendix C
IARC Group 2a

When something is listed as a carcinogen for the sake of creating fear through ignorance, the IARC monographs are often used (but rarely without full clarification). As you can see from this list, things are nowhere near as black and white as they are made to appear. Caution is advised as the materials and usages here are not necessarily carcinogenic to humans and in many cases are only toxic in large amounts over many years. As the experts at the American Cancer Society put it:

> *"Perhaps not surprisingly, based on how hard it can be to test possible carcinogens, most are listed as being of probable, possible, or unknown risk"* [1]

Or, put another way, if something isn't a known carginogenic compound, listed in "IARC Group 1" on page 364 you probably don't need to worry unduly about it and even if it is, you only need to be cautious and not lose too much sleep before speaking to an expert in the field.

- ☆ Acrylamide
- ☆ Adriamycin
- ☆ Androgenic (anabolic) steroids
- ☆ Art glass, glass containers and pressed ware (manufacture of)
- ☆ Azacitidine
- ☆ Biomass fuel (primarily wood), indoor emissions from household combustion of
- ☆ Bischloroethyl nitrosourea (BCNU)
- ☆ Bitumens, occupational exposure to oxidized bitumens and their emissions during roofing
- ☆ Captafol
- ☆ Carbon electrode manufacture
- ☆ Chloral
- ☆ Chloral hydrate
- ☆ Chloramphenicol

---

1   http://www.cancer.org/cancer/cancercauses/othercarcinogens/does-this-cause-cancer

☆ alpha-Chlorinated toluenes (benzal chloride, benzotrichloride, benzyl chloride) and benzoyl chloride (combined exposures)

☆ 1-(2-Chloroethyl)-3-cyclohexyl-1-nitrosourea (CCNU)

☆ 4-Chloro-ortho-toluidine

☆ Chlorozotocin

☆ Cisplatin

☆ Cobalt metal with tungsten carbide

☆ Creosotes

☆ Cyclopenta[cd]pyrene

☆ 333-41-5 Diazinon

☆ Dibenz[a,j]acridine

☆ Dibenz[a,h]anthracene

☆ Dibenzo[a,l]pyrene

☆ Dichloromethane (Methylene chloride)

☆ Diethyl sulfate

☆ Dimethylcarbamoyl chloride

☆ 1,2-Dimethylhydrazine

☆ Dimethyl sulfate

☆ Epichlorohydrin

☆ Ethyl carbamate (Urethane)

☆ Ethylene dibromide

☆ N-Ethyl-N-nitrosourea

☆ Frying, emissions from high-temperature

☆ Glycidol

☆ Glyphosate

☆ Hairdresser or barber (occupational exposure as a)

☆ Human papillomavirus type 68

☆ Indium phosphide

☆ IQ (2-Amino-3-methylimidazo[4,5-f]quinoline)

☆ Lead compounds, inorganic

☆ Malaria (caused by infection with Plasmodium falciparum in holoendemic areas)

☆ Malathion

☆ Mate, hot

☆ Merkel cell polyomavirus (MCV)

☆ 5-Methoxypsoralen

☆ Methyl methanesulfonate

☆ N-itro-N-nitrosoguanidine (MNNG)

☆ N-Methyl-N-nitrosourea

☆ Nitrate or nitrite (ingested) under conditions that result in endogenous nitro-

sation
- ☆ 6-Nitrochrysene 2A
- ☆ Nitrogen mustard 2A
- ☆ 1-Nitropyrene
- ☆ N-Nitrosodiethylamine
- ☆ N-Nitrosodimethylamine
- ☆ 2-Nitrotoluene
- ☆ Non-arsenical insecticides (occupational exposures in spraying and application of)
- ☆ Petroleum refining (occupational exposures in)
- ☆ Pioglitazone
- ☆ Polybrominated biphenyls
- ☆ Procarbazine hydrochloride
- ☆ 1,3-Propane sultone
- ☆ Shiftwork that involves circadian (sleep) disruption
- ☆ Silicon carbide whiskers
- ☆ Styrene-7,8-oxide
- ☆ Teniposide
- ☆ Tetrachloroethylene (Perchloroethylene)
- ☆ Tetrafluoroethylene
- ☆ 1,2,3-Trichloropropane
- ☆ Tris(2,3-dibromopropyl) phosphate
- ☆ Vinyl bromide (For practical purposes, vinyl bromide should be considered to act similarly to the human carcinogen vinyl chloride.)
- ☆ Vinyl fluoride (For practical purposes, vinyl fluoride should be considered to act similarly to the human carcinogen vinyl chloride.)

Appendix D
IARC Group 2b

Caution is advised as the materials and usages here are not necessarily carginongenic to humans and in many cases only toxic in large amounts over many years. Agents and mixtures in this group are thought to be the least likely carcinogenic to humans, although they may be carcinogenic to animals.

- ☆ A-alpha-C (2yrido[2,3-b]indole)
- ☆ Acetaldehyde
- ☆ Acetamide
- ☆ Acrylonitrile
- ☆ Auitro-2-furyl)acrylamide]
- ☆ Aflatoxin M1
- ☆ Aloe vera, whole leaf extract
- ☆ para-Aminoazobenzene
- ☆ ortho-Aminoazotoluene
- ☆ 1-Amino-2,4-dibromoanthraquinone
- ☆ 2-Aitro-2-furyl)-1,3,4-thiadiazole
- ☆ Amsacrine
- ☆ ortho-Anisidine
- ☆ Anthraquinone
- ☆ Antimony trioxide
- ☆ Aramite®
- ☆ Auramine
- ☆ Azaserine
- ☆ Aziridine
- ☆ Benz[j]aceanthrylene
- ☆ Benz[a]anthracene
- ☆ Benzo[b]fluoranthene
- ☆ Benzo[j]fluoranthene
- ☆ Benzo[k]fluoranthene
- ☆ Benzofuran
- ☆ Benzo[c]phenanthrene
- ☆ Benzophenone

- ☆ Benzyl violet 4B
- ☆ 2,2-Bis(bromomethyl)propane-1,3-diol
- ☆ Bitumens, occupational exposure to hard bitumens and their emissions during mastic asphalt work
- ☆ Bitumens, occupational exposure to straight-run bitumens and their emissions during road paving
- ☆ BK polyomavirus (BKV)
- ☆ Bleomycins
- ☆ Bracken fern
- ☆ Bromochloroacetic acid
- ☆ Bromodichloromethane
- ☆ Butylated hydroxyanisole (BHA)
- ☆ beta-Butyrolactone
- ☆ Caffeic acid
- ☆ Carbazole
- ☆ Carbon black
- ☆ Carbon nanotubes, multi-walled MWCNT-7
- ☆ Carbon tetrachloride
- ☆ Carpentry and joinery
- ☆ Carrageenan, degraded (Poligeenan)
- ☆ Catechol
- ☆ Chlordane
- ☆ Chlordecone (Kepone)
- ☆ Chlorendic acid
- ☆ Chlorinated paraffins of average carbon chain length C12 and average degree of chlorination approximately 60%
- ☆ para-Chloroaniline
- ☆ 3-Chloro-4-(dichloromethyl)-5-hydroxy-2(5H)-furanone
- ☆ Chloroform
- ☆ 1-Chloro-2-methylpropene
- ☆ Chlorophenoxy herbicides
- ☆ 4-Chloro-ortho-phenylenediamine
- ☆ Chloroprene
- ☆ Chlorothalonil
- ☆ Chrysene
- ☆ CI Acid Red 114
- ☆ CI Basic Red 9
- ☆ CI Direct Blue 15
- ☆ Citrus Red No. 2
- ☆ Cobalt and cobalt compounds

- ☆ Cobalt metal without tungsten carbide
- ☆ Cobalt sulfate and other soluble cobalt(II) salts
- ☆ Coconut oil diethanolamine condensate
- ☆ Coffee (urinary bladder)
- ☆ para-Cresidine
- ☆ Cumene
- ☆ Cycasin
- ☆ Dacarbazine
- ☆ Dantron (Chrysazin; 1,8-Dihydroxyanthraquinone)
- ☆ Daunomycin
- ☆ DDT (4,4'-Dichlorodiphenyltrichloroethane)
- ☆ N,N'-Diacetylbenzidine
- ☆ 2,4-Diaminoanisole
- ☆ 4,4'-Diaminodiphenyl ether
- ☆ 2,4-Diaminotoluene
- ☆ Dibenz[a,h]acridine
- ☆ Dibenz[c,h]acridine
- ☆ 7H-Dibenzo[c,g]carbazole
- ☆ Dibenzo[a,h]pyrene
- ☆ Dibenzo[a,i]pyrene
- ☆ Dibromoacetic acid
- ☆ Dibromoacetonitrile
- ☆ 1,2-Dibromo-3-chloropropane
- ☆ 2,3-Dibromopropan-1-ol
- ☆ Dichloroacetic acid
- ☆ para-Dichlorobenzene
- ☆ 3,3'-Dichlorobenzidine
- ☆ 3,3'-Dichloro-4,4'-diaminodiphenyl ether
- ☆ 1,2-Dichloroethane
- ☆ 1,3-Dichloro-2-propanol
- ☆ 1,3-Dichloropropene (technical-grade)
- ☆ Dichlorvos
- ☆ Diesel fuel, marine
- ☆ Diethanolamine
- ☆ Di(2-ethylhexyl)phthalate
- ☆ 1,2-Diethylhydrazine
- ☆ Diglycidyl resorcinol ether
- ☆ Digoxin
- ☆ Dihydrosafrole
- ☆ Diisopropyl sulfate

- ☆ 3,3'-Dimethoxybenzidine (ortho-Dianisidine)
- ☆ para-Dimethylaminoazobenzene
- ☆ trans-2-[(Dimethylamino)methylim5-nitro-2-
- ☆ furyl)-vinyl]-1,3,4-oxadiazole
- ☆ 2,6-Dimethylaniline (2,6-Xylidine)
- ☆ Dimethylarsinic acid
- ☆ 3,3'-Dimethylbenzidine (ortho-Tolidine)
- ☆ 1,1-Dimethylhydrazine
- ☆ 3,7-Dinitrofluoranthene
- ☆ 3,9-Dinitrofluoranthene
- ☆ 1,3-Dinitropyrene
- ☆ 1,6-Dinitropyrene
- ☆ 1,8-Dinitropyrene
- ☆ 2,4-Dinitrotoluene
- ☆ 2,6-Dinitrotoluene
- ☆ 1,4-Dioxane
- ☆ Disperse Blue 1
- ☆ Dry cleaning (occupational exposures in)
- ☆ Engine exhaust, gasoline
- ☆ 1,2-Epoxybutane
- ☆ Ethyl acrylate
- ☆ Ethylbenzene
- ☆ Ethyl methanesulfonate
- ☆ Firefighter (occupational exposure as a)
- ☆ 2-(2-Formylhydrazitro-2-furyl)thiazole
- ☆ Fuel oils, residual (heavy)
- ☆ Fumonisin B1
- ☆ Furan
- ☆ Fusarium moniliforme, toxins derived from (fumonisin B1, fumonisin B2, and fusarin C)
- ☆ Gasoline
- ☆ Ginkgo biloba extract
- ☆ Glu-P-1 (2-Amino-6-methyldipyrido[1,2-a:3',2'- d]imidazole)
- ☆ Glu-P-2 (2-Aminodipyrido[1,2-a:3',2'-d]imidazole)
- ☆ Glycidaldehyde
- ☆ Goldenseal root powder
- ☆ Griseofulvin
- ☆ HC Blue No. 1
- ☆ Heptachlor
- ☆ Hexachlorobenzene

- ☆ Hexachlorocyclohexanes
- ☆ Hexachloroethane
- ☆ 2,4-Hexadienal
- ☆ Hexamethylphosphoramide
- ☆ Human immunodeficiency virus type 2 (infection with)
- ☆ Human papillomavirus types 5 and 8 (in patients with epidermodysplasia verruciformis)
- ☆ Human papillomavirus types 26, 53, 66, 67, 70, 73, 82
- ☆ Human papillomavirus types 30, 34, 69, 85, 97
- ☆ Hydrazine
- ☆ Hydrochlorothiazide
- ☆ 1-Hydroxyanthraquinone
- ☆ Indeno[1,2,3-cd]pyrene
- ☆ Iron-dextran complex
- ☆ Isoprene
- ☆ JC polyomavirus (JCV)
- ☆ Kava extract
- ☆ Lasiocarpine
- ☆ Lead
- ☆ Magenta
- ☆ Magnetic fields, extremely low-frequency
- ☆ MeA-alpha-C (2-Amino-3-yrido[2,3-b]indole)
- ☆ Medroxyprogesterone acetate
- ☆ MeIQ (2-Amino-3,4-dimethylimidazo[4,5-f]quinoline)
- ☆ MeIQx (2-Amino-3,8-dimethylimidazo[4,5-f]quinoxaline)
- ☆ Merphalan
- ☆ Methylarsonic acid
- ☆ 2-Methylaziridine (Propyleneimine)
- ☆ Methylazoxymethanol acetate
- ☆ 5-Methylchrysene
- ☆ 4,4'-Methylene bis(2-methylaniline)
- ☆ 4,4'-Methylenedianiline
- ☆ Methyleugenol
- ☆ 2-Methylimidazole
- ☆ 4-Methylimidazole
- ☆ Methyl isobutyl ketone
- ☆ Methylmercury compounds
- ☆ 2-Methyl-1-nitroanthraquinone (uncertain purity)
- ☆ N-Methyl-N-nitrosourethane
- ☆ α-Methylstyrene

☆ Methylthiouracil
☆ Metronidazole
☆ Michler's base [4,4'-methylenebis(N,N-dimethyl)-benzenamine]
☆ Michler's ketone [4,4'-Bis(dimethylamino)benzophenone]
☆ Microcystin-LR
☆ Mirex
☆ Mitomycin C
☆ Mitoxantrone
☆ 3-Monochloro-1,2-propanediol
☆ Monocrotaline 5-(Morpholinomethyl)-3-[(5-nitrofurfurylidene)amino]-2-oxazolidinone
☆ Multi-walled carbon nanotubes MWCNT-7 (see Carbon nanotubes, multi-walled MWCNT-7)
☆ Nafenopin
☆ Naphthalene
☆ Nickel, metallic and alloys
☆ Niridazole
☆ Nitrilotriacetic acid and its salts
☆ 5-Nitroacenaphthene
☆ 2-Nitroanisole
☆ 3-Nitrobenzanthrone
☆ Nitrobenzene
☆ Nitrofen (technical-grade)
☆ 2-Nitrofluorene
☆ 1-[(5-Nitrofurfurylidene)amino]-2-imidazolidinone
☆ N-[4-(5-Nitro-2-furyl)-2-thiazolyl]acetamide
☆ Nitrogen mustard N-oxide
☆ Nitromethane
☆ 2-Nitropropane
☆ 4-Nitropyrene
☆ N-Nitrosodi-n-butylamine
☆ N-Nitrosodiethanolamine
☆ N-Nitrosodi-n-propylamine
☆ 3-(N-Nitrosomethylamino)propionitrile
☆ N-Nitrosomethylethylamine
☆ N-Nitrosomethylvinylamine
☆ N-Nitrosomorpholine
☆ N-Nitrosopiperidine
☆ N-Nitrosopyrrolidine
☆ N-Nitrososarcosine

☆ Ochratoxin A
☆ Oil Orange SS
☆ Oxazepam
☆ Palygorskite (Attapulgite) (long fibres, > 5 micrometres)
☆ Panfuran S (containing dihydroxymethylfuratrizine)
☆ Parathion
☆ Pentosan polysulfate sodium
☆ Perfluorooctanoic acid
☆ Pickled vegetables (traditional Asian)
☆ Phenazopyridine hydrochloride
☆ Phenobarbital
☆ Phenolphthalein
☆ Phenoxybenzamine hydrochloride
☆ Phenyl glycidyl ether
☆ Phenytoin
☆ PhIP (2-Amino-1-methyl-6-phenylimidazo[4,5-b]pyridine)
☆ Polychlorophenols and their sodium salts (mixed exposures)
☆ Ponceau 3R
☆ Ponceau MX
☆ Potassium bromate
☆ Primidone
☆ Printing processes (occupational exposures in)
☆ Progestins
☆ Progestogen-only contraceptives
☆ beta-Propiolactone
☆ Propylene oxide
☆ Propylthiouracil
☆ Pulegone
☆ Radiofrequency electromagnetic fields1
☆ Refractory ceramic fibres
☆ Riddelliine
☆ Safrole
☆ Schistosoma japonicum (infection with)
☆ Silicon carbide, fibrous
☆ Sodium ortho-phenylphenate
☆ Special-purpose fibres such as E-glass and '475' glass
☆ fibres
☆ Sterigmatocystin
☆ Streptozotocin
☆ Styrene

- ☆ Sulfallate
- ☆ Sulfasalazine
- ☆ Surgical implants and other foreign bodies:
- ☆ - Polymeric implants prepared as thin smooth film (with the exception of poly(glycolic acid))
- ☆ - Metallic implants prepared as thin smooth films
- ☆ - Implanted foreign bodies of metallic cobalt, metallic nickel and an alloy powder containing 66-67% nickel, 13-16% chromium and 7% iron
- ☆ Talc-based body powder (perineal use of)
- ☆ 1,1,1,2-Tetrachloroethane
- ☆ 1,1,2,2-Tetrachloroethane
- ☆ Tetranitromethane
- ☆ Includes radiofrequency electromagnetic fields from wireless phones
- ☆ Tetrachlorvinphos
- ☆ Textile manufacturing industry (work in)
- ☆ Thioacetamide
- ☆ 4,4'-Thiodianiline
- ☆ Thiouracil
- ☆ Titanium dioxide
- ☆ Toluene diisocyanates
- ☆ Toxaphene (Polychlorinated camphenes)
- ☆ Triamterene
- ☆ Trichlormethine (Trimustine hydrochloride)
- ☆ Trichloroacetic acid
- ☆ Trp-P-1 (3-Amino-1,4-diyrido[4,3-b]indole)
- ☆ Trp-P-2 (3-Amino-1-yrido[4,3-b]indole)
- ☆ Trypan blue
- ☆ Uracil mustard
- ☆ Vanadium pentoxide
- ☆ Vinyl acetate
- ☆ 4-Vinylcyclohexene
- ☆ 4-Vinylcyclohexene diepoxide
- ☆ Welding fumes
- ☆ Zalcitabine
- ☆ Zidovudine (AZT)

Appendix D
Erasing Past Mistakes

An example of Food Babe's canny technique to remove offending information is shown on the next page (Mark has further examples on page 297.) While this might not seem particularly surprising, she has already promised:

> As is traditional in print journalism, I am going to start a Corrections/Editor's Note feature on my web site.

But the Internet doesn't forget—so we can go back in time using caches such as *Archive.org* to find out what she really wrote, right? Wrong.

The entire site has been deliberately masked from caching using something called a robots directive. [1] All sites can have these; they are optional and entirely legitimate.

FoodBabe.com has a site wide cache prohibition in effect. Preventing the spiders from archiving her past—in other words, errors—particularly libelous ones—are easier to hide. Two lines are all it takes.

```
User-agent: ia_archiver
Disallow: /
```

Don't take our word for it though—you can check any site just by entering its name followed by: "/robots.txt"—so to get the robots directives for FoodBabe.com you would enter:

```
http://www.foodbabe.com/robots.txt
```

---

1   http://www.robotstxt.org

There's a group of aggressive scientists, biased doctors, skeptics, agribusiness publicists, lobbyists (and their anonymous webpages and social media sites), along with in some cases, well intended but misinformed people (influenced by propaganda) attacking our work, other consumer advocacy groups, my partners, my friends and me, personally.

Part of the reason I am responding now is because their messages have started to infiltrate the mainstream media. Seemingly reputable news organizations like NPR (in a blog post titled "Is The Food Babe A Fearmonger? Scientists Are Speaking Out") even linked to the hate groups—quoting one of their spokespeople and repeated their ridiculous and biased messages as if they have any merit.

As I expected, the people who wish to keep the status quo are attacking me personally while simultaneously trying to discredit the entire *Good Food Movement.*

Food Babe's original post, archived at the Genetic Literacy Project and dated December 8, 2014.

There's a group of aggressive scientists, biased doctors, skeptics, agribusiness publicists, lobbyists (and their anonymous webpages and social media sites), along with in some cases, well intended but misinformed people (influenced by propaganda) attacking our work, other consumer advocacy groups, my partners, my friends and me, personally.

Did you think the powerful chemical companies and food giants of the world were going to let us waltz right into their world and turn it upside down?

No—they won't and, as I expected, the people who wish to keep the status quo are attacking me personally while simultaneously trying to discredit the entire *Good Food Movement.*

This revised version (snapshot July 30, 2015) is the fourth revision listed, makes no mention of the NPR article. Rather than highlighting the unwarranted swipe with a strike through, it's silently removed without trace, apology or explanation.

Appendix E
Scientific Consensus

As authors, we often talk to people who demand to know "How do you know that?", which is a reasonable question. Even the best scientists in the world (let alone popular science writers) cannot know everything, right? As the old adage goes, there are two sides to every argument. Like weights on a scale, it's the amount of cold, hard evidence that determines which side wins out.

It's true that every once in a while, the weight shifts but in this modern age, that is an increasingly rare occurrence. There are numerous reasons why this is the case but the Internet has helped more scientists confer more easily and more quickly than has ever been possible.

Science works because lots of independent teams check each other's work in their own fields. So in other words, if you produce some new research and manage to get it published in a respected journal (not one of the self-published magazines) your findings are instantly under the strict scrutiny of all of your peers the world over.

Simple mistakes are often caught by the review process (peer review) but when this fails—as it sometimes does—so many other scientists are able to view the final article that even subtle mistakes, perhaps buried deep in esoteric data, are rapidly revealed and exposed. Sometimes these mistakes are so severe that the entire paper is retracted.

One of the most outrageous examples in recent years was the Séralini paper lead by Gilles-Éric Séralini; although since retracted, it is still produced as an example of how GM crops are dangerous (an assertion, the scientific consensus says is false).

A similar instance occurred in 1998 when Dr. Andrew Wakefield's paper connecting MMR to autism and IBD was printed in The Lancet—a prestigious medical journal. A long investigation by Sunday Times reporter Brian Deer, uncovered previously undisclosed financial conflicts of interest directly linked to Wakefield. Following this, most of the co-authors formerly withdrew their support for the paper and in the years that followed trail after trail has failed to demonstrate any causal link between the combined vaccine, autism (which is an innate, largely hereditary condition) and inflammatory bowel disorder. So the consensus (not just small majority): every respected paper since Wakefield's results were published has given MMR a clean bill of health

In early 2010 the UK's General Medical Council found against Dr. Wakefield, including 12 counts of abuse of developmentally challenged children and four more counts of dishonesty. Shortly thereafter, the Lancet officially retracted the paper with editor Richard Horton describing the paper as utterly false. Dr Wakefield was subsequently struck off the UK's medical register and barred from practice.

However, that has not prevented him from garnering a huge base of support in the United States and from celebrities such as Jenny McCarthy and Jim Carey. While he continues to this day to protest his innocence, the following quote from a longer article in the British Medical Journal should serve as some evidence of who is telling the truth.

> "The Office of Research Integrity in the United States defines fraud as fabrication, falsification, or plagiarism. [1] [Brian] Deer unearthed clear evidence of falsification. He found that not one of the 12 cases reported in the 1998 Lancet paper was free of misrepresentation or undisclosed alteration, and that in no single case could the medical records be fully reconciled with the descriptions, diagnoses, or histories published in the journal.

> "Who perpetrated this fraud? There is no doubt that it was Wakefield. Is it possible that he was wrong, but not dishonest: that he was so incompetent that he was unable to fairly describe the project, or to report even one of the 12 children's cases accurately? No. A great deal of thought and effort must have gone into drafting the paper

---

1   http://ori.hhs.gov/misconduct/definition_misconduct.shtml.

to achieve the results he wanted: the discrepancies all led in one direction; misreporting was gross." [2]

The visceral clarity of these statements and the fact that Dr. Wakefield has not chosen to challenge them in court is indicative of the scale of the problem facing society today. We want to believe what we are told and even when the evidence is stacked against that belief, we find it difficult or impossible to change our minds. Being able to doing so is the very essence of good science and a functional society.

■

---

[2]   BMJ 2011;342:c7452 & BMJ 2011;342:d1678

Appendix F
Tarte Cosmetics

Published Ingredients from the Tarte Website

Lucky

Octyldodecanol, candelilla cera/euphorbia cerifera (candelilla) wax/cire de candelilla,C12-15 alkyl ethylhexanoate, isopropyl palmitate, cyclopenta*siloxane*, silica, nylon -12, VP/eicosene copolymer, copernicia cerifera (carnauba) wax /cera carnauba/cire de carnauba, phenyl *trimethicone*, disteardimonium hectorite, hydrogenated coco-glycerides, mentha piperita (peppermint) oil, caprylic/ capric triglyceride, propylene carbonate, ethylhexyl methoxycinnamate, *dimethicone*, caprylyl glycol, sorbitan stearate, benzophenone-3, tocopheryl acetate, *sodium saccharin*, castor oil bis-hydroxypropyl *dimethicone* esters, *retinyl palmitate*, salicornia herbacea extract, dimethyl isosorbide, palmitoyl hexapeptide-14, limonene, linalool. (+/-): *Titanium dioxide* (CI 77891), iron oxides (CI 77491, CI 77492, CI 77499), red 7 lake (CI 15850), yellow 6 lake (CI 15985), red 40 lake (CI 16035).

Envy

Octyldodecanol, candelilla cera/euphorbia cerifera (candelilla) wax/cire de candelilla, C12-15 alkyl ethylhexanoate, isopropyl palmitate, cyclopenta*siloxane*, silica, nylon -12, mica, VP/eicosene copolymer, copernicia cerifera (carnauba) wax /cera carnauba/cire de carnauba, phenyl *trimethicone*, disteardimonium hectorite, hydrogenated coco-glycerides, mentha piperita (peppermint) oil, caprylic/ capric triglyceride, propylene carbonate, ethylhexyl methoxycinnamate, *dimethicone*, caprylyl glycol, sorbitan stearate, benzophenone-3, tocopheryl acetate, *sodium saccharin*, castor oil bis-hydroxypropyl *dimethicone* esters, *retinyl palmitate*, limonene, linalool, salicornia herbacea extract, dimethyl isosorbide, palmitoyl hexapeptide-14. (+/-): *Titanium dioxide*

(CI 77891), iron oxides (CI 77491, CI 77492, CI 77499), red 7 lake (CI 15850), red 40 lake (CI 16035), blue 1 lake (CI 42090).

Hope

Octyldodecanol, candelilla cera/euphorbia cerifera (candelilla) wax/cire de candelilla, C12-15 alkyl ethylhexanoate, isopropyl palmitate, cyclopenta*siloxane*, silica, nylon -12, mica, VP/eicosene copolymer, copernicia cerifera (carnauba) wax /cera carnauba/cire de carnauba, phenyl *trimethicone*, disteardimonium hectorite, hydrogenated coco-glycerides, mentha piperita (peppermint) oil, caprylic/ capric triglyceride, propylene carbonate, ethylhexyl methoxycinnamate, *dimethicone*, caprylyl glycol, sorbitan stearate, benzophenone-3, tocopheryl acetate, *sodium saccharin*, castor oil bis-hydroxypropyl *dimethicone* esters, *retinyl palmitate*, limonene, linalool, salicornia herbacea extract, dimethyl isosorbide, palmitoyl hexapeptide-14. (+/-): *Titanium dioxide* (CI 77891), iron oxides (CI 77491, CI 77492, CI 77499), red 7 lake (CI 15850), red 40 lake (CI 16035), blue 1 lake (CI 42090).

Exposed

Octyldodecanol, candelilla cera/euphorbia cerifera (candelilla) wax/cire de candelilla, C12-15 alkyl ethylhexanoate, isopropyl palmitate, cyclopenta*siloxane*, siliac, nylon-12, VP/Eicosene copolymer, mica, copernica cerifera (carnauba) wax/cera carnauba/cire de carnauba, phenyl *trimethicone*, disteardimonium hectorite, hydrogenated coco-glycerides, mentha piperita (peppermint) oil, caprylic/capric triglyceride, propylene carbonate, *dimethicone*, ethylhexyl methoxycinnamate, caprylyl glycol, sorbitan stearate, benzophenone-3, tocopheryl acetate, *sodium saccharin*, castor oil bis-hydroxypropyl *dimethicone* esters, *retinyl palmitate*, salicornia herbacea extract, dimethyl isosorbide, palmitoyl hexapeptide-14, limonene, linalool, *Titanium dioxide* (CI 77891), iron oxides (CI 77491, CI 77492, CI 77499), red 7 lake (CI 15850), red 40 lake (CI 16035), yellow 5 lake (CI 19140), red 6 lake (CI 15850).

Fiery

Octyldodecanol, candelilla cera/euphorbia cerifera (candelilla) wax/ cire de candelilla,C12-15 alkyl ethylhexanoate, isopropyl palmitate, cyclopenta*siloxane*, silica, nylon -12, VP/eicosene copolymer, copernicia cerifera (carnauba) wax /cera carnauba/cire de carnauba, phenyl *trimethicone*, disteardimonium hectorite, hydrogenated coco-glycerides, mentha piperita (peppermint) oil, caprylic/ capric triglyceride, propylene carbonate, ethylhexyl methoxycinnamate, *dimethicone*, caprylyl glycol, sorbitan stearate, benzophenone-3, tocopheryl acetate, *sodium saccharin*, castor oil bis-hydroxypropyl *dimethicone* esters, *retinyl palmitate*, salicornia herbacea extract, dimethyl isosorbide, palmitoyl hexapeptide-14, limonene, linalool. (+/-): *Titanium dioxide* (CI 77891), iron oxides (CI 77491, CI 77492, CI 77499), red 7 lake (CI 15850), yellow 6 lake (CI 15985), red 40 lake (CI 16035).

Lively

Octyldodecanol, candelilla cera/euphorbia cerifera (candelilla) wax/cire de candelilla, C12-15 alkyl ethylhexanoate, isopropyl palmitate, cyclopenta*siloxane*, silica, nylon -12, VP/eicosene copolymer, mica, copernicia cerifera (carnauba) wax /cera carnauba/cire de carnauba, phenyl *trimethicone*, disteardimonium hectorite, hydrogenated coco-glycerides, mentha piperita (peppermint) oil, caprylic/ capric triglyceride, propylene carbonate, ethylhexyl methoxycinnamate, *dimethicone*, caprylyl glycol, sorbitan stearate, benzophenone-3, tocopheryl acetate, *sodium saccharin*, castor oil bis-hydroxypropyl *dimethicone* esters, *retinyl palmitate*, salicornia herbacea extract, tin oxide, dimethyl isosorbide, palmitoyl hexapeptide-14, limonene, linalool, *Titanium dioxide* (CI 77891), red 7 lake (CI 15850), red 40 lake (CI 16035), iron oxides (CI 77492, CI 77499), red 27 lake (CI 45410).

Appendix G

E-Number Reference

E100-200 Permitted colors

E	Chemical Name	Function
E100	Curcumin	Orange-yellow color
E100(ii)	Turmeric	Orange-yellow color
E101	Riboflavin	Yellow color, vitamin B2
E101(ii)	Riboflavin- 5'- Phosphate	Yellow color, vitamin B2
E102	Tartrazine/Yellow 5	Yellow color, azo dye
E104	Quinoline Yellow	Green-yellow color, synthetic
E106	Riboflavin-5-Sodium Phosphate	Yellow color, vitamin B2
E107	Yellow 2G	Yellow color, azo dye
E110	Sunset Yellow/Yellow 6	Yellow color, azo dye
E120	Carmine, Cochineal	Red color, natural
E122	Azorubine	Red color, azo dye
E123	Amaranth / Red 2	Red color, azo dye
E124	Ponceau 4R	Red color, azo dye
E127	Erythrosine / Red 3	Red color, synthetic
E128	Red 2G / Red 11	Red color, azo dye
E129å	Allura Red AC / Red 40	Red color, azo dye
E131	Patent Blue V	Blue color, synthetic
E132	Indigotine / Blue 2	Blue color, synthetic
E133	Brilliant Blue FCF / Blue 1	Blue color, synthetic
E140	Chlorophylls	Green color, natural
E141	Copper complexes of chlorophyll	Green color, synthetic
E142	Green S	Green color, synthetic
E150a-d	Caramel	Brown color

E151	Brilliant black BN	Black color, azo dye
E153	Carbon	Natural black color
E154	Brown FK	Brown color, azo dye
E155	Brown HT	Brown color, azo dye
E160a	Alfa-, Beta- and Gamma- Carotene	Natural orange-yellow color
E160b	Annatto, Bixin, Norbixin	Natural yellow color
E160c	Bell pepper (Paprika) extract	Natural orange color
E160d	Lycopene	Natural red color
E160e	Beta-apo-8'-carotenal	Natural orange-yellow color
E160f	Ethyl ester of beta-apo-8'-carotenic acid	Natural orange-yellow color
E161a	Flavoxanthin	Natural, yellow color
E161b	Lutein	Natural, yellow color
E161c	Cryptoxanthin	Natural, yellow color
E161d	Rubixanthin	Natural, yellow color
E161e	Violaxanthin	Natural, yellow color
E161f	Rhodoxanthin	Natural, yellow color
E161g	Canthaxanthin	Natural, orange color
E161h	Citranaxanthin	Natural, yellow color
E162	Beetroot extract	Natural red color
E163	Anthocyanins	Natural red-purple colors
E170	Calcium carbonate	White color
E171	Titanium dioxide	White color
E172	Iron oxides	Natural red-brown color
E173	Aluminium	Metal (color)
E174	Silver	Metal (color)
E175	Gold	Metal (color)
E180	Lithol Rubine BK	Red color, azo dye
181	Tannins	Yellow-white color and flavor

E200-300 Preservatives

E	Chemical Name	Function
E200	Sorbic acid	Natural preservative

E201	Sodium sorbate/Sorbic acid sodium salt	Synthetic preservative
E202	Potassium sorbate	Synthetic preservative
E203	Calcium sorbate	Synthetic preservative
E210	Benzoic acid	Natural preservative
E211	Sodium benzoate/Benzoic acid sodium salt	Synthetic preservative
E212	Potassium benzoate/benzoic acid potassium salt	Synthetic preservative
E213	Calcium benzoate/Benzoic acid calcium salt	Synthetic preservative
E214	Ethyl 4-hydroxybenzoate	Synthetic preservative
E215	Ethyl 4-hydroxybenzoate sodium salt	Synthetic preservative
E216	Propyl 4-hydroxybenzoate	Synthetic preservative
E217	Sodium salt of E216	Synthetic preservative
E218	Methyl 4-hydroxybenzoate	Synthetic preservative from benzoic acid
E219	Sodium salt of E218	Synthetic preservative from benzoic acid
E220	Sulphur dioxide	Natural preservative
E221	Sodium sulphite	Synthetic preservative
E222	Sodium hydrogen sulphite	Synthetic preservative; bleach
E223	Sodium metabisulphite	Synthetic preservative; anti oxidant
E224	Potassium metabisulphite	Synthetic preservative
225	Potassium sulphite	Synthetic preservative
E226	Calcium sulphite	Synthetic preservative
E227	Calcium hydrogen sulphite	Synthetic preservative
E228	Potassium hydrogen sulphite	Synthetic preservative
E230	Biphenyl	Synthetic preservative
E231	2-hydroxybiphenyl	Synthetic preservative
E232	Sodium biphenyl-2-yl oxide	Synthetic preservative
E233	2-(Thiazol-4-yl)benzimidazole	Synthetic preservative
E234	Nisin	Natural antibiotic
E235	Pimaracin	Natural antibiotic

236	Formic acid	Natural acid, preservative
237	Sodium formate	Natural salt, preservative
238	Calcium formate	Natural salt, preservative
E239	Hexamine	Synthetic preservative
240	Formaldehyde	Preservative
E242	Dimethylcarbonate	Synthetic preservative
E249	Potassium nitrite	Natural salt, preservative
E250	Sodium nitrite	Natural salt, preservative
E251	Sodium nitrate	Natural salt, preservative
E252	Potassium nitrate	Natural salt, preservative
E260	Acetic acid	Natural acid, preservative
E261	Potassium acetate	Preservative, natural salt
E262	Sodium acetate	Preservative, natural salt
E263	Calcium acetate	Preservative, natural salt
E270	Lactic acid	Natural acid
E280	Propionic acid	Natural acid
E281	Sodium propionate	Natural salt
E282	Calcium propionate	Natural salt
E283	Potassium propionate	Natural salt
E284	Boric acid	Natural acid
E285	Sodium tetraborate	Natural acid
E290	Carbon dioxide	Natural gas
E296	Malic acid	Acid
E297	Fumaric acid	Natural acid

E300-400 Permitted Anti-oxidants, emulsifiers and stabilizers

E300	L-Ascorbic acid	Natural anti-oxidant, vitamin C
E301	Sodium L-ascorbate	Natural anti-oxidant, vitamin C
E302	Calcium L-ascorbate	Natural anti-oxidant, >vitamin C
E304	6-0-palmitoyl-L-ascorbic acid	Synthetic anti-oxidant
E306	Extracts of tocopherols	Natural anti-oxidant, vitamin E
E307	alfa- Tocopherol	Synthetic anti-oxidant, vitamin E
E308	gamma-Tocopherol	Synthetic anti-oxidant, vitamin E
E309	delta- Tocopherol	Synthetic anti-oxidant, vitamin E

E310	Propyl gallate	Synthetic anti-oxidant
E311	Octyl gallate	Synthetic anti-oxidant
E312	Dodecyl gallate	Synthetic anti-oxidant
313	Thiodipropionic acid	Synthetic anti-oxidant
314	Guaiac Gum	Natural anti-oxidant
E315	Erythorbic acid	Synthetic anti-oxidant
E316	Sodium erythorbate	Synthetic anti-oxidant
319	Butylhydroxinon	Synthetic anti-oxidant
E320	Butylated hydroxyanisole	Synthetic anti-oxidant
E321	Butylated hydroxytoluene	Synthetic anti-oxidant
E322	Lecithin	Natural emulsifier
E325	Sodium lactate	Sodium salt of lactic acid
E326	Potassium lactate	Potassium salt of lactic acid
E327	Calcium lactate	Calcium salt of lactic acid
E330	Citric acid	Acidity regulators
E331	Sodium citrates	Acidity regulators
E332	Potassium citrates	Acidity regulators
E333	Mono, di, and Tri-Calcium citrate	Acidity regulators
E334	L-(+)- tartaric acid	Natural acid
E335	mono/di Sodium L-(+)- tartrate	Salt of tartaric acid
E336	monoPotassium L-(+)- tartrate	Salt of tartaric acid
E337	Potassium sodium L-(+)- tartrate	Salt of tartaric acid
E338	Phosphoric acid	Buffers
E339	Sodium orthophosphates	Buffers
E340	Potassium orthophosphates	Buffers
E341	Calcium orthophosphates	Buffers
343	Magnesium orthophosphates	Buffers
E350	Sodium malate	Sodium salt of malic acid
E351	Potassium malate	Potassium salt of malic acid
E352	Calcium malate	Calcium salt of malic acid
E353	meta tartaric acid	Natural acid
E354	Calcium tartarate	Natural preservative
E355	Adipic acid	Natural acid

E356	Sodium adipate	Acidity regulator
E357	Potassium adipate	Acidity regulator
E363	Succinic acid	Natural acid
365	Sodium fumarate	Acidity regulator
370	1,4-Heptonolactone	Synthetic acid
375	Nicotinic acid	B vitamin, color protector
E380	triAmmonium citrate	Synthetic salt of citric acid
381	Ammonium ferric citrate	Synthetic salt of citric acid
E385	Calcium disodium ethylenediamine	Sequestrant, chelating substance
386	EDTA: Disodium ethylenediamine tetra-acetate	Synthetic stabilizer
387	Oxystearin	Stabilizer
388	Thiodipropionic acid	Synthetic anti-oxidant

E400-500 Emulsifiers and thickening agents

E400	Alginic acid	Natural thickening agent
E401	Sodium alginate	Natural thickening agent
E402	Potassium alginate	Natural thickening agent
E403	Ammonium alginate	Natural thickening agent
E404	Calcium alginate	Natural thickening agent
E405	Propane-1, 2-diol alginate	Derived of alginic acid
E406	Agar	Natural thickening agent
E407	Carrageenan	Natural thickening agent
408	Furcelleran	Natural thickening agent
E410	Locust bean gum	Natural thickening agent
E411	Oat Gum	Natural thickening agent
E412	Guar Gum	Natural thickening agent
E413	Tragacanth	Natural thickening agent
E414	Gum Arabic	Natural thickening agent
E415	Xanthan gum	Natural thickening agent
E416	Karaya gum	Natural thickening agent
E417	Tara gum	Natural thickening agent
E418	Gellan gum	Natural thickening agent
E420	Sorbitol	Natural sugar alcohol

E421	Mannitol	Natural sugar alcohol
E422	Glycerol	Natural alcohol
430	Polyoxyethylene(8) stearate	Synthetic emulsifier
E431	Polyoxyethylene (40) stearate	Synthetic emulsifier
E432	Polyoxyethylene-20-sorbitan monolaurate	Synthetic emulsifier
E433	Polyoxyethylene-20-sorbitan mono-oleate	Synthetic emulsifier
E434	Polyoxyethylene-20-sorbitan monopalmitate	Synthetic emulsifier
E435	Polyoxyethylene-20-sorbitan monostearate	Synthetic emulsifier
E436	Polyoxyethylene-20-sorbitan tristearate	Synthetic emulsifier
E440	Pectin	Natural thickening agent
441	Gelatin	Natural thickening agent
E442	Ammonium phosphatides	Synthetic emulsifier
E450	Di- and polyphosphates	Salt of phosphoric acid
E451	Triphosphates	Salt of phosphoric acid
E452	Polyphosphates	Salt of phosphoric acid
E460	Cellulose	Natural fiber, thickening agent
E461	Methyl cellulose	Semi-synthetic thickening agent
462	Ethyl cellulose	Semi-synthetic thickening agent
E463	Hydroxypropyl cellulose	Semi-synthetic thickening agent
E464	Hydroxypropylmethyl cellulose	Semi-synthetic thickening agent
E465	Methylethyl cellulose	Semi-synthetic thickening agent
E466	Carboxymethyl cellulose	Semi-synthetic thickening agent
E470	Fatty acid salts	Semi-synthetic emulsifiers
E471	Mono- and di-glycerides of fatty acids	Semi-synthetic emulsifiers
E472	Esters of mono- and diglycerides	Semi-synthetic emulsifiers
E473	Sugar esters of fatty acids	Semi-synthetic emulsifiers
E474	Sugarglycerides	Semi-synthetic emulsifiers
E475	Polyglycerol esters of fatty acids	Semi-synthetic emulsifiers

E476	Polyglycerol polyricinoleate	Semi-synthetic emulsifiers
E477	Propyleneglycol esters of fatty acids	Semi-synthetic emulsifiers
E478	Mixture of glycerol- and propyleneglycol esters of lactic acid and fatty acids	Semi-synthetic emulsifiers
E479	Esterified soy oil	Semi-synthetic emulsifiers
480	Dioctyl sodium sulphosuccinate	Synthetic emulsifier
E481	Sodium stearoyl lactate	Semi-synthetic emulsifier
E482	Calcium stearoyl lactate	Semi-synthetic emulsifier
E483	Stearyl tartrate	Semi-synthetic emulsifier
484	Stearyl citrate	Semi-synthetic emulsifier
E485	Renamed as E441	
490	Propylene glycol	solvent
E491	Sorbitane mono stearate	Semi-synthetic emulsifier
E492	Sorbitane tri stearate	Semi-synthetic emulsifier
E493	Sorbitane mono laurate	Semi-synthetic emulsifier
E494	Sorbitane mono oleate	Semi-synthetic emulsifier
E495	Sorbitane mono palmitate	Semi-synthetic emulsifier

E500-600 Additives with different functions

E500	Sodium carbonate	Base
E501	Potassium carbonate	Base
E503	Ammonium carbonate	Base
E504	Magnesium carbonate	Alkali, anti-caking agent
505	Ferro carbonate	Acidity regulator
E507	Hydrochloric acid	acid
E508	Potassium chloride	Salt substitute
E509	Calcium chloride	Sequestrant, firming agent
510	Ammonium chloride	Yeast food, flavor
E511	Magnesium chloride	Acidity regulator
E512	Stannous chloride	Anti-oxidant
E513	Sulphuric acid	Acid
E514	Sodium sulphate	Acid, diluent
E515	Potassium sulphate	Salt substitute

E516	Calcium sulphate	Firming agent
E517	Ammonium sulphate	Stabilizer
518	Magnesium sulphate	Dietary supplement
E520	Aluminium sulphate	Clarification agent
E521	Aluminium sodium sulphate	Acidity regulator
E523	Aluminium ammonium sulphate	Stabilizer
E524	Sodium hydroxide	Base, color solvent
E525	Potassium hydroxide	Base
E526	Calcium hydroxide	Firming agent
E527	Ammonium hydroxide	Base
E528	Magnesium hydroxide	Base
E529	Calcium oxide	Alkali
E530	Magnesium oxide	Anti caking agent, alkali
E535	Sodium ferrocyanide	Anti caking agent
E536	Potassium ferrocyanide	Anti caking agent
537	Ferrohexacyanomanganate	Anti-caking agent
E538	Calcium ferrocyanide	Anti-caking agent
539	Sodium thiosulphate	Anti-oxidant
540	Dicalcium pyrophosphate (now E450)	Raising agent
E541	Sodium Aluminium phosphate	Raising agent
542	Edible bone phosphate	Anti caking agent
543	Sodium calcium polyphosphate	Emulsifier
544	Calcium polyphosphates	Emulsifier
545	Ammonium polyphosphates	Emulsifier
546	Magnesium pyrophosphate	Emulsifier
550	Sodium silicates	Anti-caking agent
E551	Silicium dioxide	Anti caking agent
E552	Calcium silicate	Anti caking agent
E553	Magnesium silicate	Anti caking agent
E554	Aluminium sodium silicate	Anti caking agent
E555	Aluminium potassium silicate	Anti caking agent
E556	Aluminium calcium silicate	Anti caking agent

557	Zinc silicate	Anti caking agent
E558	Bentonite	Anti caking agent
E559	Kaolin	Anti caking agent
E570	Stearic acid	Anti caking agent
571	Ammonium stearate	Anti caking agent
572	Magnesium stearate	Anti caking agent
573	Aluminium stearate	Anti caking agent
E574	Gluconic acid	Sequestrant
E575	D-glucono-1, 5-lactone	Sequestrant
E576	Sodium gluconate	Sequestrant
E577	Potassium gluconate	Sequestrant
E578	Calcium gluconate	Firming agent, sequestrant
E579	Ferro gluconate	Colour and nutrient
E585	Ferro lactate	Nutrient

E600-700

E620	Glutamic acid	Flavor enhancer
E621	Mono sodium glutamate	Flavor enhancer
E622	Mono potassium glutamate	Flavor enhancer
E623	Calcium glutamate	Flavor enhancer
E624	Ammonium glutamate	Flavor enhancer
E625	Magnesium glutamate	Flavor enhancer
E626	Guanylic acid	Flavor enhancer
E627	Sodium guanylate	Flavor enhancer
E628	Di-potassium guanylate	Flavor enhancer
E629	Calcium guanylate	Flavor enhancer
E630	Inosinic acid	Flavor enhancer
E631	Sodium inosinate	Flavor enhancer
E632	Di-potassium inosinate	Flavor enhancer
E633	Calcium inosinate	Flavor enhancer
E634	Calcium ribonucleotides	Flavor enhancer
E635	Di-sodium ribonucleotides	Flavor enhancer
636	Maltol	Flavor enhancer
637	Ethylmaltol	Flavor enhancer

E640	Glycine and sodium glycinate	Nutrient

E700-800 Antibiotics

E710	Spiramycins	Antibiotic
E713	Tylosin	Antibiotic

E900-1300

E900	Dimethyl-polysiloxane	Anti-foaming agent
E901	Beeswax	Coating, glazing agent
E902	Candilla wax	Coating, glazing agent
E903	Canauba wax	Coating, glazing agent
E904	Lac, Shellac	Coating, glazing agent made from lice
905	Paraffine, Vaseline	Coating, glazing agent
906	Gum benzoic	Flavor, coating
907	Micro-crystalline wax	Coating, glazing agent
908	Rice bran wax	Coating, glazing agent
E912	Montan acid esters	Coating, glazing agent
913	Lanoline	Coating, glazing agent
E914	Oxidized polyethylene wax	Coating, glazing agent
915	Esters of Colophane	Stabilizer, flavor
E920	L-Cysteine	Bread enhancer
E921	L-Cystine	Bread enhancer
922	Potassium persulphate	Bread enhancer
923	Ammonium persulphate	Bread enhancer
924	Potassium bromates	Flour bleaching agent
925	Chlorine	Flour bleaching agent
926	Chlorodioxide	Bleaching agent and preservative
E927a	Azodicarbonamide	Bread enhancer
E927b	Urea	Buffer
928	Benzoylperoxide	Bread enhancer
930	Calciumperoxide	Bread enhancer
E938	Argon	Propellant
E939	Helium	Propellant
E940	Dichlorodifluormethane	Propellant, anti-freeze

E941	Nitrogen	Propellant
E942	Nitrous oxides	Propellant
E943	Butane, isobutane	Propellant
E944	Propane	Propellant
E948	Oxygen	Propellant
E949	Hydrogen	Propellant
E950	Acesulfame K	Sweetener
E951	Aspartame	Sweetener
E952	Cyclamates	Sweetener
E953	Isomalt	Sweetener
E954	Sacharine	Sweetener
E955	Sucralose	Sweetener
E957	Thaumatine	Sweetener
E959	Neohesperidin	Sweetener
E960	Stevia	Sweetener
E961	Neotame	Sweenener
E962	Salt of aspartame-acesulfame	Sweetener
E965	Maltitol	Sweetener
E966	Lactitol	Sweetener
E967	Xylitol	Sweetener
E999	Quillaia extract	Foaming agent
1000	Cholic acid	Emulsifier
E1105	Lysozyme	Preservative
E1200	Polydextrose	Thickening agent
E1201	Polyvinylpyrrolidon	Thickening agent, stabilizer
E1202	insoluble polyvinylpyrrolidon	Clarifying agent

E1400-1500 Thickening Agents

1400	Dextrins	Thickening agent
1401	Acid treated starch	Thickening agent
1402	Alkaline treated starch	Thickening agent
1403	Bleached starch	Thickening agent
E1404	Oxidized starch	Thickening agent
E1410	mono-starch phosphate	Thickening agent

1411	Di-starch glycerol	Thickening agent
E1412	Di-starch phosphates	Thickening agent
E1413	Phosphatylated di-starch phosphate	Thickening agent
E1414	Acetylated di-starch phosphate	Thickening agent
E1420	Starch acetate	Thickening agent
1421	Starch acetate	Thickening agent
E1422	Acetylated di-starch adipate	Thickening agent
E1423	Acetylated di-starch glycerol	Thickening agent
E1440	Hydroxypropylstarch	Thickening agent
1441	Hydroxypropyl-di-starchglycerol	Thickening agent
E1442	Hydroxypropyl-di-starchphosphate	Thickening agent
E1450	Starch sodium octenyl succinate	Thickening agent

E1500-1600

1501	Benzylated hydrocarbons	Flavours
1502	Butane-1,3-diol	Flavor solvent
1503	Castor Oil	Flavor and solvent
1504	Ethyl acetate	Flavor solvent
E1505	Triethyl citrate	Flavor solvent
1516	Glycerol monoacetate	Flavor solvent
1517	Glycerol diacetate	Flavor solvent
E1518	Glycerol triacetate	Flavor solvent
1520	Propylene glycol	Solvent for anti-oxidants
1525	Hydroxy ethyl cellulose	Thickening agent

E is for Allergens

Compounds known to cause problems for people allergic to aspirin, with asthma or similar conditions. Not all of these compounds cause problems for every affected person—note that colors can be mixed to achieve different hues.

Colors

E102	Yellow
E107	Yellow
E110	Yellow
E122	Red
E123	Red
E124	Red

Preservatives

E212	Potassium benzoate
E213	Calcium benzoate
E214	Ethyl 4-hydroxybenzoate
E215	Ethyl 4-hydroxybenzoate sodium
E216	Propyl 4-hydroxybenzoate
E217	Propyl 4-hydroxybenzoate sodium
E218	Methyl 4-hydroxybenzoate
E219	Methyl 4-hydroxybenzoate sodium

Anti-oxidants

E310	Propyl gallate
E311	Octyl gallate
E321	Butylated hydroxytoluene

Flavor enhancers

E621	Mono sodium glutamate
E622	Mono potassium glutamate
E623	Calcium glutamate
E627	Sodium guanylate
E631	Sodium inosinate
E635	Di-sodium ribonucleotides

E Might Be for ADHD

E Numbers thought to cause problems in susceptible individuals (ADHD). We should stress that while there is little scientific evidence to support this assumption, this information is included for those people who wish to avoid them. We have no qualms feeding them to our families in moderation.

Colors

E102	Yellow	E104	Yellow
E107	Yellow	E110	Yellow
E120	Red	E122	Red
E123	Red	E124	Red
E127	Red	E128	Red
E132	Blue	E133	Blue
E150	Brown	E154	Brown
E155	Brown		

Preservatives

E210	Benzoic acid
E211	Sodium benzoate
E220	Sulphur dioxide
E251	Sodium sulphite

Anti-oxidants

E320	Butylated hydroxyanisole
E321	Butylated hydroxytoluene

Acknowledgements

A number of people have contributed research, ideas or just been there when things got murky—these are in no particular order: *Kim Curran, Debbie Berry, Edie Diaf, William Enright, Katherine Falk, Bryleigh Goff, Cheri Kent, Alexander Huszagh, Amanda Leigh, Tricia Meyer (MeyerTech LLC), Nandu Nandini, Nina Pengelly, Emma Price Bauer, Valerie Sabo, Autumn Smith, Jason Smith, Laura Steffes, "Deep Throat", Michael Weinberg* and members of the *Banned By Food Babe* group on Facebook.

Also *Ron Johnson* and *Michelle Ashworth* of The New Horsemen.

Final artwork check and editing expertise provided by *Maxwell Katz*.

The team is grateful to them all for their contributions—even if they were only a smile and a kind word. It's hard living in a jar.

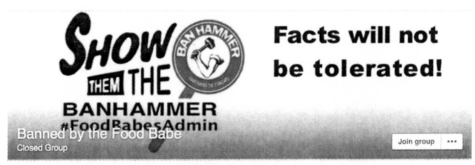

https://www.facebook.com/groups/BannedByFoodBabeOpen

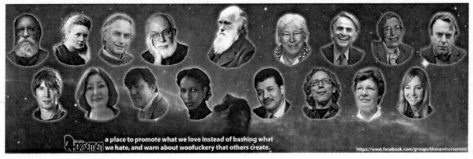

https://www.facebook.com/groups/thenewhorsemen

About the
Contributing authors

Kavin Senapathy

Kavin is a freelance writer, science popularizer, and a mom of two. She despises unscientific misinformation mongering, and devotes her time and energy to refuting myths about health and food. Kavin is the co-founder of "March Against Myths," also known as MAMyths, an international grassroots response to widespread myths about biotechnology, genetic engineering, cancer, autism, and more. She has amassed a loyal following known as the "Senapath Crew."

fb.com/Ksenapathy / @ksenapathy

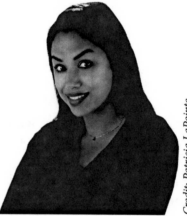

Credit: Patricia LaPointe

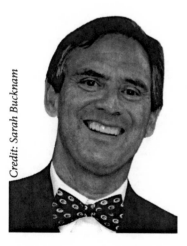

Credit: Sarah Bucknam

Mark Alsip

Mark Alsip writes the skeptical science blog Bad Science Debunked. His degree in computer science and math was put to good use as a member of the "IDEX II" project, currently on display at the Smithsonian's National Air and Space Museum. He returned to university as a pre-med student, where studies in life sciences led him to develop a deep distrust in pseudoscientists who pursue their education at the University of Google.

badscidebunked.wordpress.com
@markaaronky

Mike the Chicken Vet

Mike Petrik received his Doctorate of Veterinary Medicine (DVM) from the Ontario Veterinary College in 1998, and an MSc in animal welfare from the University of Guelph in 2014. His blog is located at:

http://mikethechickenvet.wordpress.com

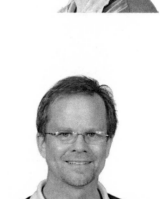

Kevin Folta, Ph.D

A scientist in a scientifically illiterate nation at a time when we need science the most. Let me know if you need guidance with a science fair project, a scientific presentation, or would like me to visit with your school, church group, or organic coop. Believe it or not, these get-togethers are always fun and we all learn something important.

http://kfolta.blogspot.com

Marc Draco

It's said Marc lives in a jar at a secret location after losing his body in a winner-takes-all strip poker game at a late-night party at Monsanto's headquarters. Donating his brain to science, he was re-booted in a cocktail of aspartame, MSG and glyphosate and is now the subject of hideous GMO experimentation where he is forced to watch hours of organic crops being tortured by scientists in chlorophyll-stained lab coats. No one knows for sure, someone probably just made that up—this is the age of the Internet after all and who can you believe?

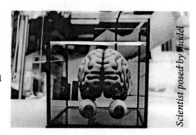

Scientist posed by model

Index

Index

CPSIA information can be obtained at www.ICGtesting.com
Printed in the USA
LVOW07*0823051016

507473LV00001B/1/P